Biological Aspects of
Reconstructive Surgery

Biological Aspects of Reconstructive Surgery

Desmond A. Kernahan, M.B., F.R.C.S.E., F.R.C.S.(C)

*Professor of Surgery,
Northwestern University Medical School;
Chief, Plastic Surgery,
Children's Memorial Hospital,
Chicago, Illinois*

•

Lars M. Vistnes, M.D., F.R.C.S.(C), F.A.C.S.

*Associate Professor of Surgery,
Stanford University School of Medicine;
Stanford, California
Chief, Surgical Service,
Veterans Administration Hospital,
Palo Alto, California*

Editors

Little, Brown and Company, Boston

Contents

Preface

The extent and application of plastic surgery have expanded rapidly in the last twenty-five years, and the concept of repair as opposed to ablation has extended into most fields of surgical endeavor. Although the development of plastic surgery was in large part pragmatic and technical—trial and too often error being the way in which the frontiers were advanced—there has been a steady increase in our knowledge of why and how our successes and failures occur. Particular instances are in our understanding of the circulatory patterns of skin flaps, the vascularization of skin grafts, and the behavior of healing tendons, to mention only a few. Much of this information still is gained only by searching for and reading the original papers. This is time-consuming for all, and often confusing for those still in training. Standard texts of pathology and surgical physiology, oriented as they are to the wider audience, do not always present in sufficient detail concepts of particular interest to the plastic surgeon.

Biological Aspects of Reconstructive Surgery brings together in one place this body of information: the basic science foundation on which reconstructive surgery builds. We have in general excluded subjects, such as hand anatomy and skin pathology, that are distinct entities covered in standard texts. Our contributing authors have concentrated on the fundamental biological processes and their impact on the practice of plastic surgery.

The conception of this book occurred when the editors were associates in the practice of plastic surgery, and the contributors largely reflect the institutions with which we have been associated. Other authors were chosen by virtue of their personal contributions in particular spheres of interest. Like most outstanding professionals, they are busy and often overcommitted. We thank them both for the quality of their contributions and for the way in which they found time to produce them.

It is a particular pleasure to thank Mr. Fred Belliveau, General Manager of the Medical Division of Little, Brown and Company, for his enthusiasm, support, and guidance in bringing the project to completion. We also thank Mr. Robert M. Davis for his many helpful suggestions and editorial supervision.

D. A. K.
L. M. V.

Contributing Authors

JOHN M. BOWMAN, M.D.

Professor of Pediatrics, University of Manitoba, Medical Faculty; Medical Director, Canadian Red Cross Blood Transfusion Center, Winnipeg, Canada
Chapter 5

HUNTER J. H. FRY, M.S., F.R.C.S., F.R.A.C.S.

Honorary Research Fellow, Department of Surgery, University of Melbourne; Plastic Surgeon, Royal Melbourne Hospital, Melbourne, Australia
Chapter 19

MARK GORNEY, M.D., F.A.C.S.

Clinical Associate Professor of Surgery, Stanford University School of Medicine, Stanford, California; Chairman, Plastic Surgery Division, Saint Francis Memorial Hospital, San Francisco, California
Chapter 16

WILLIAM C. GRABB, M.D.

Professor and Head, Section of Plastic Surgery, University of Michigan Medical School; Staff Surgeon, University Hospital, Ann Arbor, Michigan
Chapter 22

B. HEROLD GRIFFITH, M.D., F.A.C.S.

Professor of Surgery and Chief of Plastic Surgery, Northwestern University Medical School; Attending Plastic Surgeon, Northwestern Memorial Hospital and Children's Memorial Hospital, Chicago, Illinois
Chapter 11

RONALD P. GRUBER, M.D.

Clinical Instructor, Surgery, Stanford University School of Medicine, Stanford, California; Consultant Plastic Surgeon, Veterans Administration Hospital, Palo Alto, California
Chapter 8

HAROLD A. HARPER, Ph.D.

Professor of Biochemistry, Departments of Biochemistry and Surgery, University of California School of Medicine, San Francisco, California; Consulting Biochemist, Clinical Investigation Center, U.S. Naval Regional Medical Center, Oakland, California
Chapter 4

CLIFFORD M. HERMAN, M.D., CAPT., MC, USN

Professor of Surgery, Uniformed Services University of the Health Sciences, Bethesda, Maryland; Assistant

Chairman, Department of Surgery, National Naval Medical Center, Bethesda, Maryland
Chapter 10

NORMAN E. HUGO, M.D.

Associate Professor of Surgery, Northwestern University Medical School; Attending Surgeon, Northwestern Memorial Hospital,
Chicago, Illinois
Chapter 18

LAWRENCE N. HURST, M.D., F.R.C.S.(C)

Assistant Professor of Surgery, University of Western Ontario; Attending Surgeon and Chief, Division of Plastic Surgery, University Hospital, London, Canada
Chapter 21

ERNEST N. KAPLAN, M.D.

Associate Professor of Surgery, Stanford University School of Medicine; Attending Surgeon, Division of Plastic Surgery, Stanford University Hospital, Stanford, California
Chapters 13 and 15

RICHARD L. KEMPSON, M.D.

Professor of Pathology, Stanford University School of Medicine; Co-Director of Surgical Pathology, Stanford Medical Center, Stanford, California
Chapter 12

DESMOND A. KERNAHAN, M.B., F.R.C.S.E., F.R.C.S.(C)

Professor of Surgery, Northwestern University Medical School; Chief, Plastic Surgery, Children's Memorial Hospital, Chicago, Illinois
Editor; Chapter 14

TERRY R. KNAPP, M.D.

Chief Resident, Plastic and Reconstructive Surgery, Stanford University Medical Center, Stanford, California
Chapter 15

ZOLTAN J. LUCAS, M.D.

Associate Professor of Surgery, Department of Surgery, Stanford University School of Medicine, Stanford, California
Chapter 17

JOHN K. McKENZIE, M.D.

Associate Professor of Internal Medicine, University of Manitoba Medical Faculty; Attending Nephrologist and Director, Hypertension Clinic, Health Sciences Centre General, Winnipeg, Canada
Chapters 3 and 9

KEITH L. MOORE, Ph.D.

Professor and Chairman, Department of Anatomy, University of Toronto Faculty of Medicine, Toronto, Canada
Chapter 1

DONALD A. NAGEL, M.D.

Professor of Orthopedic Surgery, Stanford University School of Medicine, Stanford, California; Professor of Orthopedic Surgery, Stanford University Medical Center, Stanford, California
Chapter 20

ALLAN R. RONALD, M.D.

Associate Professor, Departments of Medical Microbiology and Medicine, University of Manitoba Medical Faculty; Acting Director, Department of Clinical Microbiology, Health Sciences Centre, Winnipeg, Canada
Chapters 7 and 9

MOHAMED H. K. SHOKEIR, M.D., Ph.D.

Professor, Department of Pediatrics, University of Saskatchewan College of Medicine, Director, Division of Medical Genetics, University Hospital, Saskatoon, Canada
Chapter 2

CHARLES F. T. SNELLING, M.D., F.R.C.S.(C)

Assistant Professor, Department of Surgery, University of Manitoba Medical Faculty; Active Staff, Department of Surgery, Health Sciences Centre, Winnipeg, Canada
Chapters 6 and 9

LARS M. VISTNES, M.D., F.R.C.S.(C), F.A.C.S.

Associate Professor of Surgery, Stanford University School of Medicine, Stanford, California; Chief, Surgical Service, Veterans Administration Hospital, Palo Alto, California
Editor; Chapters 8 and 9

I

The Predetermined Aspects

INTRODUCTION

A person's genetic and embryological constitution determines his body form. Therefore, and because the sciences of genetics and embryology have advanced significantly in the past decade and a half, Part I of this book is devoted to these disciplines.

The plastic surgeon must have a good working knowledge of genetics and embryology because he frequently treats congenitally deformed children and counsels their families. Knowing the embryological background of a lesion is often the key to successful treatment. Informed advice to parents enables them to plan their family wisely and prevent future tragedies.

The material in Chapters 1 and 2 will help the surgeon to advise a family on why a deformity occurred and provide suitable counseling when confronted with an inherited or de novo developmental anomaly. At the same time, these chapters are a current concise review of pertinent topics in two difficult and diffuse basic sciences.

1

The Embryological Basis of Congenital Defects

Keith L. Moore

EARLY HUMAN DEVELOPMENT

Development begins at fertilization when a sperm unites with an ovum to form a single cell called a *zygote* (Fig. 1-1). Fertilization restores the diploid number of 46 chromosomes and initiates preparations for the first division of the zygote. Mutant genes or abnormal numbers of chromosomes from the ovum or the sperm, or both, can cause congenital malformations (see Chapter 2).

The process of cleavage consists in repeated mitotic divisions of the zygote into cells called *blastomeres* (Fig. 1-2). By the third day a solid ball of 16 or so blastomeres, called a *morula* (Fig. 1-2D), has formed. The morula enters the uterus from the uterine tube, and fluid passes into the morula from the uterine cavity. As the fluid collects, a blastocyst cavity forms, converting the morula into a blastocyst (Fig. 1-2E). The embryo-forming cells making up the inner cell mass are surrounded by a peripheral layer of trophoblastic cells. The membranous zona pellucida degenerates as the blastocyst forms on the fourth and fifth days. The trophoblast adheres to the endometrial epithelium, and implantation of

the blastocyst begins; implantation ends during the second week (Fig. 1-3).

Differentiation of cells in the inner cell mass into an embryo begins at the end of the first week. The cells facing the blastocyst cavity become cuboid and form a single layer of endoderm; the remaining cells become columnar during the second week and form a thick layer known as the *ectoderm*. The amniotic cavity appears between the ectoderm and the trophoblast. By the end of the second week, the developing embryo consists of a bilaminar embryonic disk which is continuous peripherally with the amnion and the yolk sac (Fig. 1-3E).

The third week is a period of rapid embryonic development. The primitive streak appears as a midline thickening of the embryonic ectoderm, and cells from it spread laterally between the ectoderm and the endoderm of the embryonic disk to form mesoderm, the third germ layer of the embryo. From the thickened end of the primitive streak, called the *primitive knot*, cells extend cranially to form the notochordal process, the primordium of the notochord. To-

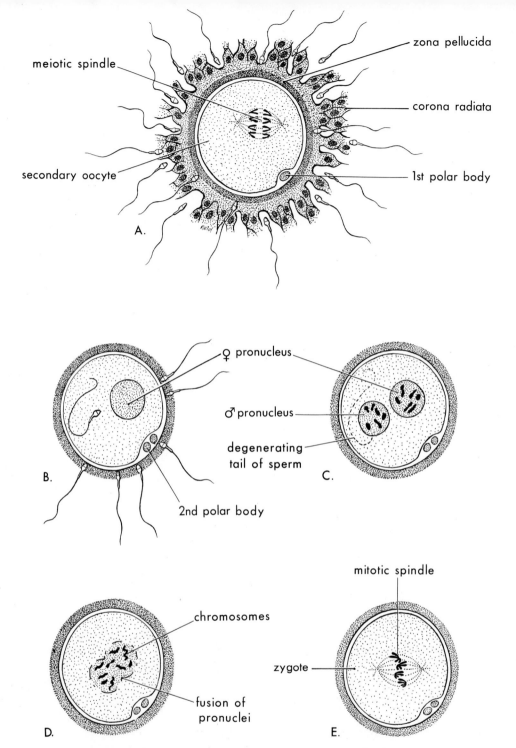

FIGURE 1-1.   *Fertilization. A. Secondary oocyte about to be fertilized (only four of the 23 chromosome pairs are shown). B. The corona radiata has disappeared, and the sperm has passed through the zona pellucida into the ovum. The second maturation division has occurred. C. The sperm head has enlarged to form the male pronucleus. D. The pronuclei are fusing. E. The chromosomes of the zygote are arranged on a mitotic spindle in preparation for the first cleavage. (From K. L. Moore,* The Developing Human *[2nd ed.]. Philadelphia: Saunders, 1977.)*

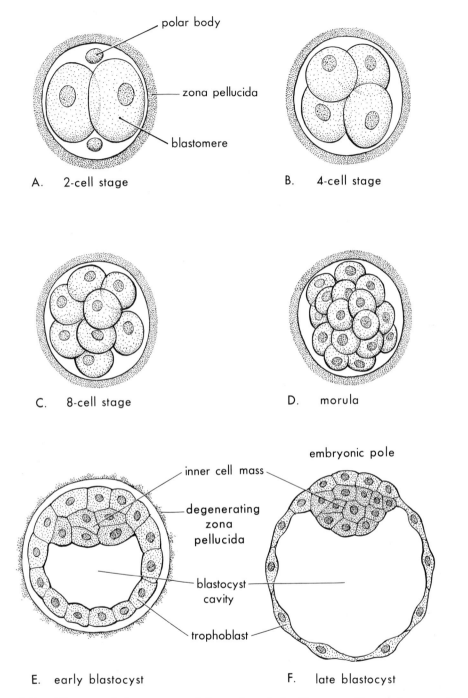

FIGURE 1-2. *Cleavage of the zygote and formation of the blastocyst. E and F are sections of blastocysts showing the inner cell mass (primordium of the embryo). (From K. L. Moore,* The Developing Human *[2nd ed.]. Philadelphia: Saunders, 1977.)*

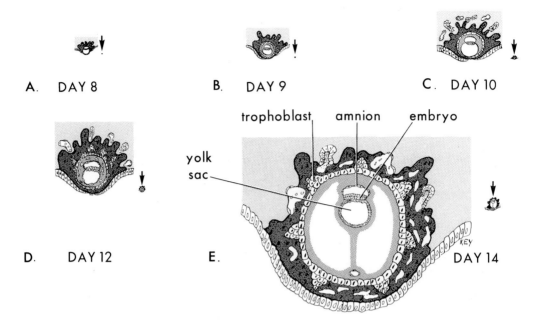

A.   DAY 8

B.   DAY 9

C.   DAY 10

D.   DAY 12

E.   DAY 14

trophoblast   amnion   embryo

yolk
sac

FIGURE 1-3.   *Sections of human blastocysts during the second week, illustrating the implantation, the rapid expansion of the trophoblast, and the relatively minute size of the embryo (×25); the sketches indicated by the arrows show the actual size of the blastocysts. (From K. L. Moore,* The Developing Human *[2nd ed.]. Philadelphia: Saunders, 1977.)*

ward the end of the third week, formation of the nervous and cardiovascular systems begins.

THE EMBRYONIC PERIOD AND TERATOGENESIS

Rapid growth and differentiation of the embryo continue throughout the embryonic period. By the end of the eighth week all the main systems of the body have formed and all major features of external body form have appeared. Exposure of an embryo to environmental teratogens (substances known to cause congenital malformations) may result in abnormal development and congenital malformations. Despite rapid advances in knowledge concerning congenital malformations in the last decade, much is still to be learned about the etiology of birth defects. It is estimated that about 10 percent of malformations are caused by environmental factors and another 10 percent by genetic and

chromosomal factors. Probably many of the remaining abnormalities result from a complex interaction of genetic and environmental factors. For a review of the causes of human malformations, see Moore [9] and Persaud and Moore [11].

FOURTH WEEK.   Initially the embryo is almost straight, but longitudinal and lateral folding resulting from rapid growth of the embryo, especially of the brain and spinal cord, produces a somewhat cylindrical embryo. The main external features of four-week embryos are shown in Figure 1-4.

FIFTH WEEK (FIG. 1-5).   Growth of the head is extensive and results mainly from rapid development of the brain. Other external changes are minor compared with those occurring during the fourth week. The limbs, especially the arm buds, show considerable regional differentiation.

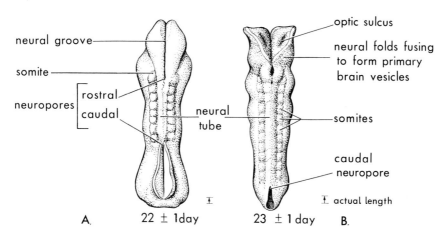

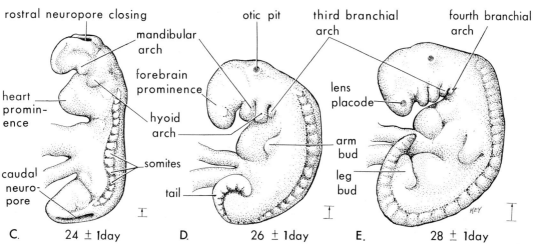

FIGURE 1-4. *Four week embryos. A and B. Dorsal views. C, D, and E. Lateral views. (From K. L. Moore,* The Developing Human *[2nd ed.]. Philadelphia: Saunders, 1977.)*

SIXTH AND SEVENTH WEEKS (FIG. 1-6). The cervical flexure of the brain causes the head to bend over the chest. The intestines enter the umbilical cord, and short webbed fingers are present. The somites are no longer recognizable; the tail is still present but much shorter.

EIGHTH WEEK (FIG. 1-7). The embryo now has unquestionably human characteristics (Fig. 1-7B). By the end of the week, the head is more rounded and the digits are clearly defined. The beginnings of all major external and internal structures are now formed.

THE FETAL PERIOD

From the ninth week until birth the developing human is referred to as a *fetus*. Changes that take place during this period (Fig. 1-8) are not so dramatic as those in the embryonic period but these changes are very important. The fetus is far less vulnerable to the teratogenic or deforming effects of drugs, viruses, and radiation, but these agents may interfere with normal functional development, especially of the brain. Development during the fetal period is primarily concerned with growth and maturation of tissues and organs that appeared during the embryonic period. Few new structures appear in the fetal period. The rate of body growth is remarkable, especially between the twelfth and sixteenth weeks, and weight gain is phenomenal during the terminal months.

Factors Influencing Fetal Growth

Glucose is the primary source of energy for fetal metabolism and growth. This and other nutrient substances are derived from the mother via the placenta. Insulin secreted by the fetal pancreas appears to be the primary growth-regulating hormone.

Severe maternal malnutrition resulting from a poor-quality diet is known to reduce fetal growth. Poor nutrition and faulty food habits are common, and they are not restricted to mothers belonging to poverty groups.

The growth rate for fetuses of mothers who smoke heavily is less than normal during the last six to eight weeks of pregnancy. The effect is greater on fetuses whose mothers also eat a poor-quality diet.

Maternal placental circulation may be reduced by a variety of conditions that decrease uterine blood flow (e.g., severe hypotension and renal disease). Chronic reduction of uterine blood flow can cause fetal starvation and fetal growth retardation.

Placental defects can also cause intrauterine fetal growth retardation. These placental changes reduce the total surface area available for exchange of nutrients between the fetal and maternal bloodstreams.

Structural and numerical chromosomal aberrations are associated with cases of retarded fetal growth. Intrauterine growth retardation is pronounced in Down's syndrome

FIGURE 1-5. *Lateral views of five week embryos showing their external characteristics. (From K. L. Moore,* The Developing Human *[2nd ed.]. Philadelphia: Saunders, 1977.)*

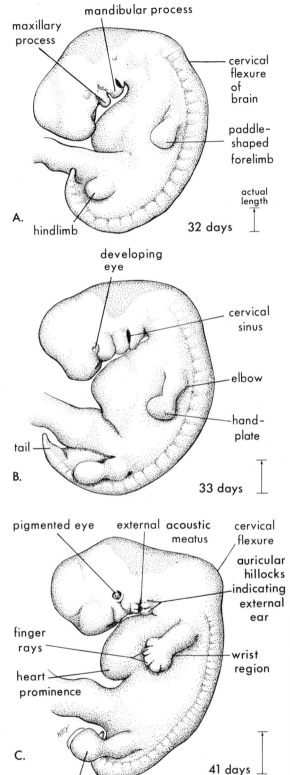

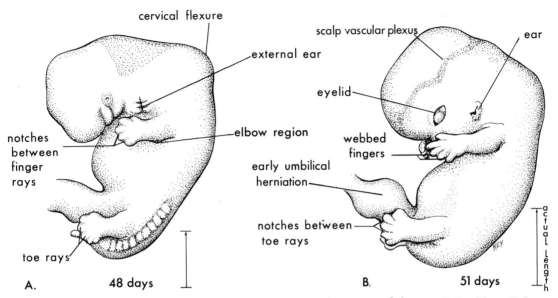

FIGURE 1-6.   *Lateral views of six week embryos showing their external characteristics. (From K. L. Moore,* The Developing Human *[2nd ed.]. Philadelphia: Saunders, 1977.)*

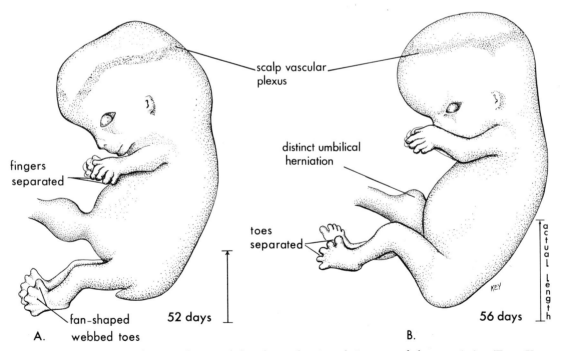

FIGURE 1-7.   *Lateral views of seven week embryos showing their external characteristics. (From K. L. Moore,* The Developing Human *[2nd ed.]. Philadelphia: Saunders, 1977.)*

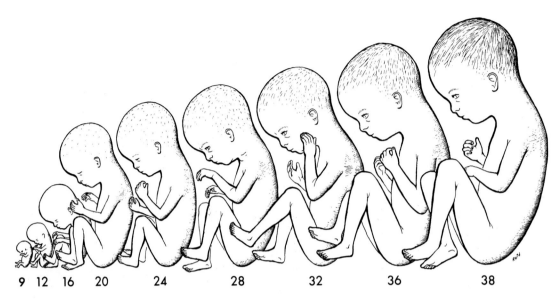

9 12 16   20   24   28   32   36   38

FIGURE 1-8. *Human fetuses about one-fifth actual size. Head hair begins to appear at about 20 weeks. Eyebrows and eyelashes are usually recognizable by 24 weeks, and the eyes open by 28 weeks. There is no sharp limit of development, age, or weight at which a fetus automatically becomes viable or beyond which survival is assured, but experience has shown that it is unusual for a baby to survive whose weight is less than 1000 gm or whose gestation age is less than 26 weeks. (From K. L. Moore,* The Developing Human *[2nd ed.]. Philadelphia: Saunders, 1977.)*

and is a characteristic of trisomy 18 or E syndrome.

The Branchial Apparatus and Its Derivatives

The branchial apparatus consists of branchial arches, pharyngeal pouches, branchial grooves (clefts), and branchial (closing) membranes (Fig. 1-9). The cranial region of an early human embryo somewhat resembles that of a fish embryo of a comparable stage, but these ancestral structures become rearranged and adapted to new functions or disappear.

The Branchial Arches

Branchial arches develop during the fourth week and appear as ridges on the future head and neck region (Fig. 1-9B–G). The arches are separated from each other by branchial grooves. The mouth initially appears as a slight depression of the surface ectoderm, called the *stomodeum* or primitive mouth (Fig. 1-9D–G). At first this cavity is separated from the primitive pharynx by a bilaminar membrane, the thin oropharyngeal (buccopharyngeal) membrane. The membrane ruptures during the fourth week, bringing the digestive tract into communication with the amniotic cavity.

FATE OF THE BRANCHIAL ARCHES.   The first branchial arch is involved with development of the face. During the fifth week the second (hyoid) arch overgrows the third and fourth arches, forming an ectodermal depression known as the *cervical sinus* (Fig. 1-10A–D). Gradually, the second to fourth branchial grooves and the cervical sinus are obliterated, giving the neck a smooth contour (Fig. 1-10F, G).

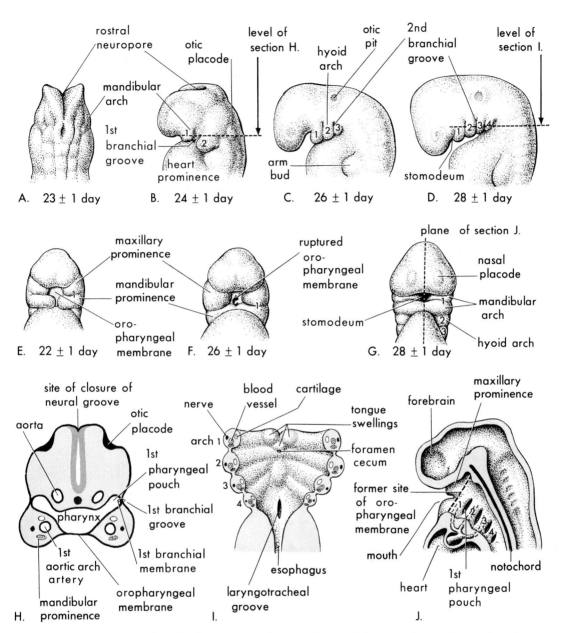

FIGURE 1-9.   *Human branchial apparatus. A. Dorsal view of the cranial part of an early embryo. B–D. Lateral views showing later development of the branchial arches. E–G. Facial views illustrating the relationship of the first arch to the stomodeum or primitive mouth. H. Transverse section through the cranial region of an embryo. I. Horizontal section through the cranial region of an embryo, illustrating the branchial arch components and the floor of the primitive pharynx. J. Sagittal section of the upper region of an embryo illustrating the openings of the pharyngeal pouches in the lateral wall of the primitive pharynx. (From K. L. Moore,* The Developing Human *[2nd ed.]. Philadelphia: Saunders, 1977.)*

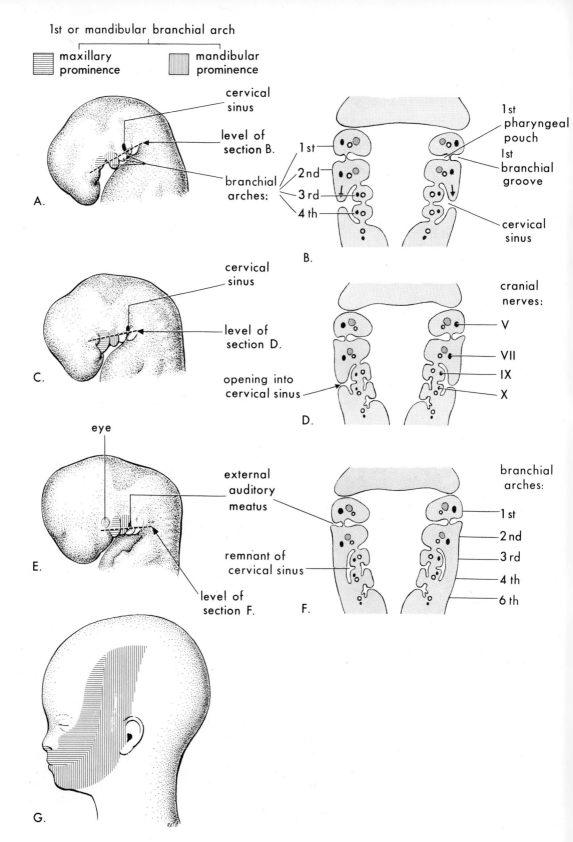

1st or mandibular branchial arch

maxillary prominence

mandibular prominence

cervical sinus

level of section B.

branchial arches:
1st
2nd
3rd
4th

A.

1st pharyngeal pouch

1st branchial groove

cervical sinus

B.

cervical sinus

level of section D.

opening into cervical sinus

C.

cranial nerves:
V
VII
IX
X

D.

eye

external auditory meatus

remnant of cervical sinus

level of section F.

E.

branchial arches:
1st
2nd
3rd
4th
6th

F.

G.

DERIVATIVES OF THE BRANCHIAL ARCH CARTILAGES (FIG. 1-11). The dorsal end of the first arch (Meckel's cartilage) becomes ossified to form two middle ear bones, the malleus and the incus. The intermediate portion of the cartilages regresses and its perichondrium forms the anterior ligament of the malleus and the sphenomandibular ligament also forms. The ventral portion of Meckel's cartilage largely disappears as the mandible develops around it by intramembranous ossification.

The dorsal end of the second arch (Reichert's cartilage) also ossifies and forms the stapes of the middle ear and the styloid process of the temporal bone. The portion of cartilage between the styloid process and the hyoid bone regresses, and its perichondrium forms the stylohyoid ligament. The ventral end of Reichert's cartilage ossifies to form the lesser cornu and upper part of the body of the hyoid bone.

The third arch cartilage is located in the ventral portion of the arch and ossifies to form the greater cornu and lower part of the body of the hyoid bone. The fourth and sixth arch cartilages are in the ventral regions of the arches and form the laryngeal cartilages.

The Pharyngeal Pouches

The primitive pharynx is wide cranially and narrow caudally. The endoderm of the pharynx lines the inner aspects of the branchial arches and passes into balloon-like outgrowths called *pharyngeal pouches* (Figs. 1-9, 1-10). There are four well-defined pairs of pouches.

DERIVATIVES OF THE PHARYNGEAL POUCHES. The first pharyngeal pouch expands into an elongate tubotympanic recess which gives rise to the tympanic cavity and antrum (Fig. 1-12). Its connection with the pharynx gradually elongates to form the pharyngotympanic (eustachian) tube. The endoderm of the second pharyngeal pouch proliferates and forms buds. The central parts of these buds break down, forming the tonsillar crypts. The pouch endoderm forms the surface epithelium and the lining of the crypts of the palatine tonsil. The mesenchyme surrounding the crypts differentiates into lymphoid tissue (lymph nodules).

The third pharyngeal pouch expands into a solid dorsal bulbar portion and a hollow ventral elongate part. Each dorsal bulbar portion differentiates into an inferior parathyroid and thymus. The thymus and parathyroid glands migrate caudally. Later the parathyroid glands separate from the thymus and come to lie on the dorsal surface of the thyroid gland, which has descended from the foramen cecum of the tongue (Fig. 1-12C).

The fourth pharyngeal pouch also expands into a dorsal bulbar portion and a ventral elongate part. Each dorsal portion develops into a superior parathyroid gland. The ventral elongate part of each fourth pouch develops into an ultimobranchial body which becomes incorporated into the thyroid gland as the parafollicular (C) cells. These cells produce thyrocalcitonin, a hormone involved in the regulation of the normal calcium level in body fluids.

Development of the Face

The five facial primordia appear around the stomodeum, or primitive mouth, early in the fourth week (Fig. 1-13). The unpaired maxillary processes of the first branchial arch form

FIGURE 1-10. *A. Lateral view of the head and neck region of a 30 day embryo showing the branchial arches and the cervical sinus. B. Horizontal section through the embryo illustrating the growth of the second branchial arch over the third and fourth arches. C. A 33 day embryo. D. Horizontal section through the embryo illustrating closure of the cervical sinus. E. A 35 day embryo. F. Horizontal section through the embryo showing the transitory cystic remnant of the cervical sinus. G. A 20 week fetus, illustrating the areas of the face and neck derived from the first three branchial arches. (From K. L. Moore,* The Developing Human *[2nd ed.]. Philadelphia: Saunders, 1977.)*

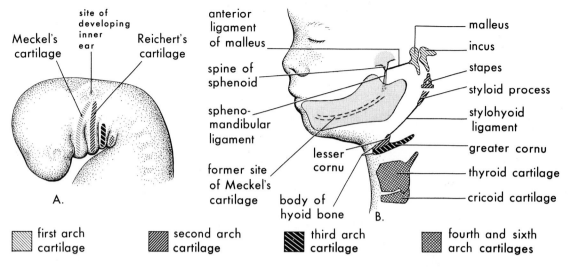

FIGURE 1-11.   *A. Head and neck region of a four week embryo, illustrating the location of the branchial arch cartilages. B. A 24 week fetus, illustrating the adult derivatives of the branchial arch cartilages. (From K. L. Moore,* The Developing Human *[2nd ed.]. Philadelphia: Saunders, 1977.)*

the lateral boundaries, or sides, of the stomodeum, and the paired mandibular processes of this same arch constitute the lower boundary of the stomodeum.

Bilateral oval-shaped thickenings of the surface ectoderm, called *nasal placodes*, develop on each side of the lower part of the frontonasal prominence (Fig. 1-13B). Horseshoe-shaped medial and lateral nasal prominences or processes develop at the margins of the nasal placodes (Fig. 1-13C, D), causing the placodes to lie in depressions called *nasal pits*. The maxillary prominences grow rapidly and approach each other and the medial nasal prominences (Fig. 1-13D, E).

During the sixth and seventh weeks, the medial nasal prominences merge with each other and the maxillary prominences (Fig. 1-13F, G). As the medial nasal prominences merge with each other, they form an intermaxillary segment of the upper jaw (Fig. 1-13H). This segment gives rise to the middle portion of the upper lip, called the *philtrum*, the middle portion of the upper jaw and its associated gingiva, and the primary palate. The lateral parts of the upper lip, the upper jaw, and the secondary palate form from the

maxillary prominences (Fig. 1-13H, I). The frontonasal elevation forms the forehead and the dorsum and apex of the nose. The sides or alae of the nose are derived from the lateral nasal prominences.

The mandibular prominences merge with each other in the fourth week, and the groove between them disappears during the fifth week. The mandibular prominences give rise to the lower jaw, the lower lip, and the lower part of the face. Final development of the face occurs slowly and results mainly from changes in the proportion and relative position of the facial components.

Development of the Palate

The primary palate (median palatine process) develops at the end of the fifth week from the innermost part of the intermaxillary segment of the upper jaw. It forms a wedge-shaped mass of mesoderm between the maxillary prominences of the developing upper jaw (Fig. 1-14B).

The secondary palate develops from two horizontal projections from the maxillary prominences (Fig. 1-14B). These processes initially project downward on each side of the

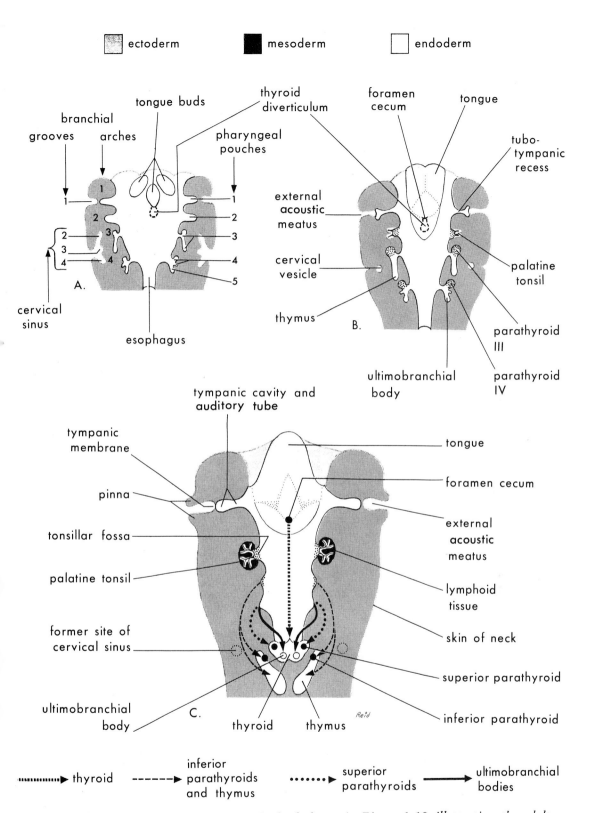

ectoderm   mesoderm   endoderm

A.

branchial grooves
arches
tongue buds
thyroid diverticulum
pharyngeal pouches

1
2
3
4

2
3
4

1
2
3
4
5

cervical sinus

esophagus

B.

foramen cecum
tongue
tubo-tympanic recess

external acoustic meatus

cervical vesicle

thymus

palatine tonsil

parathyroid III

parathyroid IV

ultimobranchial body

C.

tympanic cavity and auditory tube

tympanic membrane

pinna

tonsillar fossa

palatine tonsil

former site of cervical sinus

ultimobranchial body

thyroid   thymus

tongue

foramen cecum

external acoustic meatus

lymphoid tissue

skin of neck

superior parathyroid

inferior parathyroid

Reid

thyroid   inferior parathyroids and thymus   superior parathyroids   ultimobranchial bodies

FIGURE 1-12. *Horizontal sections at the level shown in Figure 1-10 illustrating the adult derivatives of the pharyngeal pouches. A. Five weeks. B. Six weeks. C. Seven weeks. (From K. L. Moore,* The Developing Human *[2nd ed.]. Philadelphia: Saunders, 1977.)*

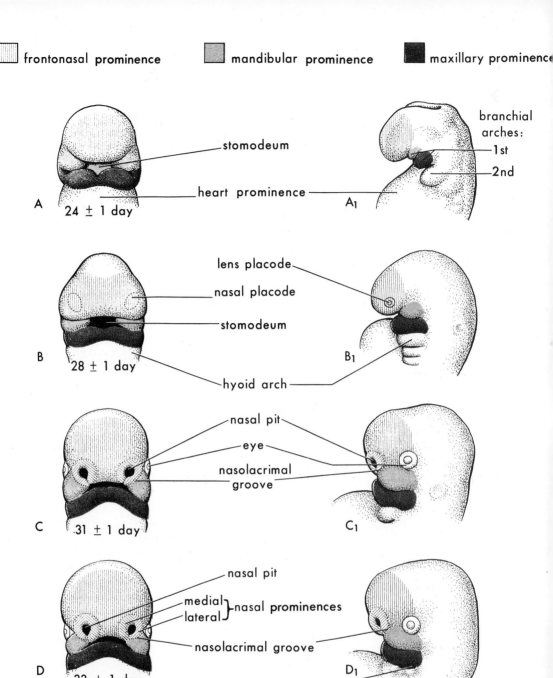

frontonasal prominence   mandibular prominence   maxillary prominence

stomodeum

branchial arches:
—1st
—2nd

heart prominence — A_1

A 24 ± 1 day

lens placode

nasal placode

stomodeum

B_1

B 28 ± 1 day

hyoid arch

nasal pit
eye
nasolacrimal groove

C 31 ± 1 day C_1

nasal pit
medial } nasal prominences
lateral
nasolacrimal groove

D 33 ± 1 day D_1

first branchial groove

medial nasal prominence
lateral nasal prominence
external ear

E 35 ± 1 day E_1

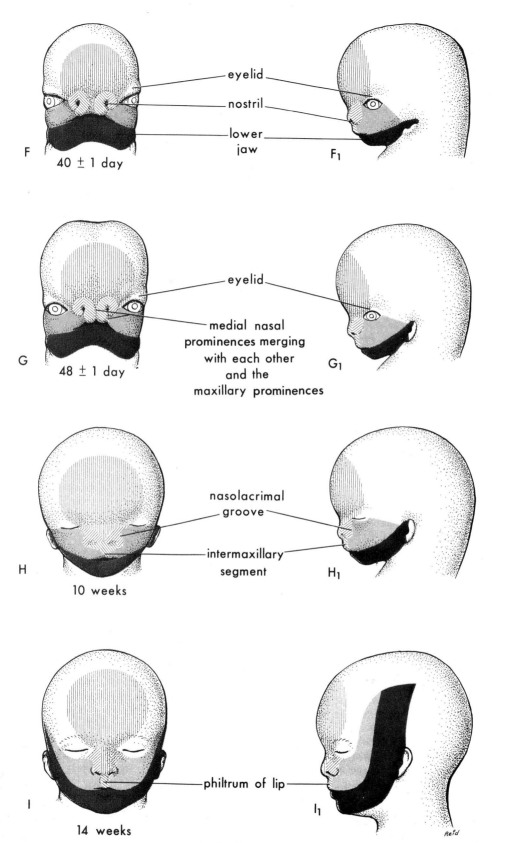

FIGURE 1-13.   *Progressive stages in the development of the human face. (From K. L. Moore,* The Developing Human *[2nd ed.]. Philadelphia: Saunders, 1977.)*

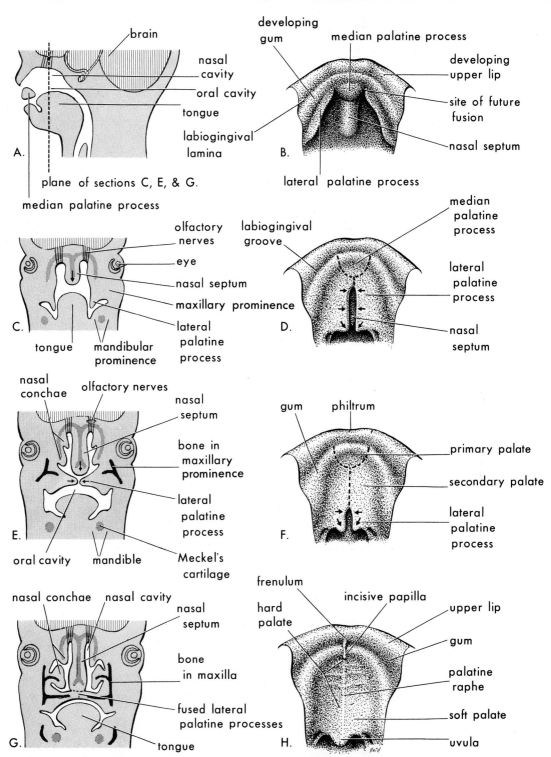

FIGURE 1-14.   A. *Sagittal section of the embryonic head at the end of the sixth week showing the primary palate. B, D, F, and H. Roof of the mouth from sixth to twelfth weeks illustrating development of the palate. The broken lines in D and F indicate sites of fusion of the palatine processes; the arrows indicate medial and posterior growth of the lateral palatine processes. C, E, and G. Frontal sections of the head illustrating fusion of the lateral palatine processes with each other and with the nasal septum, and separation of the nasal and oral cavities. (From K. L. Moore,* The Developing Human *[2nd ed.]. Philadelphia: Saunders, 1977.)*

tongue (Fig. 1-14C), but as the jaws develop the tongue moves downward and the lateral palatine processes gradually grow toward each other and fuse (Fig. 1-14E, G). They also fuse with the primary palate and the nasal septum. The fusion begins anteriorly during the ninth week and is complete posteriorly by the twelfth week. The palatine raphe indicates the line of fusion of the lateral palatine processes (Fig. 1-14H).

Congenital Malformations of the Head and Neck

Abnormalities of the head and neck mainly originate during transformation of the branchial apparatus into adult structures.

Congenital Auricular Pits and Cysts

Small blind pits or cysts in the skin are commonly found in a triangular area anterior to the ear (Fig. 1-15F). Although often claimed to be remnants of the first branchial cleft, they probably represent ectodermal folds which become isolated during formation of the external ear.

Branchial or Lateral Cervical Sinus

Branchial sinuses are uncommon; they open externally on the side of the neck and result from failure of the second branchial cleft or groove to obliterate (Fig. 1-15C, D). Often there is an intermittent discharge of mucus from the opening. Branchial sinuses which open into the pharynx (usually into the tonsillar fossa) are very rare (Fig. 1-15D, F). They probably result from persistence of part of the second pharyngeal pouch.

Branchial Fistula

A branchial fistula opens externally on the side of the neck and internally in the pharynx (Fig. 1-15E, F). It usually results from persistence of parts of the second branchial groove and the second pharyngeal pouch. The fistula ascends through the subcutaneous tissue, the platysma muscle, and the deep fascia and passes between the internal and external carotid arteries on its way to the tonsillar fossa.

Branchial, or Lateral, Cervical Cyst

Remnants of the cervical sinus, the second branchial groove, or the second pharyngeal pouch may persist and form cysts (Fig. 1-15F). Although they are sometimes associated with branchial sinuses and drain through them, they often lie free in the neck just below the angle of the jaw.

The First Arch Syndrome

A pattern of multiple malformations resulting from abnormal transformation of first branchial arch components into various adult derivatives is often referred to as the *first arch syndrome*. In the Treacher Collins syndrome (mandibulofacial dysostosis) there are malar hypoplasia with downslanting palpebral fissures, defects of the lower lid, deformed external ear, and sometimes abnormalities of the middle and inner ear. In the Pierre Robin syndrome, striking hypoplasia of the mandible, cleft palate, and defects of the eye and ear are found.

Cleft Lip and Cleft Palate

Although often associated, cleft lip and cleft palate are embryologically and etiologically distinct malformations. They originate at different times during development and involve different developmental processes.

CLEFT LIP. Cleft of the upper lip, with or without cleft palate, occurs about once in 900 births; the defect may be unilateral or bilateral. The clefts vary from a small notch to a complete division of the lip and alveolar process. Unilateral cleft lip results from a deficiency of mesenchyme causing failure of the maxillary prominence on the affected side to merge with the intermaxillary segment formed by the merged medial nasal prominences (Fig. 1-16). Bilateral cleft lip results from a mesenchymal deficiency causing failure of the maxillary prominences to meet and merge with the medial nasal prominences. In complete bilateral cleft of the upper lip and alveolar process, the intermaxillary segment hangs free and projects anteriorly.

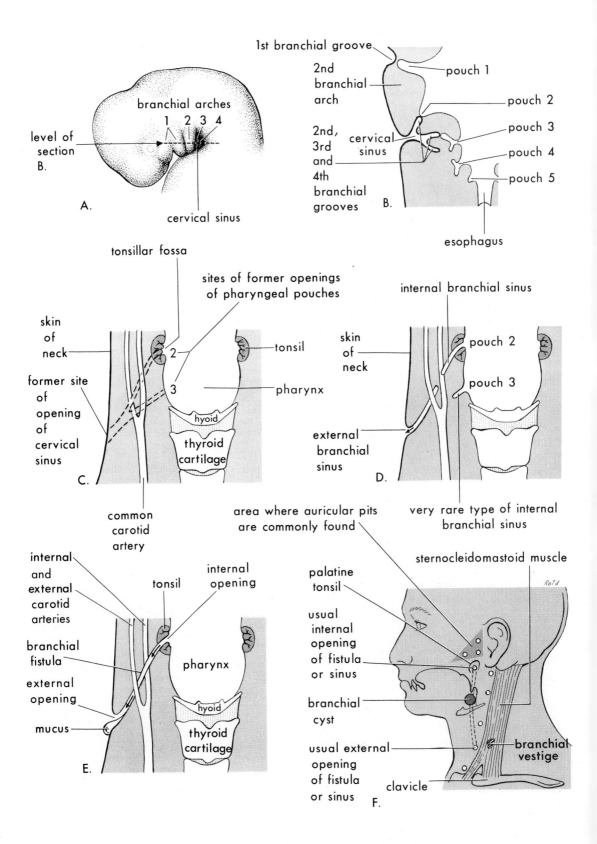

A.

branchial arches
1 2 3 4

level of
section
B.

cervical sinus

B.

1st branchial groove

2nd
branchial
arch

pouch 1

pouch 2

2nd,
3rd
and
4th
branchial
grooves

cervical
sinus

pouch 3

pouch 4

pouch 5

esophagus

C.

tonsillar fossa

sites of former openings
of pharyngeal pouches

skin
of
neck

tonsil

former site
of
opening
of
cervical
sinus

pharynx

hyoid

thyroid
cartilage

common
carotid
artery

D.

internal branchial sinus

skin
of
neck

pouch 2

pouch 3

external
branchial
sinus

very rare type of internal
branchial sinus

E.

internal
and
external
carotid
arteries

tonsil

internal
opening

branchial
fistula

external
opening

mucus

pharynx

hyoid

thyroid
cartilage

F.

area where auricular pits
are commonly found

sternocleidomastoid muscle

palatine
tonsil

usual
internal
opening
of fistula
or sinus

branchial
cyst

usual external
opening
of fistula
or sinus

branchial
vestige

clavicle

CLEFT PALATE.   Cleft palate, with or without cleft lip, occurs in about one in 2500 births; the cleft may be unilateral or bilateral (Fig. 1-17). A cleft may involve only the uvula, or it may extend through the soft and hard palates. In severe cases associated with cleft lip, the cleft in the anterior and posterior palate extends through the alveolar process and lip on both sides. The embryological basis of cleft palate is failure of the mesenchymal masses of the lateral palatine processes to meet and fuse with each other, with the nasal septum, and/or with the median palatine process.

Facial Clefts

Various types of facial cleft occur, but they are all extremely rare. Severe clefts are usually associated with gross malformations of the head. In median cleft of the mandible (Fig. 1-18B), there is a deep cleft resulting from failure of the mandibular prominences of the first branchial arch to merge completely with each other.

Oblique facial clefts are often bilateral and extend from the upper lip to the medial margin of the orbit (Fig. 1-18C). They are caused by failure of the maxillary prominences to merge with lateral and medial nasal prominences. Lateral or transverse facial clefts run from the mouth toward the ear. Bilateral clefts leave the mouth very large, a condition called *macrostomia* (Fig. 1-18D); this abnormality is due to failure of the maxillary and mandibular prominences to merge.

Other Rare Facial Malformations

Congenital microstomia (small mouth) is caused by excessive merging of the maxillary and mandibular prominences of the first arch (Fig. 1-18E). A single nostril results when only one nasal placode forms. Bifid nose results from failure of the medial nasal prominences to merge completely (Fig. 1-18F).

Development of the Limbs

The general features of early limb development are illustrated in Figures 1-4 to 1-7. The limb buds first appear toward the end of the fourth week as small elevations of the ventrolateral body wall. The early stages of limb development are alike for the upper and lower limbs (Figs. 1-19, 1-20), except that appearance of the arm buds precedes that of the leg buds by a few days. The arm buds develop opposite the caudal cervical segments, and the leg buds form opposite the lumbar and upper sacral segments. Each limb bud consists of a mass of mesenchyme covered by a layer of ectoderm. The apical ectodermal ridge exerts an inductive influence on this mesenchyme (Fig. 1-21B), promoting growth and development of the limb bones. The ends of the flipper-like limb buds flatten into paddle-like hand or foot plates, and digits differentiate at the margins of these plates (Fig. 1-19).

As the limbs elongate and the bones form, muscle-forming cells (myoblasts) aggregate and develop into a large muscle mass in each extremity. This muscle mass separates into dorsal (extensor) and ventral (flexor) components. Initially the limbs are directed caudally, but soon they extend ventrally. Subsequently the developing arms and legs rotate in opposite directions and to different degrees (Fig. 1-20). Originally the flexor aspect of the limbs is ventral and the extensor aspect dorsal. The arm buds rotate laterally through 90 degrees on their longitudinal axes; thus

---

FIGURE 1-15.   *A. Head and neck region of a five week embryo. B. Horizontal section through the embryo illustrating the relationship of the cervical sinus to the branchial arches and pharyngeal pouches. C. Adult neck region, indicating the former sites of openings of the cervical sinus and the pharyngeal pouches. The broken lines indicate possible courses of branchial fistulas. D. Embryological basis of various types of branchial sinus. E. Branchial fistula resulting from persistence of parts of the second branchial cleft and the second pharyngeal pouch. F. Possible sites of branchial cysts and openings of branchial sinuses and fistulas. A cartilaginous branchial vestige is also illustrated. (From K. L. Moore,* The Developing Human *[2nd ed.]. Philadelphia: Saunders, 1977.)*

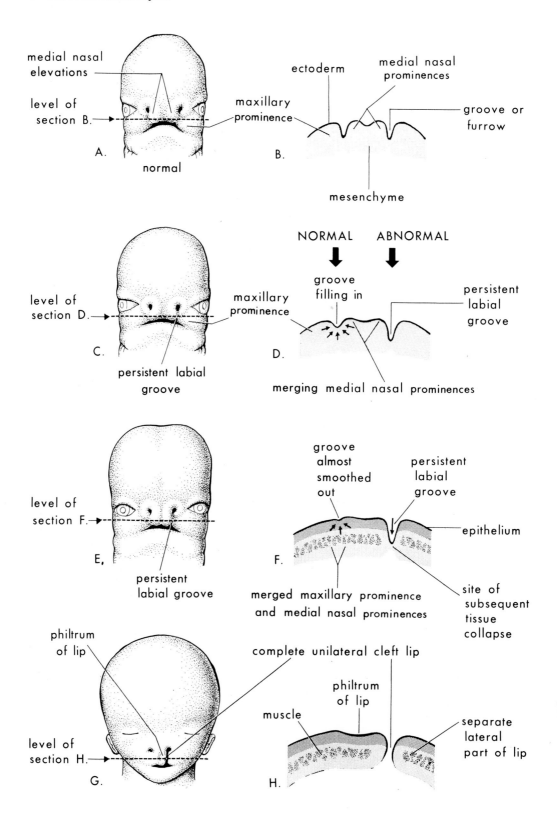

A. normal

medial nasal elevations

level of section B.

maxillary prominence

B.

ectoderm

medial nasal prominences

groove or furrow

mesenchyme

C.

level of section D.

maxillary prominence

persistent labial groove

NORMAL   ABNORMAL

D.

groove filling in

persistent labial groove

merging medial nasal prominences

E,

level of section F.

persistent labial groove

F.

groove almost smoothed out

persistent labial groove

epithelium

merged maxillary prominence and medial nasal prominences

site of subsequent tissue collapse

G.

philtrum of lip

level of section H.

complete unilateral cleft lip

H.

philtrum of lip

muscle

separate lateral part of lip

the future elbows point backward, or dorsally, and the extensor muscles come to lie on the outer and dorsal aspect of the arm. The leg buds rotate medially through 90 degrees on their longitudinal axes; thus the future knees point forward, or ventrolaterally, and the extensor muscles lie on the ventral aspect of the leg. It should also be clear that the radius and tibia and the ulna and fibula are homologous bones, just as the thumb and the big toe are homologous digits.

During the sixth week, the mesenchymal primordia of bones in the limb buds undergo chondrification to form hyaline cartilage models of the future limb bones (Fig. 1-21D, E). The models in the upper limb bones appear slightly before those in the lower limbs, and the models of each extremity appear in a proximodistal sequence. Ossification begins in the long bones by the end of the embryonic period, and primary ossification centers have appeared in nearly all limb bones by the end of the first trimester. Secondary centers of ossification appear after birth.

The musculature of the limbs develops from the mesenchyme surrounding the developing bones. This mesenchyme is derived from the somatic mesoderm. It is now generally believed that there is no migration of mesenchyme from the somites to form limb muscles.

Limb Malformations

Minor limb defects are relatively common, but major malformations are usually rare; however, an "epidemic" of limb deformities occurred from 1957 to 1962 as a result of maternal ingestion of thalidomide.

Cleft Hand and Foot

In the rare defect often called the *lobster-claw deformity* there is absence of one or more central digits (Fig. 1-22E, F). Thus the hand or foot is divided into two parts that oppose each other like lobster claws. The remaining digits are partially or completely fused (syndactyly).

Brachydactyly

Abnormal shortness of the fingers or toes is uncommon (Fig. 1-23A). It results from reduction in the size of the phalanges. It is usually inherited as a dominant trait and is often associated with shortness of stature.

Polydactyly or Supernumerary Digits

Supernumerary fingers or toes are common (Fig. 1-23C, D). Often the extra digit is incompletely formed and useless. If the hand is affected, the extra digit is ordinarily ulnar or radial in position rather than central. In the foot, the extra toe is usually in the fibular position. Polydactyly is inherited as a dominant trait.

Syndactyly or Webbed Digits

Fusion of the fingers or toes is a common limb malformation (Fig. 1-24). Webbing of the skin between the fingers or toes results from failure of the tissue to break down between the digits during development. Syndactyly is most frequently observed between

---

FIGURE 1-16. *Embryological basis of complete unilateral cleft lip. A. Five week embryo. B. Horizontal section through the head illustrating the grooves between the maxillary processes and the merged medial nasal elevations. C. Six week embryo showing a persistent labial groove on the left side. D. Horizontal section through the head showing the disappearance of the groove on the right side because of proliferation of the mesenchyme (arrows). A deficiency of mesenchymal proliferation on the left side has resulted in persistence of the labial groove. E. Seven week embryo. F. Horizontal section through the head showing that the epithelium on the right has been almost pushed out of the groove between the maxillary process and the medial nasal elevation. G. Ten week fetus with a complete unilateral cleft lip. H. Horizontal section through the head following stretching of the epithelium and breakdown of the tissues in the floor of the persistent labial groove on the left side. (From K. L. Moore,* The Developing Human *[2nd ed.]. Philadelphia: Saunders, 1977.)*

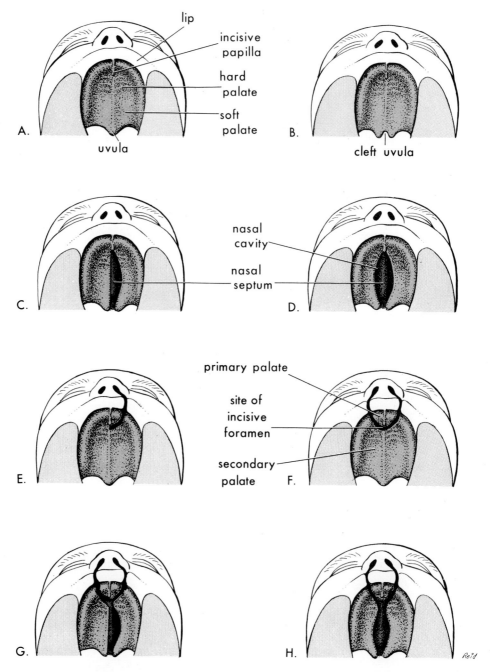

FIGURE 1-17.   *Various types of cleft lip and palate. A. Normal lip and palate. B. Cleft uvula. C. Unilateral cleft of the posterior or secondary palate. D. Bilateral cleft of the posterior palate. E. Complete unilateral cleft of the lip and alveolar process with a unilateral cleft of the anterior or primary palate. F. Complete bilateral cleft of the lip and alveolar process with bilateral cleft of the anterior palate. G. Complete bilateral cleft of the lip and alveolar process with bilateral cleft of the anterior palate and unilateral cleft of the posterior palate. H. Complete bilateral cleft of the lip and alveolar process with complete bilateral cleft of the anterior and posterior palate. (From K. L. Moore,* The Developing Human *[2nd ed.]. Philadelphia: Saunders, 1977.)*

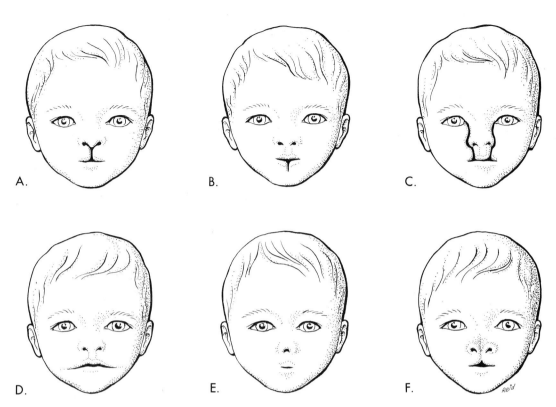

FIGURE 1-18.   *Rare malformations of the face. A. Median cleft lip. B. Median cleft of the lower lip and jaw. C. Bilateral oblique facial clefts with complete bilateral cleft lip. D. Macrostomia or lateral facial cleft. E. Single nostril and microstomia; these malformations are not usually associated. F. Bifid nose and incomplete median cleft lip. (From K. L. Moore,* The Developing Human *[2nd ed.]. Philadelphia: Saunders, 1977.)*

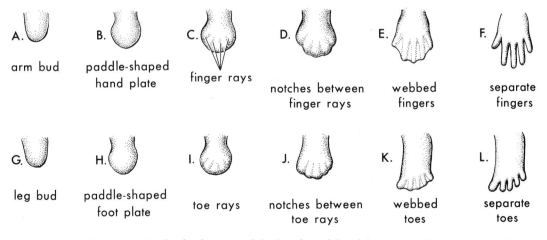

FIGURE 1-19.   *Stages in the development of the hands and feet during the embryonic period. (From K. L. Moore,* The Developing Human *[2nd ed.]. Philadelphia: Saunders, 1977.)*

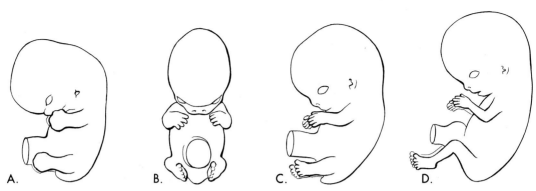

FIGURE 1-20.   *Positional changes of the developing limbs. A. About 37 days, showing the extremities extending ventrally and the hand and foot plates facing each other. B. About 41 days, showing the arms bent at the elbows and the hands curved over the thorax. C. About 43 days, showing the soles of the feet facing each other. D. About 48 days; note that the elbows now point caudally and the knees cranially. (From K. L. Moore,* The Developing Human *[2nd ed.]. Philadelphia: Saunders, 1977.)*

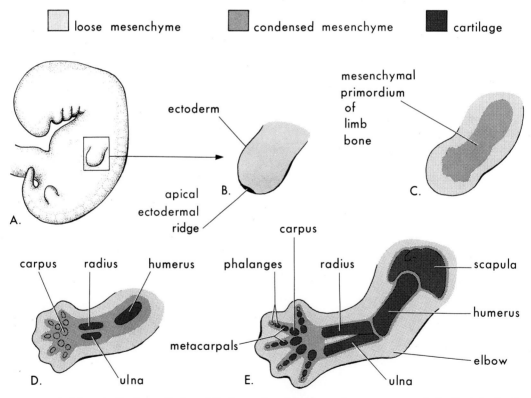

FIGURE 1-21.   *A. Embryo of about 28 days, showing the early appearance of the limb buds. B. Longitudinal section through an early arm bud. The apical ectodermal ridge has an inductive influence on the loose mesenchyme in the limb bud; it promotes growth of the mesenchyme and appears to give it the ability to form specific cartilaginous elements. C. Arm bud at 33 days, showing the mesenchymal primordium of a limb bone. D. Forelimb at six weeks, showing the completed cartilaginous models of the bones of the upper limb. E. Later in the sixth week, showing the completed cartilaginous models of the bones of the upper limb. (From K. L. Moore,* The Developing Human *[2nd ed.]. Philadelphia: Saunders, 1977.)*

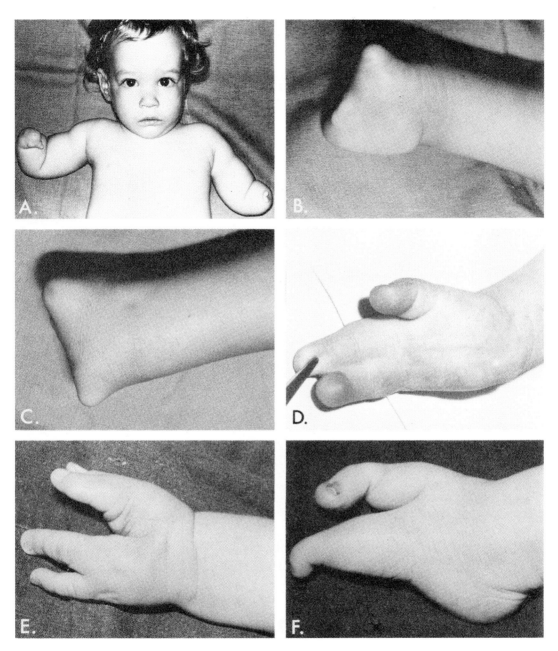

FIGURE 1-22.   *Various types of meromelia (partial absence of a limb or limbs). A. Absence of the hands and most of the forearms. B. Absence of the phalanges. C. Absence of the hand. D. Absence of the fourth and fifth phalanges and metacarpals; there is also syndactyly. E. Absence of the third phalanx, resulting in a cleft hand (lobster claw). F. Absence of the second and third toes, resulting in a cleft foot. (From K. L. Moore,* The Developing Human *[2nd ed.]. Philadelphia: Saunders, 1977.)*

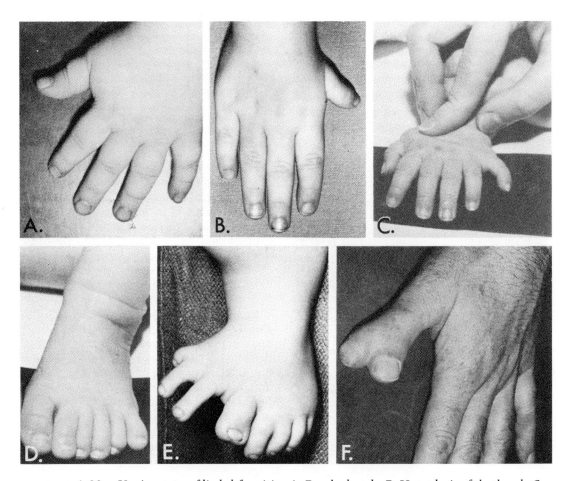

FIGURE 1-23. *Various types of limb deformities. A. Brachydactyly. B. Hypoplasia of the thumb. C. Polydactyly showing a supernumerary finger. D. Polydactyly showing a supernumerary toe. E. Partial duplication of the foot. F. Partial duplication of the thumb. (From K. L. Moore,* The Developing Human *[2nd ed.]. Philadelphia: Saunders, 1977.)*

third and fourth fingers and second and third toes. It is inherited as a simple dominant or simple recessive trait.

Clubfoot or Talipes Equinovarus

Talipes equinovarus is relatively common and is about twice as frequent in males (Fig. 1-24C). The sole of the foot is turned medially, and the foot is adducted and plantar-flexed at the midtarsal joint. Although it is often stated that the condition results from abnormal positioning or restricted movement of the lower extremities in utero, the evidence for this hypothesis is inconclusive.

Hereditary factors are involved in some cases, but environmental factors seem also to be involved in most cases.

Development of the Urinary System
The Kidney and Ureter

Three successive sets of excretory organs develop: the pronephros, the mesonephros, and the metanephros. The third set remains as the permanent kidneys. The pronephros on each side is a transitory, nonfunctional structure which appears in the cervical region early in the fourth week (Fig. 1-25). The pronephros soon degenerates, but most of its

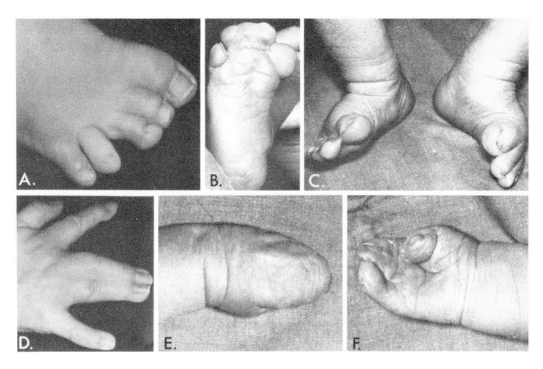

FIGURE 1-24. *Various types of limb deformities. A. Syndactyly showing skin webs between the first and second and second and third toes. B. Syndactyly involving fusion of all the toes except the fifth. C. Syndactyly associated with clubfoot (talipes equinovarus). D. Syndactyly involving webbing of the third and fourth fingers. E and F. Dorsal and palmar views of a child's right hand showing syndactyly or fusion of the second to fifth fingers. (From K. L. Moore,* The Developing Human *[2nd ed.]. Philadelphia: Saunders, 1977.)*

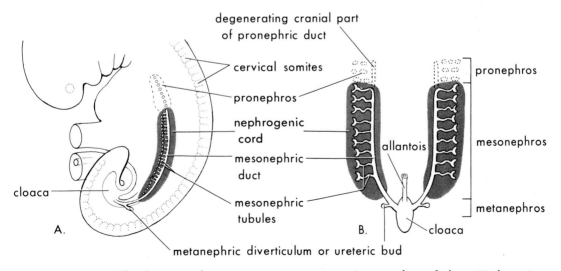

FIGURE 1-25. *The three sets of excretory structures present in an embryo of about 29 days. A. Lateral view. B. Ventral view. (From K. L. Moore,* The Developing Human *[2nd ed.]. Philadelphia: Saunders, 1977.)*

duct is utilized by the next kidney or mesonephros.

The mesonephros appears later in the fourth week caudal to the rudimentary pronephros (Fig. 1-25). It may function while the permanent kidney is developing, but by the embryonic period it has degenerated and disappeared, except for its duct and a few tubules.

The metanephros or permanent kidney appears early in the fifth week and begins to function about three weeks later. It develops from two sources: the metanephric diverticulum or ureteric bud, and the metanephric mass of mesoderm (Fig. 1-26). The metanephric diverticulum grows from the mesonephric duct into the mass of metanephric mesoderm (Fig. 1-26B). The stalk of the diverticulum becomes the ureter, and its ex-

panded cranial end forms the renal pelvis. The pelvis is divided into major and minor calyces, from which collecting tubules soon grow. Each collecting tubule undergoes repeated branching, forming successive generations of collecting tubules. Near the blind end of each arched collecting tubule, clusters of mesenchymal cells develop into metanephric tubules (Fig. 1-27). The blind ends of these tubules are invaginated by an ingrowth, or tuft, of fine branches of the renal artery, to form a glomerulus and a double-layered cup called a *glomerular* (Bowman's) *capsule*. The renal corpuscle and its associated tubules form a nephron. The distal convoluted tubule of the nephron contacts an arched collecting tubule and becomes confluent.

Initially the kidneys are in the pelvis, but they gradually come to lie in the abdomen. As

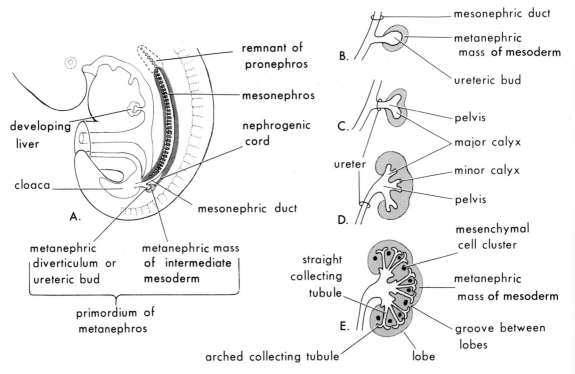

FIGURE 1-26.   A. *Lateral view of a five week embryo showing the primordium of the metanephros or permanent kidney. B–E. Successive stages of development of the ureteric bud into the ureter, pelvis, calyces, and collecting tubules. (From K. L. Moore,* The Developing Human *[2nd ed.]. Philadelphia: Saunders, 1977.)*

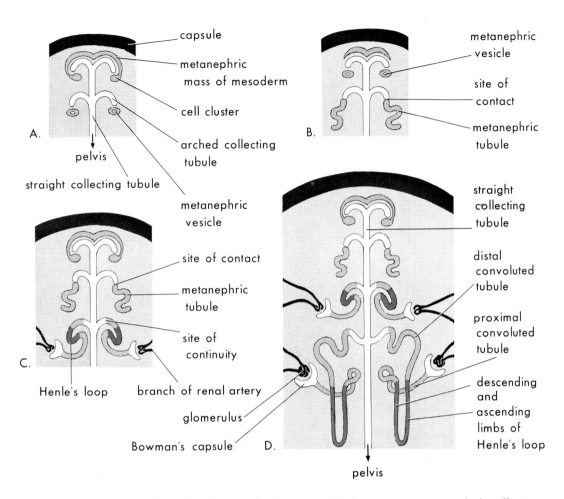

FIGURE 1-27. *Stages in the development of nephrons, which become continuous with the collecting tubules to form uriniferous tubules. (From K. L. Moore,* The Developing Human *[2nd ed.]. Philadelphia: Saunders, 1977.)*

the kidneys move out of the pelvis, they are supplied by arteries at successively higher levels. The caudal arteries normally degenerate as the kidneys ascend and new vessels form.

The Bladder and Urethra

Division of the cloaca by the urorectal septum into a dorsal rectum and a ventral urogenital sinus is illustrated in Figure 1-28. The urinary bladder and urethra are derived from the urogenital sinus and adjacent splanchnic mesenchyme. As the bladder enlarges, the caudal portions of the mesonephric ducts are incorporated into its dorsal wall. During this process the ureters come to open separately into the urinary bladder.

Development of the Reproductive System

The genetic sex of an embryo is determined by the kind of sperm that fertilizes the ovum, but there is no morphological indication of sex in the organs until the seventh week, when the gonads (future ovaries or testes) begin to acquire sexual characteristics. The early genital system is similar in both sexes, and initially all normal human embryos are potentially bisexual.

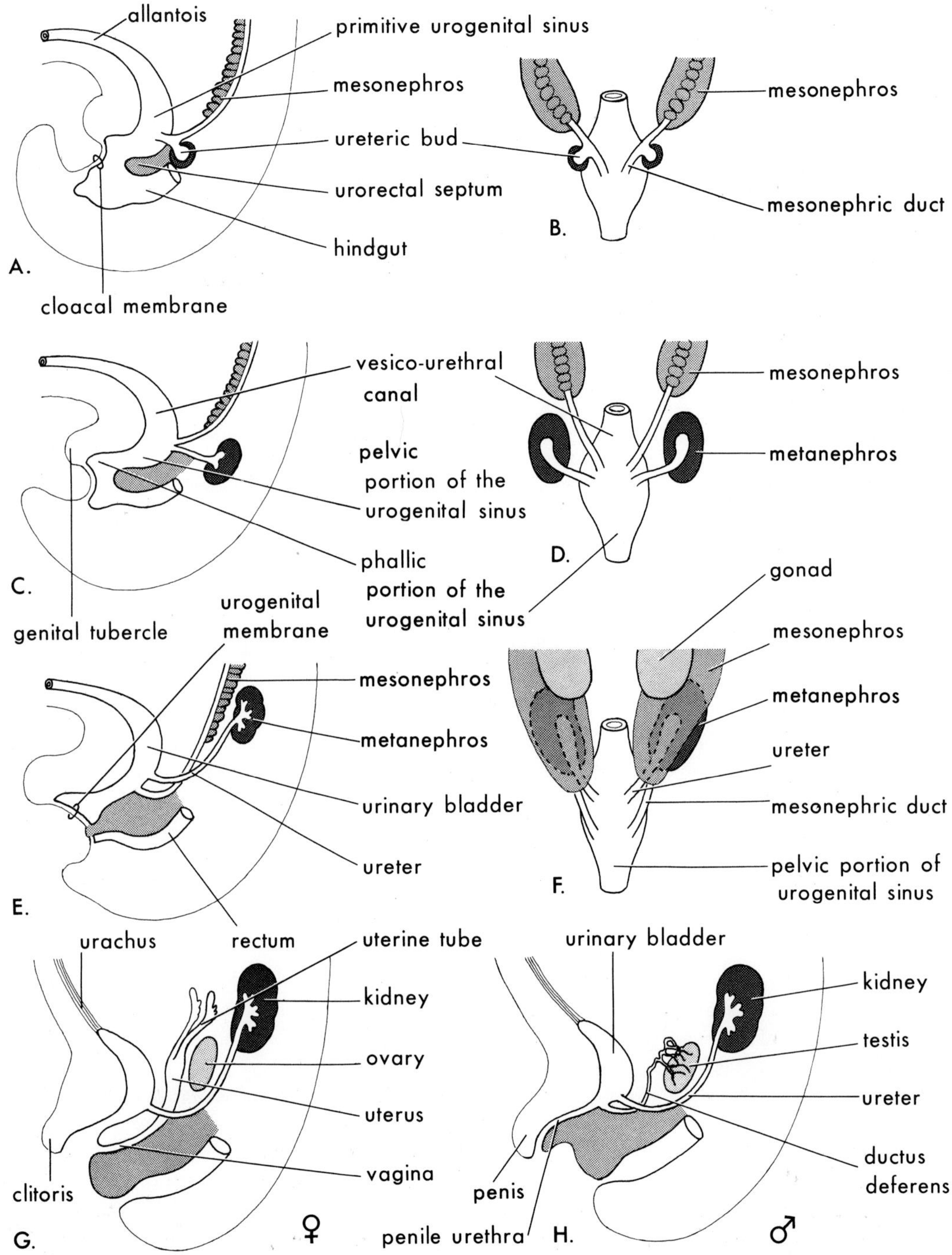

FIGURE 1-28. *Diagrams showing (1) division of the cloaca into the urogenital sinus and the rectum, (2) absorption of the mesonephric ducts, (3) development of the urinary bladder, urethra, and urachus, and (4) changes in the location of the ureters. A. Lateral view of the caudal half of a five week embryo. B, D, and F. Dorsal views. C, E, G, and H. Lateral views. The stages shown in G and H are reached by about 12 weeks. (From K. L. Moore,* The Developing Human *[2nd ed.]. Philadelphia: Saunders, 1977.)*

Gonadal development is first indicated during the fifth week, when a thickened area of germinal epithelium forms a gonadal ridge on the medial aspect of the urogenital ridge (Fig. 1-29C). Epithelial cords, called *primary sex cords*, soon grow into the underlying mesenchyme. Large spherical primitive sex cells, called *primordial germ cells*, are visible early in the fourth week on the wall of the yolk sac. Later they migrate along the dorsal mesentery of the hindgut to the gonadal ridges (Fig. 1-29) and become incorporated in the primary sex cords.

Development of Testes

In embryos with a Y chromosome, the primary sex cords undergo branching, and their ends anastomose to form the rete testis (Fig. 1-30B, D). The primary sex cords, now called *seminiferous*, or testicular, *cords*,

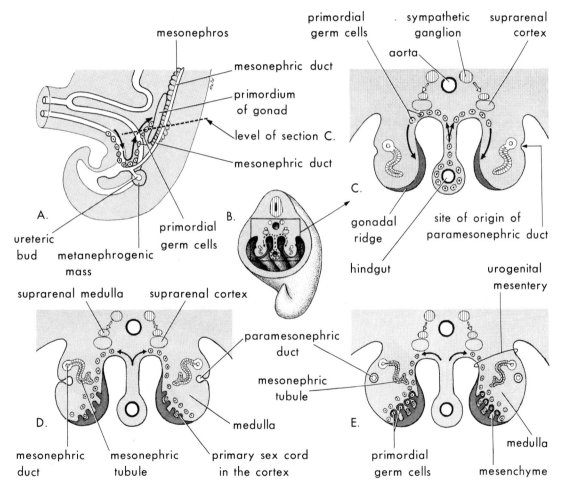

FIGURE 1-29.   *A. Five week embryo, illustrating the migration of primordial germ cells. B. Caudal region of a five week embryo, showing the location and extent of the gonadal ridges on the medial aspect of the urogenital ridges. C. Transverse section showing the primordium of the adrenal glands, the gonadal ridges, and the migration of primordial germ cells. D. Transverse section through a six week embryo showing the primary sex cords and the developing paramesonephric ducts. E. Similar section at later stage showing the indifferent gonads and the mesonephric and paramesonephric ducts. (From K. L. Moore,* The Developing Human *[2nd ed.]. Philadelphia: Saunders, 1977.)*

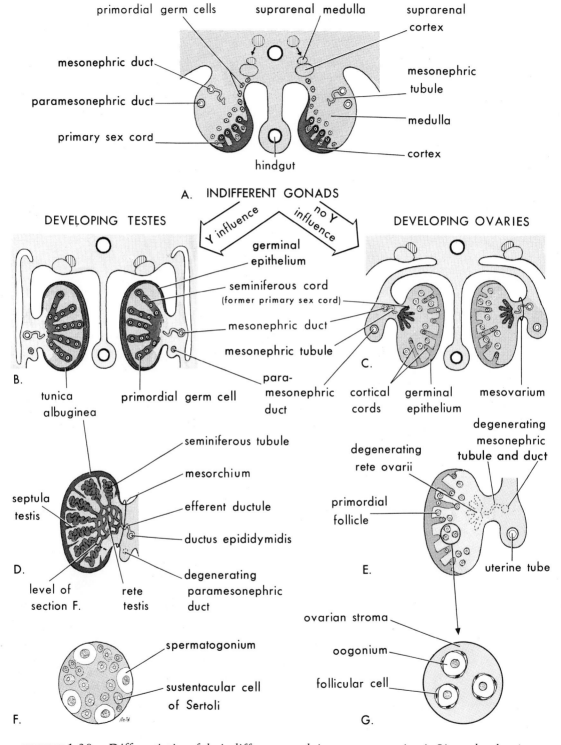

FIGURE 1-30.   *Differentiation of the indifferent gonads into testes or ovaries. A. Six weeks, showing the bipotential gonads composed of an outer cortex and an inner medulla. B. Seven weeks, showing*

lose their connections with the germinal epithelium as a thick fibrous capsule, called the *tunica albuginea*, develops. The seminiferous cords develop into the seminiferous tubules, the tubuli recti, and the rete testis. The walls of the seminiferous tubules are composed of two kinds of cells (Fig. 1-30F): supporting, or sustentacular, cells of Sertoli derived from the germinal epithelium, and spermatogonia derived from the primordial germ cells.

Development of Ovaries

In embryos lacking a Y chromosome, gonadal development occurs very slowly (Fig. 1-30C, E, G). The ovaries do not show distinguishing characteristics until the tenth week, when the cortex begins to develop. The primary sex cords degenerate and form a rudimentary rete ovarii, which soon disappears.

During the fetal period cortical cords extend from the germinal epithelium into the underlying mesenchyme (Fig. 1-30C). As these cords increase in size, primordial germ cells are incorporated into them. The cords break up into isolated cell clusters called *primordial follicles*, consisting of an oogonium derived from a primordial germ cell surrounded by a layer of follicular cells (Fig. 1-30E, G). Active mitosis of oogonia occurs during fetal life, producing thousands of these primitive germ cells. No oogonia form postnatally.

Development of the Genital Ducts

Two pairs of genital ducts develop in both sexes: mesonephric ducts and paramesonephric ducts (Fig. 1-31). The paramesonephric ducts come together in the midline and fuse into a Y-shaped uterovaginal primordium or canal. The uterovaginal primordium projects into the dorsal wall of the urogenital sinus and produces an elevation called the *sinus*, or *Müller's, tubercle*.

DEVELOPMENT OF MALE GENITAL DUCTS. The fetal testes produce at least two hormones: One stimulates development of the mesonephric duct into the male genital tract; the other suppresses development of the paramesonephric ducts. When the mesonephros degenerates, some mesonephric tubules near the testis persist and are transformed into efferent ductules, or ductuli efferentes (Fig. 1-32A). These ductules open into the mesonephric duct, which becomes the ductus epididymidis in this region. Beyond the epididymis, the mesonephric duct becomes the ductus deferens. A lateral outgrowth from the caudal end of each mesonephric duct gives rise to a seminal vesicle. The part of the mesonephric duct between the duct of this gland and the urethra becomes the ejaculatory duct.

DEVELOPMENT OF THE FEMALE GENITAL DUCTS. In embryos with ovaries, the mesonephric ducts regress and the parame-

---

testes developing under the influence of a Y chromosome. Note that the primary sex cords have become seminiferous cords and that they are separated from the germinal epithelium by the tunica albuginea. C. Twelve weeks, showing ovaries beginning to develop in the absence of a Y chromosome influence. Cortical (secondary sex) cords have extended from the germinal epithelium, displacing the primary sex cords centrally into the mesovarium, where they form the rudimentary rete ovarii. D. Testis at 20 weeks, showing the rete testis and the seminiferous tubules derived from the seminiferous cords. An efferent ductule has developed from a mesonephric tubule, and the mesonephric duct has become the ductus epididymidis. E. Ovary at 20 weeks, showing the primordial follicles formed from the cortical cords. The rete ovarii derived from the primary sex cords and the mesonephric tubule and duct are regressing. F. Section of a seminiferous tubule from a 20 week fetus. Note that no lumen is present at this stage and that the seminiferous epithelium is composed of two kinds of cells. G. Section from the ovarian cortex of a 20 week fetus showing three primordial follicles. (From K. L. Moore, The Developing Human *[2nd ed.]. Philadelphia: Saunders, 1977.)*

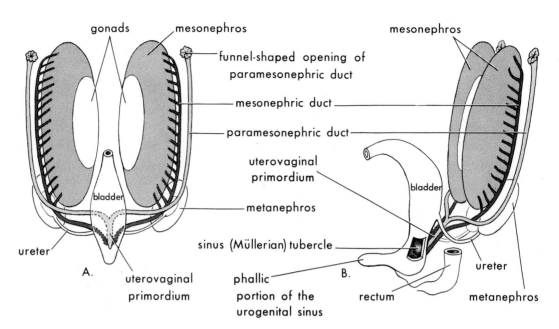

gonads   mesonephros   mesonephros

funnel-shaped opening of
paramesonephric duct

mesonephric duct

paramesonephric duct

uterovaginal
primordium

bladder

metanephros

bladder

sinus (Müllerian) tubercle

ureter

ureter

A.   uterovaginal
primordium

phallic
portion of the
urogenital sinus

rectum

B.

metanephros

FIGURE 1-31.   *A. Frontal view of the posterior abdominal wall of a seven week embryo showing the two pairs of genital ducts present during the indifferent stage. B. Lateral view of a nine week fetus showing the sinus (Müller's) tubercle on the posterior wall of the urogenital sinus. (From K. L. Moore,* The Developing Human [*2nd ed.*]. *Philadelphia: Saunders, 1977.)*

sonephric ducts develop into the female genital tract. The cranial unfused portions of the ducts develop into the uterine tubes, and the fused portions (or uterovaginal primordium) give rise to the epithelium and glands of the uterus (Fig. 1-32B, C). The endometrial stroma and the myometrium are derived from the adjacent mesenchyme.

The epithelium of the vagina is derived from the endoderm of the urogenital sinus, and its fibromuscular wall develops from the uterovaginal primordium (Fig. 1-32B). A solid cord of endodermal cells, called the *vaginal plate*, forms from cells which grow from the urogenital sinus. The central cells of this plate later break down and form the lumen of the vagina. Until late fetal life, the lumen of the vagina is separated from the cavity of the

urogenital sinus by the hymen (Fig. 1-32C and 1-33).

Descent of the Testes

Inguinal canals develop and later form pathways for the testes to descend through the abdominal wall into the scrotum. Descent of the testes through the inguinal canals usually begins during the twenty-eighth week and takes about three days. About four weeks later the testes enter the scrotum, and the inguinal canals contract.

Development of the External Genitalia

The external genitalia also pass through a stage that is not distinguishable as male or female. Early in the fourth week a genital tubercle develops ventral to the cloacal

FIGURE 1-32.   *Development of the male and female reproductive systems from the primitive genital ducts. Vestigial structures are also shown. A. Reproductive system in a newborn male. B. Female reproductive system in a 12 week fetus. C. Reproductive system in a newborn female. (From K. L. Moore,* The Developing Human [*2nd ed.*]. *Philadelphia: Saunders, 1977.)*

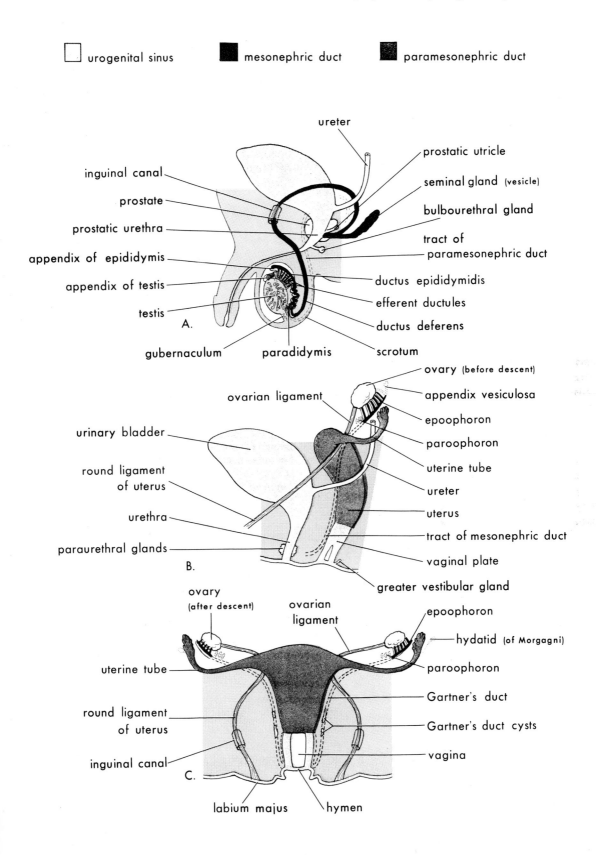

☐ urogenital sinus   ■ mesonephric duct   ■ paramesonephric duct

ureter

prostatic utricle

seminal gland (vesicle)

bulbourethral gland

tract of
paramesonephric duct

inguinal canal

prostate

prostatic urethra

appendix of epididymis

appendix of testis

testis

ductus epididymidis

efferent ductules

ductus deferens

A.

gubernaculum   paradidymis   scrotum

ovary (before descent)

appendix vesiculosa

epoophoron

paroophoron

uterine tube

ureter

uterus

tract of mesonephric duct

vaginal plate

greater vestibular gland

ovarian ligament

urinary bladder

round ligament
of uterus

urethra

paraurethral glands

B.

ovary
(after descent)

ovarian
ligament

epoophoron

hydatid (of Morgagni)

paroophoron

Gartner's duct

Gartner's duct cysts

vagina

uterine tube

round ligament
of uterus

inguinal canal

C.

labium majus   hymen

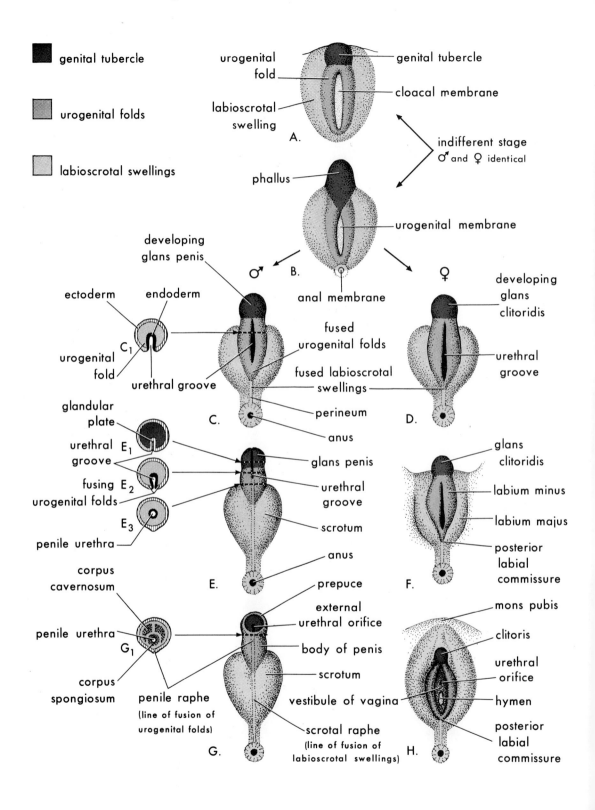

membrane, and labioscrotal swellings and urogenital folds develop on each side of the cloacal membrane (Fig. 1-33). The genital tubercle soon elongates to form a phallus; initially it is as large in females as in males. A urethral groove forms on the ventral (under) surface of the phallus.

The development of male external genitalia from the indifferent external genitalia is caused by androgens produced by the fetal testes (Fig. 1-33C, E, G). As the phallus elongates to form the penis, the urogenital folds fuse with each other along the ventral (under) surface of the penis from behind forward to form the penile urethra. As a result, the external urethral orifice moves progressively toward the glans penis. At the tip of the glans, an ectodermal ingrowth forms a cellular cord called the *glandular plate.* Subsequent splitting of this plate makes a groove on the ventral surface of the glans that is continuous with the external urethral orifice to the tip of the glans and joins the two parts of the penile urethra.

The development of female external genitalia from the indifferent external genitalia occurs in the absence of hormones. The phallus becomes the relatively small clitoris, developing like the penis except that the urogenital folds do not fuse. The unfused urogenital folds form the labia minora. The labioscrotal folds largely remain unfused and form the labia majora.

Congenital Malformations of the Urinary System

Abnormalities of the kidney and ureter occur in 3 to 4 percent of the population and include variations in blood supply, abnormal positions, and duplications. Duplications of the ureter and pelvis are relatively common,

but a supernumerary kidney is rare. These abnormalities result from division of the metanephric diverticulum or ureteric bud. Formation of two ureteric buds or division of a ureteric bud produces a supernumerary kidney if the divided portions of the bud are widely separated (Fig. 1-34C, F). Unilateral absence of a kidney is relatively common (Fig. 1-34A). Renal agenesis is probably due to failure of the ureteric bud to develop.

One or both kidneys may be in an abnormal position (simple renal ectopia, Fig. 1-34B). Pelvic kidney results from failure of the kidneys to ascend. Pelvic kidneys may fuse to form a round mass known as a *discoid,* or pancake, *kidney* (Fig. 1-34E). During ascent a kidney may cross to the opposite side (crossed renal ectopia, Fig. 1-34D) and fuse with the other kidney, producing a single large kidney. Pelvic kidneys fuse across the midline in 2 out of about 600 persons, producing a horseshoe kidney. The large U-shaped kidney usually lies at the level of the lower lumbar vertebrae and seldom gives rise to symptoms.

Protrusion of the posterior wall of the urinary bladder (exstrophy of the bladder, Fig. 1-35) results from a deficiency of mesenchyme and failure of the cells to migrate between the surface ectoderm and the urogenital sinus during the fourth week. Thus no muscle forms in the portion of the anterior abdominal wall over the urinary bladder, and this thin wall subsequently ruptures.

Congenital Malformation of the Reproductive System

Intersexuality

Because an early embryo has the potential to develop into a male or female, errors in sex development result in various degrees of in-

FIGURE 1-33. *A and B. Development of the external genitalia during the indifferent stage. C, E, and G. Stages in the development of the male external genitalia at about 9, 11, and 12 weeks, respectively. To the left are transverse sections (C_1, E_1–E_3, and G_1 through the developing penis illustrating formation of the penile urethra. D, F, and H. Stages in the development of female external genitalia at 9, 11, and 12 weeks, respectively. (From K. L. Moore,* The Developing Human *[2nd ed.]. Philadelphia: Saunders, 1977.)*

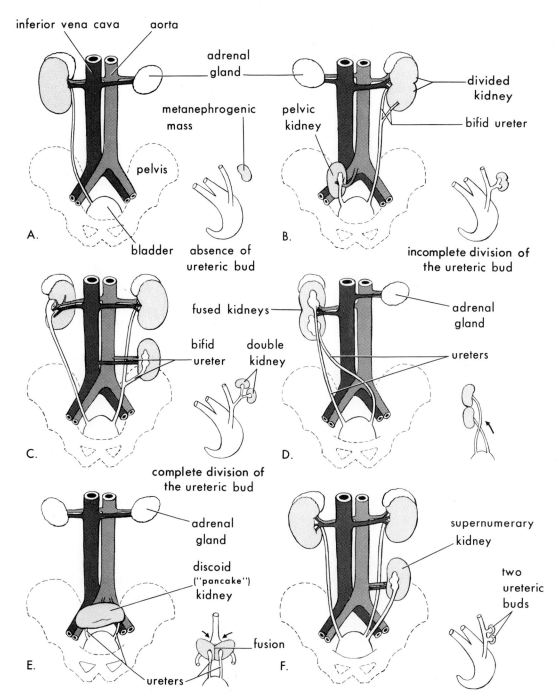

FIGURE 1-34.   *Various abnormalities of the upper urinary tract. The small sketch to the lower right of each drawing illustrates the probable embryological basis of the malformation. A. Unilateral renal agenesis. B. Right side, pelvic kidney; left side, bifid ureter. C. Right side, malrotation of the kidney; left side, bifid ureter and two kidneys. D. Crossed renal ectopia. The left kidney crossed to the right side and fused with the right kidney. E. "Pancake" or discoid kidney resulting from fusion of the unascended kidneys. F. Supernumerary left kidney resulting from the development of two ureteric buds. (From K. L. Moore,* The Developing Human *[2nd ed.]. Philadelphia: Saunders, 1977.)*

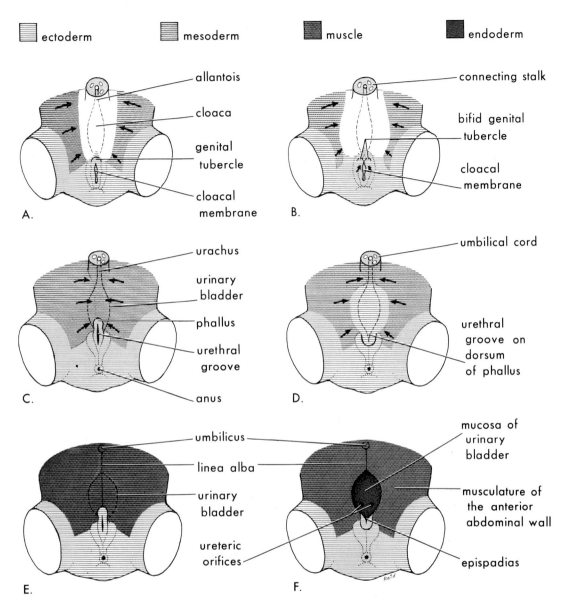

FIGURE 1-35.   *A, C, and E. Normal stages in the development of the infraumbilical body wall and the penis during the embryonic period. Note that mesoderm and later muscle reinforce the ectoderm of the developing anterior abdominal wall. B, D, and F. Probable stages in the development of exstrophy of the bladder and epispadias. In B and D, note that mesoderm (mesenchyme) fails to extend into the anterior abdominal wall anterior to the urinary bladder. Also note that the genital tubercle is located in a more caudal position than usual and that the urethral groove has formed on the dorsal (upper) surface of the penis. In F, the surface ectoderm and the endodermal anterior wall of the bladder have ruptured, resulting in exposure of the bladder mucosa. Note that the musculature of the anterior abdominal wall is present on each side of the defect. Failure of these muscle layers to meet and fuse in the midline caused rupture of the anterior abdominal wall and bladder. (Based on Patten and Berry, 1952. From K. L. Moore,* The Developing Human *[2nd ed.]. Philadelphia: Saunders, 1977.)*

termediate sex, a condition known as intersexuality, or *hermaphroditism.* A person with ambiguous external genitalia is called a *hermaphrodite.* Intersexual conditions are classified according to the histological appearance of the gonads. True hermaphrodites have both ovarian and testicular tissue. Pseudohermaphrodites with testes are called *male pseudohermaphrodites;* those with ovaries are known as *female pseudohermaphrodites.*

FEMALE PSEUDOHERMAPHRODITES. Female pseudohermaphrodites have a 46, XX chromosome constitution. The most common single cause of female pseudohermaphroditism is the adrenogenital syndrome, resulting from congenital virilizing adrenal hyperplasia. There is no ovarian abnormality, but the excessive production of androgens by the adrenal glands causes masculinization of the external genitalia, varying from enlargement of the clitoris to almost masculine genitalia. As a rule there is a clitoral hypertrophy and partial fusion of the labia majora. Persons with this syndrome are the most frequently encountered group of intersexes, accounting for about half of all cases of ambiguous external genitalia. Congenital virilizing adrenal hyperplasia is caused by recessive mutant genes.

Female pseudohermaphrodites who do not have congenital virilizing adrenal hyperplasia are very rare. The administration of certain hormones to a mother during pregnancy may cause ambiguous external genitalia.

MALE PSEUDOHERMAPHRODITES. Male pseudohermaphrodites have a 46, XY chromosome constitution. The external and internal genitalia are variable, resulting from varying degrees of development of the phallus and the paramesonephric ducts. Either an inadequate amount of androgenic hormones is produced, or they are formed after the period of maximum tissue sensitivity of the sexual structures has passed.

TRUE HERMAPHRODITES. Persons with true hermaphroditism, an extremely rare condition, usually have a 46, XX chromosome constitution. Both ovarian and testicular tissues are present, either in the same or in opposite gonads. The physical appearance may be male or female, but the external genitalia are usually ambiguous. The condition results from an error in sex determination that is poorly understood at present.

Testicular Feminization

Persons with the rare condition of testicular feminization (related to intersexuality) appear as normal females despite the presence of testes and XY sex chromosomes. Normal breast development occurs at puberty. The vagina ends blindly, and the other internal genitalia are absent or rudimentary. The testes are usually intra-abdominal or inguinal, but they may descend into the labia majora. Embryologically, these females represent an extreme form of male pseudohermaphroditism, but they are not intersexes because they have normal feminine external genitalia. Although testes develop and secrete androgens, masculinization of the genitalia fails to occur, apparently because the indifferent external genitalia are insensitive to androgens.

Hypospadias

Once in about every 300 males the external urethral orifice is on the ventral (under) surface of the penis instead of at the tip of the glans. The glandular and penile types of hypospadias constitute about 80 percent of cases. Hypospadias results from an inadequate production of androgens by the fetal testes; this causes failure of fusion of the urogenital folds. Differences in the timing and degree of hormonal failure account for the variety of types of hypospadias.

Epispadias

Once in about 30,000 infants the urethra opens on the dorsal (upper) surface of the penis. Although epispadias may occur as a separate entity, it is often associated with exstrophy of the bladder (Fig. 1-35F).

Cryptorchidism of Undescended Testes

Cryptorchidism occurs in about 3 percent of male infants. A cryptorchid testis may be located in the abdominal cavity or anywhere along the usual path of descent of the testis; ordinarily it lies in the inguinal canal. The cause of most cases of cryptorchidism is unknown, but failure of normal androgen production appears to be a factor.

Uterovaginal Malformations

Various types of uterine duplication stem from failure of the paramesonephric ducts to fuse completely with each other during formation of the uterus. Double uterus is caused by failure of fusion of the lower parts of the paramesonephric ducts and may be associated with a double or a single vagina. If the doubling involves only the upper portion of the body of the uterus, the condition is called *bicornuate* (double-horn) *uterus*. In some cases the uterus is divided internally by a thin septum. Very rarely, one paramesonephric duct degenerates or fails to form; the result is a *unicornuate* (single-horn) *uterus*.

One in about 4000 females lacks a vagina because the vaginal plate failed to develop. When the vagina is absent, the uterus is usually also absent. Failure of canalization of the vaginal plate causes vaginal atresia.

REFERENCES

1. Austin, C. R.   The egg and fertilization. *Science* (Lond.) 6:37, 1970.
2. Edwards, R. G., and Fowler, R. E. Human embryos in the laboratory. *Sci. Am.* 223:44, 1970.
3. Federman, D. D.   *Abnormal Sexual Development: A Genetic and Endocrine Approach to Differential Diagnosis.* Philadelphia: Saunders, 1967.
4. Fraser, F. C.   Etiologic Agents: II. Physical and Chemical Agents. In Rubin, A. (Ed.), *Handbook of Congenital Malformations.* Philadelphia: Saunders, 1967. Pp. 365–371.
5. Gray, S. W., and Skandalakis, J. E.   *Embryology for Surgeons. The Embryological Basis for the Treatment of Congenital Defects.* Philadelphia: Saunders, 1972.
6. Jones, H. W., Jr., and Scott, W. W. *Hermaphroditism, Genital Anomalies and Related Endocrine Disorders.* Baltimore: Williams & Wilkins, 1958.
7. Kernahan, D. A., and Stark, R. B.   A new classification for cleft lip and cleft palate. *Plast. Reconstr. Surg.* 22:435, 1958.
8. Moore, K. L.   Sex determination, sexual differentiation and intersex development. *Can. Med. Assoc. J.* 97:292, 1967.
9. Moore, K. L.   *The Developing Human: Clinically Oriented Embryology.* (2nd ed.). Philadelphia: Saunders, 1977.
10. Morton, W. R. M.   Development of the Urogenital Systems. In Rashad, M. N. and Morton, W. R. M. (Eds.), *Selected Topics on Genital Anomalies and Related Subjects.* Springfield, Ill.: Thomas, 1969. Pp. 14–35.
11. Persaud, T. V. N., and Moore, K. L. Causes and prenatal diagnosis of congenital abnormalities. *J. Obstet. Gynecol. Nurs.* 3:50, 1974.
12. Rafferty, K. A., Jr.   The Beginning of Development. In Barnes, A. C. (Ed.), *Intra-Uterine Development.* Philadelphia: Lea & Febiger, 1968. Pp. 1–25.
13. Smith, D. W.   *Recognizable Patterns of Human Malformation: Genetic, Embryologic, and Clinical Aspects.* Philadelphia: Saunders, 1970.
14. Swinyard, C. A. (Ed.).   *Limb Development and Deformity: Problems of Evaluation and Rehabilitation.* Springfield, Ill.: Thomas, 1969.
15. Warkany, J.   *Congenital Malformations: Notes and Comments.* Chicago: Year Book, 1971.

2

Genetic Abnormalities and Congenital Malformations

Mohamed H. K. Shokeir

The realization of the role of genetic disorders in the production of congenital malformations has prompted a search into possible means of their identification, prevention, and management. Plastic surgeons are increasingly concerned with the diagnosis and management of patients with congenital malformations.

PREVALENCE OF CONGENITAL MALFORMATIONS

About 1 of every 35 live-born infants (2.8 percent) suffers from an anomaly or malformation that is either partially or entirely genetic in etiology. Chromosomal abnormalities such as Down's syndrome account for 0.8 percent of the disorders, single-gene disorders such as Apert's and Treacher Collins syndromes make up 1 percent, and approximately 1 percent have a multifactorial etiology with a substantial genetic contribution such as cleft lip and palate and congenital dislocation of the hip.

The prevalence of congenital malformations varies both as regards the overall rate and for every individual malformation, according to racial and ethnic groups, sex, and environmental circumstances.

REVIEW OF GENETIC DETERMINATION AND MODES OF INHERITANCE

Most of the abnormalities, perhaps with the exception of those of traumatic and inflammatory etiology, are determined, at least in part, genetically (Table 2-1). Some are *entirely genetic* in their etiology, such as Apert's syndrome and Crouzon's syndrome, and in others *genetics plays a major role but not an exclusive role*, such as meningomyelocele [4, 7] and cleft lip and palate. In the latter category, the inherited component in the causation may vary considerably among different disorders.

If the defect in the genetic information which accounts partly or exclusively for an observed anomaly is restricted to one segment of the genome (i.e., *one locus*), the pattern of inheritance is described as *single-factor* or *monogenic* inheritance. Alternatively, several loci scattered throughout the genome may collectively contribute to the causation

TABLE 2-1.   *Summary of Congenital Malformations of Plastic Surgical Interest and Their Modes of Genetic Determination* [6, 9]

Autosomal Dominant	Autosomal Recessive	X-Linked
Achondroplasia	Ellis-van Creveld syndrome	Agammaglobulinemia
Acrocephalosyndactyly	Limb-girdle muscular	(Bruton's disease)[a]
(several types includ-	dystrophy	Hemophilia A[a]
ing Apert's syndrome)	Sickle cell anemia (of	Hemophilia B[a]
Angioneurotic edema	interest as a compli-	Muscular dystrophy
Aniridia	cating factor or spe-	(Duchenne's and
Basal cell nevus syndrome	cifically for compli-	Becker's types)
Branchial cleft anomalies	cating indolent ulcers)	Ectodermal dysplasia
Cleft lip ("lip sinuses"	Xeroderma pigmentosum	(anhidrotic)
type)		
Cleidocranial dysostosis		
Crouzon's craniofacial dysostosis		
Ectodermal dysplasia (hi-		
drotic)		
Ehlers-Danlos syndrome		
Facioscapulohumeral mus-		
cular dystrophy		
Keloids (?)		
Mandibulofacial dysostosis		
Treacher Collins syndrome		
Myotonic dystrophy		
Neurofibromatosis		
Oculodentodigital (ODD)		
syndrome		
Osteochondromas, multiple		
(metaphyseal aclasis)		
Polydactyly		
Ptosis		
Retinoblastoma		
Split hand anomaly (lob-		
ster hand)		
Symphalangism		
Syndactyly (several types,		
with or without metacar-		
pal or metatarsal fusion)		
Whistling face (craniocarpo-		
tarsal dystrophy; Freeman-		
Sheldon syndrome)		

[a]Predisposing to surgical complications.

of the anomaly, in which case the genetic component of the etiology is described as *polygenic.* Where environment also plays a major part in an anomaly, the etiology is referred to as *multifactorial with polygenic genetic component.* Whereas genetically speaking a clear dichotomy can be established among individuals in the former case (single-factor inheritance), it is believed that in the case of multifactorially determined traits all individuals in the population are distributed in a continuum with only those exceeding a certain *threshold* affected. The threshold is set by genetic and environmental factors and may be influenced by exposure to deleterious agents or therapy.

In addition to single-factor inheritance and multifactorially determined traits, *chromo-*

somal anomalies, whether numerical or structural, contribute to the etiology of a sizable number of congenital malformations.

Single-Factor Inheritance

The disorders follow typical mendelian inheritance, the pattern of transmission for a given disorder depending upon whether the determinant gene is autosomal or X-linked and whether it is dominant or recessive. In the case of autosomal loci both sexes are affected with equal or nearly equal frequency and severity (see item 4 below) whereas X-linked loci display different expression in the two sexes, males being the sole or more severely affected victims. The problem of dominance and recessivity is a little more involved. In a dominantly transmitted disorder, a *single mutant gene* (allele) is sufficient to cause a clinically significant abnormality whereas recessively transmitted disorders require a *pair* of mutant alleles *at the same locus*. As a rule of thumb, to which some exceptions can be found, dominant anomalies are *structural*, such as Marfan's syndrome or osteogenesis imperfecta, and recessive abnormalities are *functional,* such as phenylketonuria and galactosemia.

1. In autosomal dominant disorders, with certain exceptions, every individual who is affected has a parent who is affected, and the risk of appearance of the disorder in subsequent siblings or in an offspring, regardless of sex, is 50 percent. Because individuals in several generations are affected, inspection

of the pedigree in a representative family imparts a *vertical* impression to the observer (Fig. 2-1). The exceptions referred to include cases in which the condition is recognized de novo in the affected individual with *no previous family history.* If illegitimacy can be confidently excluded, this situation may be ascribed either to *impenetrance* of the expression of the culpable gene in a carrier parent because of the masking effect of the rest of the genome and/or environment or to a new mutation.

2. In autosomal recessive disorders, affected individuals have unaffected parents, grandparents, and more distant relatives. Although the patient may be the only affected member in the sibship (i.e., a sporadic case), sometimes one or more sibs are also affected. The appearance of such cases in the absence of affected individuals in antecedent generations gives, on inspection of a pedigree representative of autosomal recessive inheritance, a *horizontal* impression (Fig. 2-2).

3. X-linked inheritance is usually indicated by preponderance of one sex or the other among the affected individuals in a family. X-linked *recessive disorders* are transmitted to males through their carrier but *unaffected* mothers. For highly deleterious disorders, such as hemophilia and anhidrotic ectodermal dysplasia, the patients are almost exclusively males. However, in milder and less rare conditions such as color blindness both sexes are affected though males largely predominate (Fig. 2-3A). X-linked *dominant conditions* are more prevalent (nearly twice as

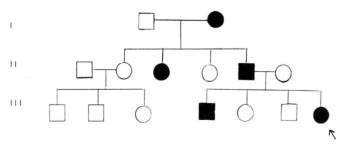

FIGURE 2-1. *Autosomal dominant disorder in the female. The three-generation pedigree imparts a vertical impression.*

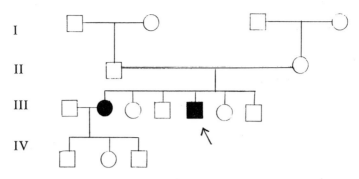

FIGURE 2-2.   *Autosomal recessive disorder with pedigree imparting a horizontal impression.*

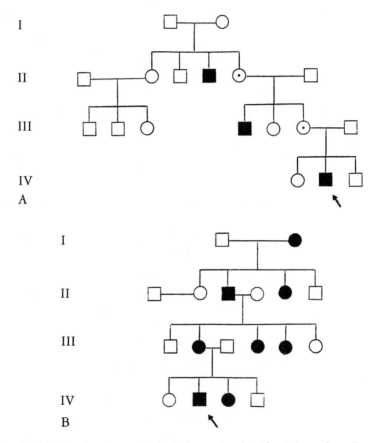

FIGURE 2-3.   *A. Pedigree showing an X-linked recessive disorder. The males only are affected. The carriers are the nonaffected females. B. Pedigree showing an X-linked dominant disorder. Both males and females of all generations are affected.*

common), though milder, in females. Representative examples include otopalatodigital (OPD) syndrome, orofaciodigital syndrome (OFD, type 1), Albright's syndrome, amelogenesis imperfecta, and vitamin D–resistant hypophosphatemic rickets (Fig. 2-3B).

4. Although the disorder may be determined by gene(s) at an autosomal locus, its expression may be confined to one sex—*sex*

limitation. For example, transverse septum of the vagina is frequently an autosomal recessive condition whose expression is obviously restricted to females. Moreover, an autosomally determined trait may be dominant in one sex (e.g., pattern baldness in males) while recessive in the other. The phenomenon is termed *sex influence.*

5. To recognize patterns of single-gene inheritance, two requirements must be met: clinical description and an adequate (preferably diagrammed) family history. Appearance of the condition in roughly equal proportions in both sexes in successive generations with approximately 50 percent of the offspring and sibs of patients affected indicates autosomal dominant transmission.

a. If the sex ratio is *lopsided*, with all the daughters of male patients affected but none of the sons, whereas approximately 50 percent of the sons and daughters of female patients are affected, one is dealing with an *X-linked dominant trait.*

b. If the disorder shows *clustering* in a single sibship (perhaps both sexes affected), with both parents and further ancestors and other relatives free of the condition, then *autosomal recessive inheritance* is the most likely mode of transmission. Consanguinity of the parents is another strong evidence for autosomal recessive inheritance.

c. If there is an *imbalance* in the sex ratio among patients, with males either predominantly or exclusively affected, *X-linked recessive inheritance* is the probable mode of transmission. (If male-to-male transmission occurs, neither X-linked dominant nor recessive inheritance can be invoked, since fathers do not give their X, but only Y, chromosomes to their sons.)

MODES OF PRESENTATION

Just as congenital malformations may or may not be genetic in etiology, so *genetic disorders may or may not be expressed at birth.* Therefore, problems either partially or exclusively of genetic causation can first present themselves to the surgeon for management at any time in the patient's life. However, the major proportion of these ought to be evident and should be sought and recognized in the neonate and young infant.

Conditions such as cleft lip, Goldenhar's syndrome, polydactyly, and the grosser limb malformations are self-evident. Malformations such as Apert's syndrome, Pierre Robin anomaly, isolated cleft palate, ambiguous genitalia, and hypospadias are readily amenable to detection on thorough clinical examination. Disorders with less manifest features such as subtle forms of Treacher Collins syndrome and Waardenburg's syndrome require not only awareness of the entity but frequently specialized investigations for confirmation of the diagnosis.

Sequelae and complications of the malformation may be responsible for the recognition of the disorder or the first indication of its existence. Failure to thrive, feeding difficulties with choking spells, and projectile vomiting are frequently the manifestations of trisomy E, tracheoesophageal fistula, and pyloric stenosis, respectively.

DIAGNOSIS (INCLUDING ANTENATAL DIAGNOSIS)

As in other fields of medicine, the first requirement in the management of genetic problems is accurate diagnosis. Unlike other areas, however, history, examination, and more complicated investigations are not confined to the patient alone; parents, sibs, offspring, and less close relatives are frequently clinically examined and subjected to elaborate forms of investigation before a definitive diagnosis is arrived at for the individual who first came for management.

Apart from complete and thorough examination, particular investigative aids are often utilized in diagnosing or excluding genetic disorders.

1. Chromosomal studies are frequently called for when certain anomalies are observed. For instance, cleft lip and palate in a newborn infant may be an isolated anomaly whose correction and subsequent supportive management will result in an essentially nor-

mal function and undiminished longevity. On the other hand, the deformity may be an integral and a prominent feature of trisomy D, a lethal disorder, associated with major internal anomalies in the brain, heart, kidneys, and other viscera. In view of the inevitable and prompt death of the victim, surgical intervention is not indicated. Distinction between these two different etiological disorders can be readily achieved, following clinical suspicion, by chromosomal studies. Recent and substantial advances in cytogenetics have made possible the identification of every individual human chromosome and smaller segments thereof. Subtle structural anomalies of chromosomes can now be easily detected by means of these newer methods.

2. Buccal smear is a much simpler form of investigation which pertains to the sex chromosome *complement* of the individual. No information relevant to autosomes (chromosomes that are equally common to both sexes and have no direct role in sex determination) is, however, available from buccal smear examination. Until recently the technique yielded information on the number and, to a lesser extent, structure of the X chromosomes. For instance, in a normal XX female a single X-chromatin body is visible in 25 to 30 percent of the cells of the buccal mucosal lining. The X-chromatin or the Barr body (named after Professor Murray Barr of London, Ontario, who first described it in 1949) represents the functionally inactivated X chromosome. In a normal XY male no such body can be discerned. In an XXX female, however, two X-chromatin bodies can usually be seen in those interphase nuclei in which the bodies are visible. As a rule, the number of X-chromatin bodies equals the number of X chromosomes minus 1. More recently, fluorescence technique has made it possible for the Y chromosome also to be visualized. Thus both the number and structure of the Y chromosomes can be ascertained with buccal smear technique, obviating the need for routine chromosomal studies.

3. Biochemical studies are essential for the diagnosis of genetic disorders involving metabolic errors. They are conducted either as a screening procedure—for example, in the case of phenylketonuria (PKU)—or when specific suspicion arises. The latter may be prompted by clinical manifestations exhibited by the patient or by known previous familial occurrence. Few of the biochemical genetic disorders are of surgical interest. Lesch-Nyhan syndrome, in which purine metabolism is affected with marked hyperuricemia and which is inherited in an X-linked recessive fashion, thus appearing almost exclusively in boys, affords some opportunities for surgical management. Because of the metabolic derangement and the consequent neurological involvement, the affected boys are given to compulsive self-mutilating behavior. The resultant facial, ocular, and hand injuries may require plastic surgical procedures.

4. Immunological studies are required in a number of disorders involving the immune system, both cellular and humoral, that are known to be inherited. Assay of immunoglobulins and of the activity of the immune-competent cells is necessary for their diagnosis.

5. Radiological studies are frequently employed for the diagnosis of congenital malformations involving both osseous and nonosseous tissues. Cranial synostosis, Apert's syndrome, Crouzon's syndrome, platybasia, holoprosencephaly, Treacher Collins syndrome, and Goldenhar's syndrome are abnormalities of the skull that are amenable to radiological diagnosis. Congenital hip dislocation is an example of skeletal anomalies wherein radiological studies are essential. In soft tissue disorders such as tracheoesophageal fistula, imperforate anus, and many others radiological studies play an important role. Occasionally radiographic findings, quickly obtained, may provide critical evidence which could influence surgical management, as in the case of duodenal atresia in a newborn infant who is suspected

of having Down's syndrome. Since chromosome studies, which will provide the definitive answer, require a few days to be completed, x-ray films of the hips and hands may afford strong support to the clinical impression. This information is of considerable weight in determining the advisability of possible surgery.

6. Pathological examination is sometimes resorted to in order to corroborate clinical diagnosis and less invasive investigations, as in the case of muscular dystrophy. Moreover, specimens from various tissues may be used as the basis for chromosomal studies. The most commonly used tissue, in this regard, is the skin.

7. Prenatal diagnosis has been possible in the last few years with an increasing number of disorders. The procedure adopted depends on the disorder suspected. However, three techniques are currently in use: radiography, ultrasound [2, 10], and amniocentesis [1]. A fourth, and still largely experimental, technique is direct visualization of the fetus in utero by fetoscopy [8].

APPROACH TO GENETIC PROBLEMS

Obtaining an obstetric and family history is mandatory for evaluation of congenital malformations. The effect of maternal age is well recognized in the increased frequency of chromosomal abnormalities among children of older mothers. Among children born to older fathers, an increased incidence of disorders determined by fresh autosomal dominant mutations (Apert's syndrome, for example) has been observed. Special attention should be paid to the administration of drugs (other than iron and vitamins), exposure to x-rays (whether diagnostic or therapeutic), and displaying or being exposed to fevers, especially in the first trimester of pregnancy.

The occurrence of a similar malformation in any related individual in the same sibship or in either the maternal or paternal side of the family is important information. Also, consanguinity (blood relationship) between

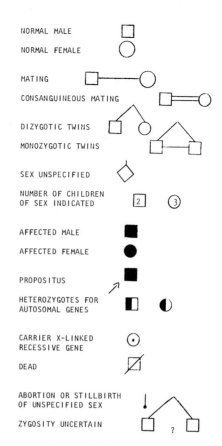

FIGURE 2-4. *Symbols used in the creation of a pedigree and their genetic meaning.*

the parents is significant. Rarely does the birth order influence the appearance of an anomaly in an infant (with the possible exception of pyloric stenosis in males and congenital dislocation of the hip in females), but the information is useful in ascertaining what happened to the other sibs.

It is best to depict the family history on a brief diagram (Fig. 2-4).

PRINCIPLES OF GENETIC COUNSELING

Although a substantial proportion of patients with congenital malformations merit detailed genetic studies and the respective families expert genetic counseling, the surgeon should be capable and willing to provide preliminary counseling in all such cases and the entire counseling in the simpler examples in which he feels competent, such as common single defects; for instance, cleft lip and palate, clubfoot, pyloric stenosis and congenital dislocation of the hip.

1. The physician should answer the parents' questions regarding causation. There is likely to be considerable concern over the possible relevance of drug intake during pregnancy or exposure to radiation or fever. In most cases the malformation would have arisen independently of such insults. The communication of this information should allay a great deal of the guilt feeling connected with the appearance of anomalies in the offspring.

The next concern relates to the risk of recurrence in future offspring. This, of course, depends on the nature of the abnormality, the mode of genetic determination, and in the case of multifactorially determined disorders the sex of the patient and the history of previous occurrence of the malformation in earlier sibs. For example, when one of the parents has features of Treacher Collins syndrome and an infant is born with it, the risk for a future offspring, regardless of sex, is 50 percent—an autosomal dominant pattern. On the other hand, if no such history exists and examination proves that both parents and perhaps other relatives are free of it, the parents should be reassured that the risk to future offspring is negligible, since the disorder in the infant is probably due to fresh mutation—a nonrepeating event in the same sibship. The parents of a newborn infant with Ellis-van Creveld syndrome should expect a recurrence risk of one in four based on autosomal recessive inheritance. The mother of a boy with anhidrotic ectodermal dysplasia (an X-linked recessive disorder) may be informed that recurrence is confined only to her future sons with a chance of 50 percent and none to her daughters. Moreover, her normal brothers or sons have no risk of transmitting the condition to any of their offspring since they lack the responsible gene.

Multifactorially determined disorders, such as cleft lip, present a slightly more complicated situation. They occur more frequently in one or the other sex. Appearance in the more rarely affected sex implies a strong genetic predisposition and a higher risk in subsequent offspring. The following example by Carter [3] for pyloric stenosis illustrates the point.

The risk for sibs and offspring expressed as multiples of population risks for the same sex are as follows:

Male relatives of male patients $\times$ 10
Female relatives of male patients $\times$ 25
Male relatives of female patients $\times$ 35
Female relatives of female patients $\times$ 80

(Population frequency of pyloric stenosis for male births = 0.005 and for female births = 0.001.)

Recurrence risk is increased if more than one individual is affected in the sibship. For instance, whereas the risk of recurrence of cleft lip and palate (CL/CP) is 4 to 6 percent if one child is affected, it rises to 10 percent if two are and 15 percent if three are. Moreover, when a parent and a child are affected, the risk of CL/CP for other children is between 11 and 14 percent. On the whole, the risk of recurrence for sibs and offspring of an individual with a multifactorially determined trait is 4 to 5 percent [3].

Frequently people are not aware of what questions to ask or of the availability or certainty of the answers to their questions. The physician should be prepared to suggest the appropriate questions to them and provide the pertinent answers. When areas of doubt exist, he should not hesitate to point them out, and if he deems that more expert opinion is useful, he should refer the case for further counseling (Table 2-2).

2. Apart from supplying information, the physician in a counseling situation should be willing to provide the necessary emotional support for the parents to handle the anxiety, denial, guilt, and anger usually provoked by

TABLE 2-2.   *Risk Table for Common Disorders with Genetic Components* [a]

Anomaly	Risk for Any Subsequent Child (%)	
	With Unaffected Parents and One Affected Child	With One Parent Affected and No Previous Affected Children
Cleft lip	4.5	4.5
Cleft lip and palate	4.5	4.5
Cleft palate	2.0	6.0
Congenital heart disease	3.0	3.0
Congenital dislocation of the hip	0.8 (males) 6.5 (females)	
Congenital clubfoot Talipes equinovarus Talipes calcaneovalgus	6.0	
Metatarsus adductus	2.0	
Congenital pyloric stenosis	5.0 (males) 2.0 (females)	Affected father, 5.0 Affected mother, 18.0
Hirschsprung's disease	5.0 (males) 2.0 (females)	
Central nervous system malformations: Anomalies of closure of neural tubes Anencephaly Meningomyelocele Spina bifida	5.5	3.0

[a]No entry indicates risk is not known.

the occurrence of a genetic problem in their offspring [5]. Mitigation of denial and guilt and articulation of anger are the prerequisites for acceptance of the individual with the malformation and compliance with the therapeutic regimen, which could be long, painful, and expensive.

3. Assistance must be given in rational planning for the future. When adequate opportunity has been provided for the parents to vent their feelings, inquiries, and misgivings, an attempt has to be made to grapple with the problem and reach a decision. The decision will pertain to the case itself—regarding whether surgical intervention should be withheld or instituted and, if the latter, what form of surgery will be carried out. Moreover, the question of care of a child during the course of surgical treatment and the possibility of institutionalization or foster home care may have to be settled. Decisions

regarding future reproduction based on the parents' desire and convictions and the risk of recurrence will also have to be made. The support and guidance of the physician in this area are invaluable. Finally, he may be called upon to arrange for the implementation of the decisions the parents themselves arrive at. Measures such as contraception, sterilization, artificial insemination, and adoption may be outside the domain of plastic surgery, but the surgeon can help the parents explore these possible avenues and refer them to the appropriate service.

REFERENCES

1. Brock, D. J. H., and Sutcliffe, R. G. Alpha-fetaprotein in the antenatal diagnosis of anencephaly and spina bifida. *Lancet* 2:197, 1972.
2. Campbell, S., Johnstone, F. D., Holt, E. M., and May, P. Anencephaly: Early ultrasonic diagnosis and active

management. *Lancet* 2:1226, 1972. (An example of the utilization of ultrasound technique in diagnosing a congenital abnormality.)

3. Carter, C. O.   The inheritance of common congenital malformation. *Prog. Med. Genet.* 4:59, 1965. (An expert and early description of the etiology of common congenital malformations.)

4. Clarke, C. A., McKendrick, O. M., and Sheppard, P. M.   Spina bifida and potatoes. *Br. Med. J.* 3:251, 1973.

5. Emery, A. E. H.   Genetic counselling. *Scott. Med. J.* 14:335, 1969. (A very useful review of factual information and attitudes related to genetic counseling for dominant, recessive, X-linked, and multifactorial disorders.)

6. McKusick, V. A.   *Mendelian Inheritance in Man* (3rd ed.). Baltimore: Johns Hopkins Press, 1971.

7. Renwick, J. H.   Hypothesis: Anenceph-aly and spina bifida are usually preventable by avoidance of a specific but unidentified substance present in certain potato tubers. *Br. J. Prev. Soc. Med.* 26:67, 1972.

8. Scrimgeour, J. B.   Fetoscopy. *Heredity* (Lond.) 28:272, 1972.

9. Smith, D. W.   *Recognizable Patterns of Human Malformations*. (Vol. VII, Major Problems in Clinical Pediatrics Series.) Philadelphia: Saunders, 1970.

10. Sunden, B.   Diagnostic value of ultrasound in obstetrics and gynecology. *Acta Obstet. Gynecol. Scand.* 43, Suppl. 6, 1964.

11. Warkany, J.   *Congenital Malformations.* Chicago: Year Book, 1971. (A bit lengthy and discursive but comprehensive coverage of malformations whether genetically or environmentally determined—best described by the subtitle "Notes and Comments.")

II

The Internal Environment:
Normal Maintenance
and Disorders

INTRODUCTION

The roots of plastic surgery are the same as those of general surgery. To treat major surgical problems effectively, the plastic surgeon must have a firm grasp of fluid and electrolyte physiology and parenteral fluid therapy. He must understand "normal" metabolism and the metabolic response to injury. Knowledge of the physiology of blood, oxygen transport, bleeding, and coagulation is required. The plastic surgeon may legitimately be called upon to manage complicated surgical situations involving any or all of these areas.

Many present-day plastic surgeons choose to renounce their general surgical background and refuse to undertake the management of difficult problems such as acute burns, pediatric fluid management, and post-traumatic and septic shock, even when these conditions complicate the care of their own patients. By doing so, they render themselves merely technicians.

Part II provides a fundamental background in fluids and electrolytes, metabolism, and blood and its components to plastic surgeons seeking to maintain their level of competence in surgical patient care.

3

Fluids and Electrolytes

John K. McKenzie

BODY FLUIDS IN HEALTH

Water accounts for between 45 and 60 percent of body weight. Intracellular fluid (ICF) has a larger volume than extracellular fluid (ECF). The latter is made up of interstitial fluid, including lymph, which surrounds cells outside the vascular system, and plasma, inside the blood vessels. Transcellular fluids include fluids in the eye, cerebrospinal fluid, and gastrointestinal secretions. Some water and sodium are locked away in bone and connective tissue and are so slowly accessible that they are not usually regarded as part of the effective extracellular fluid space (see Fig. 3-1).

The composition of these fluids can be quite similar but in the case of ICF and ECF is very different. Nevertheless, their compositions and volumes are maintained remarkably constant in health, either by active metabolism or by osmotic factors. To understand such processes, we should first define units for these activities.

UNITS OF MEASUREMENT

A *mole* (M) of a substance is its molecular weight in grams. Thus a mole of sodium

weighs 23 gm. A mole of glucose ($C_6H_{12}O_6$) weighs 180 gm. A *millimole* (mM) is the molecular weight in milligrams (see Table 3-1).

For ionized particles, the *equivalent* (Eq) weight is the weight that will combine with or displace 1 gm of hydrogen ion (H^+). Thus for sodium ion, Na^+, the equivalent weight = atomic weight = 23 gm. For calcium ion, Ca^{++}, the equivalent weight is half the atomic weight, or 20 gm. *Milliequivalents* (mEq) are equivalent weights in milligrams. Laboratories may express concentrations in milligrams per 100 ml of solution. To convert electrolyte solutions from milligrams per 100 ml to milliequivalents per liter the equation is

$$\frac{mg/100 \text{ ml} \times 10 \times \text{valence}}{\text{atomic weight}} = mEq/liter$$

Osmoles (Osm) and *milliosmoles* (mOsm) depend simply on the number of dissolved particles in solution. For substances that do not dissociate, 1 osmole will be similar to 1 mole. For substances that dissociate into two or more particles, osmoles will depend on the number of particles. Thus, 1 liter of "normal"

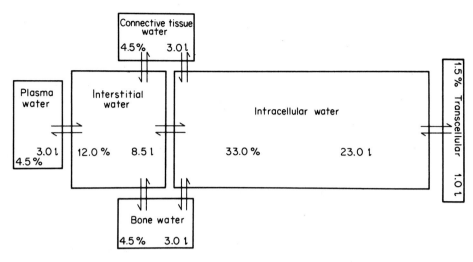

FIGURE 3-1.   *Body water compartments in an average 70 kg man shown as percentage of body weight and in liters. (Adapted from F. S. Edelman and J. Leibman,* Am. J. Med. *27:256, 1959.)*

saline solution contains 154 mM of NaCl, or 154 mEq of Na$^+$ and 154 mEq of Cl$^-$ and thus 308 mOsm of solute, approximately (see Table 3-1).

Tonicity of a solution refers to osmolality. Thus, *isotonicity* is a quality of solutions with osmolality equal to normal serum osmolality.

METHODS OF MEASUREMENT

In order to obtain information about fluid compartments, their size has to be calculated in experimental and clinical situations. A knowledge of the measurement methods used helps one assess the accuracy of information obtained and the validity of theories deduced.

The dilution principle is utilized in all methods. A material that can be easily measured and is distributed only in a particular compartment is introduced into the body, usually intravenously, and allowed to equilibrate within that compartment. Losses by excretion or metabolism are subtracted, and the volume of the compartment is determined thus:

$$V_F = \frac{C_1 V_1 - C_E V_E}{C_F}$$

where C_1 = the initial concentration of the material in the test solution

V_1 = volume of test solution introduced

TABLE 3-1.   *Units of Measurement—Relationship*

Substance	Formula	Atomic or Molecular Weight	Moles (M)	Equivalents (Eq)	Osmoles (Osm)
Sodium	Na	23	1	1	1
Chloride	Cl	35.5	1	1	1
Sodium chloride	NaCl	58.5	1	2	2
Calcium	Ca	40	1	2	1
Calcium chloride	CaCl$_2$	111	1	4	3
Glucose	C$_6$H$_{12}$O$_6$	180	1		1
Urea	CO(NH$_2$)$_2$	60	1		1

C_E = concentration excreted in urine

V_E = volume of urine before equilibration

C_F = concentration of material in the body fluid after equilibration

V_F = volume of the fluid compartment in which it is distributed.

If breakdown or excretion is small, C_E and V_E can be omitted, giving

$$V_F = \frac{C_1 V_1}{C_F}$$

The accuracy of measurement depends on several factors. The tracer material must distribute only in the compartment measured, and its distribution must be even throughout that compartment.

Extracellular Fluid Volume

For measurements of ECF volume especially, no tracer is ideal. Bromide and chloride do penetrate cells to some extent and give falsely large estimations [6], while inulin and mannitol, which are excluded from cells, equilibrate very slowly, with relatively large amounts being excreted during equilibration [12]. The volumes of distribution of tracers used to measure ECF thus vary considerably (Table 3-2), inulin having the smallest volume of distribution and bromide the largest. Radiosulfate, $^{35}SO_4$, lies between these extremes.

Total Body Water

In the past, body water was measured clinically by the analgesic antipyrine, but of recent years deuterated or tritiated water (D_2O or THO) has commonly been used [7, 20, 30].

Plasma and Blood Volume

Plasma is measured by albumin labeled either with Evans blue dye (T-1824) or with the ^{131}I radioisotope. Total blood volume can then be calculated by multiplying by a factor involving the venous hematocrit. Thus:

TABLE 3-2. *Extracellular Fluid Volumes in Men by Various Methods*

Method	Volume (% body weight)
Inulin	15.6
Mannitol	16.6
Thiosulfate	16.3
$^{35}SO_4$	18.0
Br	28.4
^{36}Cl	26.8
^{24}Na	26.2

Source: From Hays, R. M. Dynamics of Body Water and Electrolytes. In Maxwell, M. H., and Kleeman, C. R. (Eds.), *Clinical Disorders of Fluid and Electrolyte Metabolism* (2nd ed.). New York: McGraw-Hill, 1972.

$$\text{Plasma volume} \times \frac{100}{100-Hct} = \text{total blood volume}$$

However, this does not take into account plasma trapped between red cells or differences between "central" hematocrit in the great veins and peripheral hematocrit in capillaries, where streaming out of the red cells occurs. Venous hematocrit therefore overestimates red cell mass and total blood volume. Tagging of red cells with ^{51}Cr to measure red cell mass and combining this estimate with ^{131}I albumin estimation of plasma volume—the "summation" method—is the most accurate measurement available but is still subject to errors of 5 to 8 percent in reproducibility [21].

Compartment Sizes

Total body water (TBW) is greater in male adults than in females on account of the larger amounts of body fat in women. TBW is very high in infancy (up to 80 percent of body weight at 1 day) and decreases to approximately 60 to 65 percent by 1 year. Over age 60, TBW has declined to 51 percent in males and 45 percent in females (see Table 3-3).

For a 70 kg man with a total body water of 42 liters (60 percent body weight), plasma volume is approximately 3 liters (4.5 percent body weight), and interstitial volume is 11 liters (16 percent), making total ECF volume 14 liters (21 percent). This ECF estimate is a

TABLE 3-3. *Total Body Water at Various Ages (as Percent Body Weight)*

Age	Male	Female
1 day	80	77
1 year	58	57
1–5 years	63	64
9–10 years	63	60
10–16 years	59	57
17–39 years	61	50
40–59 years	55	47
60 + years	52	46

Source: Adapted from Hays, R. M. Dynamics of Body Water and Electrolytes. In Maxwell, M. H., and Kleeman, C. R. (Eds.), *Clinical Disorders of Fluid and Electrolyte Metabolism* (2nd ed.). New York: McGraw-Hill, 1972.

"functional" one and excludes bone water and transcellular water. Intracellular water obtained by subtraction of total ECF (including bone and transcellular water) from the total body water is 23 liters (33 percent body weight) (see Fig. 3-1).

Both ICF and ECF volumes depend on the accuracy of ECF estimation. Thus absolute values may be very questionable. Nevertheless, serial measurements of compartment volumes, using a standard technique, probably yield valid estimates of changes in the compartment size.

It should be remembered that, in the short term, changes in weight accurately reflect changes in body water. Lever scales are cheaper, simpler, and more accurate than body water measurements!

Composition of Compartments

Plasma and interstitial fluid are very similar in composition, with sodium (142–145 mEq per liter) and chloride (104–114 mEq per liter) being the predominant cation and anion respectively (Fig. 3-2). The main difference in composition is the 7 gm per 100 ml or 13 mEq per liter of protein in serum. This protein is retained for the most part in the vascular space by the semipermeable, but leaky, vascular endothelium. The relative impermeability to protein, which is negatively charged at pH 7.4 and has a small osmotic effect, forces a redistribution of cations and anions until concentration, electrical, and osmotic forces are in dynamic equilibrium. Such a distribution is called a *Gibbs-Donnan equilibrium* (see below).

The ICF is of vastly different composition. It tends to vary somewhat among different types of cell, but skeletal muscle is usually chosen as representative. Na^+ and Cl^- are present in only small amounts (10 and 2 mEq per liter H_2O), while potassium (156 mEq per liter H_2O) and phosphate (95 mEq per liter H_2O) are the principal ions. Magnesium (26 mEq per liter H_2O) and sulfate (20 mEq per liter H_2O) also contribute significantly. Protein concentration is high, with a chemical equivalent of 55 mEq per liter water. The difference in composition is possible not only because of selective permeability of the cell membranes, which prevents loss of proteins, organic phosphates, etc., but also because of active pumping mechanisms which extrude sodium and in some cells actively take up potassium.

Maintenance of Volume and Composition of Compartments

Osmolalities of intracellular and interstitial fluids are the same. The total number of chemical equivalents is greater intracellularly (Fig. 3-2) because each protein molecule contributes only one unit to the osmotic pressure but has a large number of ionic charges. On the other hand, the osmolality of plasma is greater than that of interstitial fluid because of the Gibbs-Donnan equilibrium.

Thus, if two fluids containing ionized solute are separated by a membrane that is impermeable to an anion present on only one side of the membrane, a rearrangement of the diffusible ions will occur according to several conditions:

1. Electrical neutrality on either side of the membrane will be maintained.
2. There will be a higher concentration of diffusible cation on the same side as the im-

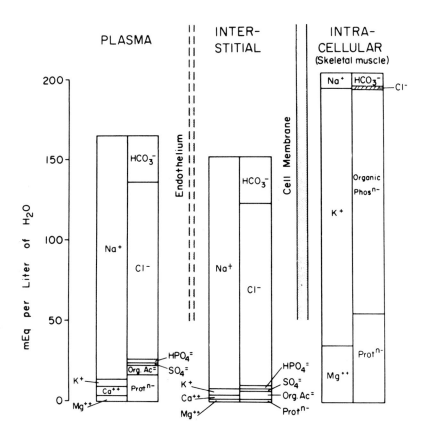

FIGURE 3-2. *Solute composition of body fluids. (From H. Valtin,* Renal Function: Mechanisms Preserving Fluid and Solute Balance in Health. *Boston: Little, Brown, 1973.)*

permeable anion and a higher concentration of diffusible anion on the opposite side, so that where protein in capillaries is the impermeable anion, and Na^+ and Cl^- are the main ions diffusing across the endothelial membrane,

$$\frac{(Na^+) \text{ intravascular}}{(Na^+) \text{ interstitial}} = \frac{(Cl^-) \text{ interstitial}}{(Cl^-) \text{ intravascular}}$$

3. There will be a higher osmotic pressure on the side of the impermeable anion. In this case the increment in osmotic pressure is known as the *oncotic pressure* and is normally balanced by hydrostatic pressure in the blood vessel.

Osmotic forces are much more potent than hydrostatic forces and determine in large

measure the distribution of water between compartments. Water movements are rapid, except for bone and transcellular water. If some solutes are excluded from compartments, either actively or by permeability barriers, an increase in the mass of such a solute (e.g., Na^+) in the ECF space will mean a redistribution of volume to ECF in preference to the ICF from which the Na^+ is excluded.

For example, if 3 liters of NaCl solution with osmolality 290 mOsm per liter H_2O (isosmolal with ECF) is given intravenously, the ECF should be expanded by 3 liters, while ICF will remain constant (assuming no renal excretion). On the other hand, if 3 liters of 5% dextrose in water is given, the dextrose will be metabolized, and if no loss of water occurs renally or by sweating or insensible loss, the water will be distributed equally throughout accessible body water, increasing total body water from an average of 42 to 45 liters. Osmolality of all compartments should be decreased to 42/45 of its original osmolality—that is, by 1/15 of 290 mOsm to 270 mOsm per liter approximately. It can be seen that low ECF electrolyte concentrations are at least as likely to be due to disturbances of water balance as of electrolyte balance, though both may participate.

MAINTENANCE OF INTRACELLULAR VOLUME AND COMPOSITION

In spite of its large size, the intracellular fluid space is difficult to study. Instead of being in continuity like the ECF and monitored by organs such as the kidney for its integrity, the ICF is composed of tiny individual aliquots of variable composition, each maintained by an individual cell. What we lump together as ICF is in reality an enormous number of tiny droplets. The constituents are hard to measure, and, as Leaf [13] has pointed out, the normal volumes of cells may be impossible to assess.

Maintenance by Active Processes

It has been shown that, in the presence of cooling [13], metabolic inhibitors, and hypoxia [5], cell swelling takes place; it is usually reversible after removal of the inhibiting agent. This effect is most obvious clinically in cerebral edema, which may occur after quite transient cerebral ischemia.

Water is normally excluded from the cell because sodium is actively extruded. Chloride also tends to be kept extracellular by the electronegativity of the cell interior, while potassium retention is favored (Fig. 3-3). Active processes also specifically accumulate potassium in many cells [25].

When cells have their metabolism interfered with, they not only gain sodium and chloride and lose potassium but tend to gain hydrogen ion, especially in an acidotic environment—for example, where lactic

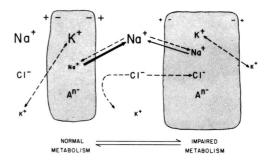

FIGURE 3-3.   *A normally functioning cell and one with inhibited function. Note the cell swelling, gain in intracellular Na^+ and Cl^-, and loss of cellular K^+. (From A. Leaf, Regulation of intracellular fluid volume and disease. Am. J. Med. 49:291, 1970.)*

acid, etc., is accumulating. The result is further harm to the intracellular machinery. These changes can be shown in healing wounds [26], while the loss of potassium from burn surfaces is greater than the normal ECF concentration [19] and suggests loss of K^+ from injured cells. Other intracellular constituents, such as phosphate, may also be lost, particularly in organs such as the liver.

Tissue Wasting and Catabolism

For the cell to maintain its internal environment, it must be supplied with suitable nutriment and oxygen. Where there are large energy requirements and inadequate calorie intake, as with fever and sepsis, and in burns, protein is converted to calories by gluconeogenesis. This includes cell proteins as well as plasma proteins. Thus, the intracellular space actually decreases as intracellular constituents are released and excreted, if renal function is adequate. ECF volume tends to be maintained so that the total body sodium-to-potassium ratio rises [21]. Nevertheless, each cell may have its normal complement of potassium. This is therefore a "lost cell" phenomenon rather than a "sick cell" phenomenon, and the potassium loss is a pseudo depletion rather than a true depletion. If renal function is inadequate, marked nitrogen and potassium retention occurs in the ECF because of catabolism and may lead to lethal hyperkalemia.

Passive Processes in the Maintenance of ICF Volume

Osmotic Pressure

The ICF participates in any changes in water balance, as discussed above. In total water depletion or water overload, the cells shrink or swell, and susceptible cells, such as brain cells, may show obvious functional impairment. Quite frequently, however, water shifts occur from ICF to ECF or vice versa. The shift occurs usually because of infusion of a relatively impermeable solute into the ECF or because such a solute is rapidly removed from the ECF. These situations are examples of "dysequilibrium syndromes." For instance, when the blood urea is rapidly lowered from a high level by hemodialysis, the cerebral cellular level of urea and other solute may remain high and cause a relative increase in the intracellular osmotic pressure. Water then moves into the cell causing swelling, which leads to confusion, convulsions, and other central nervous system phenomena. On the other hand, when cerebral swelling has occurred because of trauma, it may be counteracted by increasing ECF osmolality with infusions of mannitol and urea, in order to produce water movement out of the brain cells and reduce swelling.

Interrelated Effects of K^+ and H^+

For some years it has been known that rapid infusion of acid will produce an egress of potassium from muscle cells in exchange for H^+ ion, which reduces intracellular pH [31]. In situations of true potassium depletion, sodium tends to be retained in the body and may be taken up in cells along with H^+ [2]. The movement of H^+ into cells helps to produce the extracellular alkalosis of potassium depletion. In addition, H^+ is preferentially lost in the urine in potassium depletion, causing alkalosis. Conversely, metabolic alkalosis due to loss of H^+ from pyloric stenosis or gastric suction may lead to ac-

cumulation of potassium in cells [3]. Renal tubular cells will therefore be rich in K^+ rather than H^+ and so tend to lose K^+ rather than H^+ along the electrical gradient produced by distal tubular sodium reabsorption. This loss leads to potassium depletion seen in metabolic alkalosis. Normally, cells appear to have an acid interior though the degree of acidity is disputed [1, 9].

About 0.5 mEq per liter change in ECF K^+ concentration usually occurs with each decimal point change in extracellular pH (e.g., from pH 7.4 to 7.3, ECF K^+ may rise approximately 0.5 mEq per liter). Rapid reversal of extracellular acidosis will thus lead to shift of K^+ from the extracellular to the intracellular space. A serum K^+ of 4.0 mEq per liter may fall to the potentially dangerous level of 2.5 mEq per liter, with change of ECF pH from 7.1 to 7.4.

Potassium content and external potassium balance are shown in Table 3-4.

MAINTENANCE OF EXTRACELLULAR VOLUME AND COMPOSITION

Because sodium is the dominant cation and is for the most part excluded from ICF, almost all changes in volume, except those due to pure water depletion or overload, are tied

TABLE 3-4. *Potassium Content and Balance*

(a) *Body Content of Potassium*

	mEq	% Total K
Total	3850	100
Muscle	2530	66
Skin	500	13
Plasma and ECF	92	2.5

(b) *External Balance of Potassium*

Routes of:		Total (mEq/day)
1. Intake	Food	100–200
2. Output	Stool	10–15
	Sweat	0–20
	Urine	85–190

Source: From Black, D. A. K. Potassium Metabolism. In Maxwell, M. H., and Kleeman, C. R. (Eds.), *Clinical Disorders of Fluid and Electrolyte Metabolism* (2nd ed.). New York: McGraw-Hill, 1972.

to sodium ion. The vascular space is involved in all the volume changes of the ECF, and it is likely that many of the sensing mechanisms for homeostatic feedback are located in, or in relation to, the vascular space. Thus central venous and atrial pressure, aortic and carotid pressure, and renal afferent arteriolar pressure directly or indirectly determine the rate of antidiuretic hormone (ADH), renin, and aldosterone release, which leads to appropriate water and sodium handling.

Rapid and severe changes in ECF volume, especially depletion, produce rapid responses by the sympathetic nervous system as well as general and local hormonal activity. Slower, less severe changes, with maintenance of reasonable perfusion and blood pressure, will be in considerable measure compensated by changes in input and particularly excretion.

Water Balance

Table 3-5 demonstrates external balance figures for input and output of water. Those labeled obligatory are a result of other necessary processes, such as water of oxidation, in providing energy, plus skin and lung losses associated with cooling and humidification. Obligatory losses may be grossly increased by fever, vomiting, and diarrhea, or with losses through raw wound areas—burns, for example.

The facultative or variable input will in normal man depend on oral fluid intake and the sensation of thirst. Facultative output will depend on renal handling of water. This is for the most part under the control of the renal medullary concentrating mechanism and an-

tidiuretic hormone but will also be dependent on other factors, such as glomerular filtration and the solute content of the urine.

Thirst and ADH Regulation

Thirst requires consciousness for completion of the feedback loop, which is interrupted in coma or inability of the organism to drink. Nevertheless, the stimuli are very similar to those for release of ADH and are sensed in the same general area of the hypothalamus. They will be considered together [11].

1. *Osmotic stimuli:* Increased extracellular osmolality leads to contraction of the hypothalamic osmoreceptors, which then stimulate posterior pituitary release of ADH and the sensation of thirst.
2. *Nonosmotic stimuli:*
   a. Decreased arterial or left atrial pressure arising from a fall in cardiac output or intravascular volume.
   b. Emotion or pain.
   c. Blood temperature.
   d. Cholinergic and β-adrenergic agents (α-adrenergic agents inhibit).
   e. Other drugs—morphine, nicotine, barbiturates (alcohol, Dilantin, and anticholinergic drugs inhibit).

The potpourri of influences labeled b to e are not usually prime factors but obviously may have important effects in wounding, shock, and surgical operation. In most instances, volume considerations plus stress and pain will override osmotic changes in stimulating ADH. Thus, quite marked hypo-osmolality

TABLE 3-5. *External Water Balance*

	Input (ml)			Output (ml)	
Obligatory	Food	750	Obligatory	Skin	500
	Water of oxidation	300		Lungs	400
				Feces	150
Facultative	Fluid ingestion	500–1700	Facultative	Urine	500–1700
Total		1550–2750	Total		1550–2750

and water retention routinely occur after operation, especially when hypotonic solutions have been given intravenously.

Glomerular filtration is also important in water balance.

In summary, with a normally functioning kidney that is not subject to an osmotic load, and with a normal hypothalamus and pituitary, the body adjusts with great sensitivity to water load or water depletion. A change of osmolality of only 2 percent is required to elicit changes in ADH secretion [11].

Sodium Balance

External balance for sodium is extraordinarily flexible. In general, bowel and sweat losses are small, and balance is easily achieved with good kidney function.

Since 90 percent of cation in the ECF is sodium, this element, with its salts, dominates the control of ECF volume. As discussed above, the concentration of sodium is much more a matter of water balance than of sodium balance. The volume of ECF is a better indicator of sodium depletion or excess than sodium concentration. Water balance is normally so effective both externally and internally that ingestion or infusion of saline solutions with free access to water and normal kidneys will not change the plasma concentration of sodium but only the ECF volume. The response to increase in dietary sodium is quite sluggish, with urinary losses taking several days to "catch up" to intake. In the process, some ECF volume is accumulated or lost, but a new balance is reached (Fig. 3-4).

How is the change in volume perceived? Changes in intravascular volume may be perceived in relation to the heart and great vessels, as seen in the control of ADH. Maneuvers such as carotid occlusion alter renin secretion [16] and aldosterone activity. A receptor may exist intracranially for aldosterone, but evidence so far is not very good.

The best evidence indicates that the kidney may be the main sensor and controller of

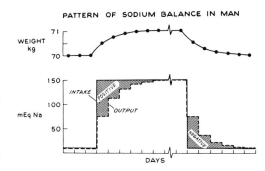

PATTERN OF SODIUM BALANCE IN MAN

FIGURE 3-4. *Sudden increase in dietary sodium from 10 to 150 mEq per day is accompanied by weight gain and a slow increase in sodium excretion until balance is regained. The reverse process is also sluggish. (From L. E. Earley, in M. H. Maxwell and C. R. Kleeman [Eds.], Clinical Disorders of Fluid and Electrolyte Metabolism [2nd ed.]. New York: McGraw-Hill, 1972.)*

sodium metabolism, with some help from adrenals and possibly hypothalamus.

Renal Mechanisms for Control of Sodium Balance

FIRST FACTOR: GLOMERULAR FILTRATION RATE (GFR). GFR for normal man is approximately 180 liters per 24 hours or 120 ml per minute. Each liter of filtrate contains approximately 140 mEq of sodium, yet final urine output is only about 1.5 liters per 24 hours (1 ml per minute), containing about 100 mEq of sodium. Ninety-nine percent of GFR is thus reabsorbed. If no compensatory tubular changes were to occur, an increase of GFR of 1 percent would double urine flow rate and sodium excretion, while an increase of 20 percent would increase urine volume to about 30 liters per day and sodium losses to 3000 mEq or almost the normal total body sodium content.

The term *glomerulotubular balance* is used to indicate the interrelationship of GFR and tubular reabsorption. It can be shown that reduction of GFR does not cause sodium to disappear from the urine, but only to diminish in amount [22], while increase in GFR causes little or no increase in urinary sodium excretion [14]. Apparently, then, tubular reabsorption of sodium varies in tune with GFR to dampen effects on urine sodium and water excretion.

SECOND FACTOR: ALDOSTERONE. Aldosterone is probably the main adrenal sodium-retaining hormone in man. It is secreted by the zona glomerulosa of the adrenal. The renin-angiotensin system and the serum potassium are probably the two major stimuli to aldosterone release.

Renin is released from the renal juxta-glomerular apparatus (JGA) by a fall in afferent arteriolar pressure and/or by a fall in the sodium load passing the macula densa area in the distal tubule [32]. Renin release is modulated by the sympathetic nervous system in two ways: first by α-adrenergic effects on afferent arterioles causing constriction and a fall in JGA perfusion pressure and second by direct β-adrenergic stimulation of the JGA itself [33].

Renin acts on its substrate, an α_2-globulin produced by the liver, to form angiotensin I, a decapeptide, which in turn is "converted" to an octapeptide, angiotensin II, in the lungs and kidneys. Angiotensin II stimulates the secretion of aldosterone. In essence, a fall in ECF volume will lead to a fall in perfusion pressure at the JGA as well as to decreased filtered sodium. The decreased sodium load passing the macula densa could also stimulate renin secretion and in turn aldosterone secretion (Fig. 3-5).

Aldosterone acts on the distal tubular segment, in the main, promoting sodium reabsorption and also H^+ and K^+ secretion, which tends to repair the ECF volume deficit.

A high serum potassium concentration stimulates aldosterone secretion, whereas a low serum potassium inhibits it.

Control of Sodium Intake

Intake of sodium is relatively uncontrolled, but a number of experiments suggest that salt

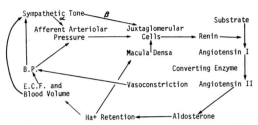

FIGURE 3-5. *The renin-angiotensin-aldosterone feedback loops showing the interrelationships of blood pressure, sodium status, and sympathetic tone on renin secretion.*

appetite exists. For instance, the normal human finds isotonic saline unpalatable and even emetic, but in states of shock and volume depletion, as in burns, subjects will drink large volumes of isotonic or hypertonic saline.

MAINTENANCE OF THE VASCULAR SPACE

The integrity of the blood volume is largely dependent on fluid exchanges at the capillary level. Plasma protein is for the most part maintained in the vascular space although some does leak out and is carried away by the lymphatics. It has been suggested that two routes of passage may exist, one consisting of small numbers of larger holes or clefts between cells, allowing a constant escape of larger molecules by bulk flow, while the other allows water and smaller molecules to escape through smaller pores or by diffusion through endothelial cells [10]. As we shall see later, injury, thermal or anoxic, increases the vascular permeability to large molecules and allows considerable losses of protein into the interstitium of the burned or injured area.

In the normal state the difference in protein concentration between lumen and interstitium around the capillary sets up an average oncotic pressure gradient of 25 mm Hg. As Starling first suggested, fluid exchange is dependent on the difference between hydrostatic and oncotic pressures. As shown in Figure 3-6, blood flow into the capillary is controlled by a precapillary sphincter which may shunt blood away from capillaries and into arteriovenous connections. Functionally, as demonstrated by Mellander and Lewis [18], there are also postcapillary or venular sphincters. If both sphincters are open, hydrostatic pressure tends to be high (about 35 mm Hg) at the arteriolar end of the capillary but falls along the capillary until at the venular end it is only 15 mm Hg. Outward flow of water and solute will therefore occur at the arteriolar end because of the hydrostatic pressure excess, while at the venous end inward flow will occur because of excess oncotic pressure.

Changes in precapillary and postcapillary sphincter tone will greatly affect inward and outward movements. Photographic studies of the microvasculature suggest that in any area the sphincters are constantly opening and closing, probably under local influences. Flow in any particular capillary is therefore normally intermittent, with uptake of tissue fluid occurring when flow ceases and outflow to the tissue when flow resumes. A generalized increase in precapillary and postcapillary sphincter tone such as takes place initially in hypovolemic shock reduces capillary hydrostatic pressure and allows influx of

interstitial fluid, which helps to repair the volume. This also produces the well-known fall in hematocrit in the early hours after hemorrhage.

When tissue has been damaged, changes in permeability will tend to reduce the oncotic pressure differences and cause marked losses from the vascular space. Any condition that reduces plasma protein concentration will also tend to allow net loss of fluid from capillaries.

General Controlling Mechanisms for the Vascular Space

A normal circulation should maintain perfusion to all vascular beds according to their needs. Arterial blood pressure has for many years been taken as a prime indicator of adequacy of circulation and blood volume. However, because it is simply a resultant of cardiac output and peripheral resistance, it may tell little about adequacy of perfusion. For example, the patient with a pheochromocytoma may have a very high blood pressure with a normal or increased cardiac output and high peripheral resistance. Yet it is plain from the pallor and coldness of his extremities and skin that perfusion is re-

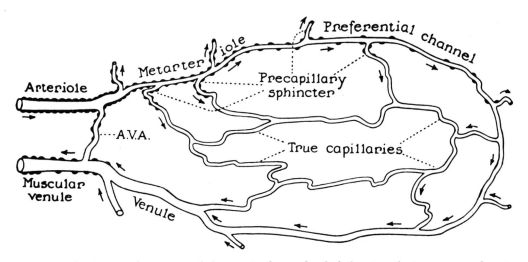

FIGURE 3-6. *Proposed anatomy of the terminal vascular bed showing the importance of various sphincter sites in controlling flow and hydrostatic pressure. (From B. W. Zweifach, as illustrated in R. F. Pitts,* Physiology of the Kidney and Body Fluids *[3rd ed.]. Chicago: Year Book, 1974.)*

duced. Again, because peripheral resistance is usually high in shock, the blood pressure may be well maintained in spite of very poor peripheral perfusion. Urine output and the skin circulation will usually tell more about adequacy of circulation than the blood pressure. The best way to improve circulation is to correct the blood volume. If volume is not replaced, a number of processes occur, which help to maintain perfusion to vital organs such as brain and heart but are eventually damaging to other organs.

Sympathetic Nervous System Stimulation

From the baroreceptors in the aorta and carotid sinus and from right and left atrial receptors, a reduction in arterial and venous pressure is sensed after, say, a hemorrhage. Increased activity from the medullary vasomotor center produces venoconstriction and reduction in the volume of the venous capacitance vessels as well as a rise in venous pressure, while cardiac rate and emptying are increased by sympathetic activity. Finally, selective peripheral arteriolar constriction occurs with marked effects on limb, renal, and splanchnic blood flow [4, 15, 24, 27]. There is relatively little effect on cerebral resistance, and in the coronary bed vasodilatation may actually occur [4]. The increase of renal resistance does not necessarily reverse with reinfusion of the lost volume [4]. In this bed, if perfusion has been poor for long enough, a prolonged state of increased resistance and low GFR may occur associated with acute renal failure.

Catecholamines

Not only does sympathetic activity increase, but the adrenal medulla is also stimulated by hypovolemia [34]. Blood and urinary concentrations of epinephrine and norepinephrine rise. The rise in norepinephrine is in large part from peripheral sympathetic nerve endings, but the epinephrine increase is primarily from adrenal medulla. The effects are like those of the sympathetic nervous system, mainly constriction of venous capacitance vessels as well as arterial and arteriolar resistance vessels.

Renin-Angiotensin

Circulating renin and angiotensin rise to high levels in hypovolemia [17, 28]. Angiotensin II, the vasoconstrictor principle, has rather more effect on arterioles than venules [23]. It is an extremely potent constrictor affecting particularly renal, splanchnic, and skin circulations. As discussed in the section on ECF volume, angiotensin also stimulates aldosterone secretion, which leads to sodium retention by the kidneys.

ADH

ADH, an octapeptide, is released in large amounts by many stimuli (see above) but must be circulating at levels at least 10 to 20 times normal before vasoconstrictor as opposed to antidiuretic effects occur. The most marked effects are on the splanchnic system and on skin and limbs [29].

Adrenal Cortical Steroids

Adrenal cortical steroids are released in considerable amounts by the stress of circulatory insufficiency. Hume and Egdahl have found that, where the stress is a wound or burn, the release of ACTH-mediated corticoid is dependent on an intact nerve supply to the damaged area [8]. Glucocorticoids reach high circulating levels in shock, and it is doubtful that in the absence of adrenal, pituitary, or hypothalamic insufficiency any exogenous steroid is required. In septic shock (see Chapter 10) there is some evidence that huge doses of glucocorticoids may be protective.

Mineralocorticoid secretion is stimulated mainly by the renin-angiotensin system. The retention of sodium and hence water is an important compensatory mechanism.

Local Factors

If local blood flow becomes very poor or if local wounding or burns have occurred, a number of vasodilating factors may be released; histamine, serotonin, kinins, and prostaglandins will cause local dilatation, mostly of the precapillary sphincters, or constriction of the postcapillary sphincters. This leads to a secondary rise in hydrostatic pressure in the capillaries, which together with an increased capillary permeability, causing a fall in oncotic pressure, will result in net fluid loss. Activation of the coagulation-fibrinolytic system may also occur, with thrombosis, microembolization, and sometimes further bleeding.

REFERENCES

1. Campion, D. S., Carter, N. W., Rector, F. C., and Seldin, D. W. Intracellular pH in chronic potassium deficiency in the rat. *Clin. Res.* 16:379, 1968.
2. Cooke, R. E., Segar, W. E., Cleek, D. B., Coville, F. E., and Darrow, D. C. The extrarenal correction of alkalosis associated with potassium deficiency. *J. Clin. Invest.* 31:789, 1952.
3. Davies, H. E. F., Jepson, R. P., and Black, D. A. K. Some metabolic sequels of gastric surgery in patients with and without pyloric stenosis. *Clin. Sci.* 15:61, 1956.
4. Dedichen, H. Hemodynamic changes in experimental hemorrhagic shock. *Acta Chir. Scand.* 138:129, 1972.
5. Dick, D. A. T. *Cell Water.* London: Butterworth, 1966.
6. Edelman, F. S., and Leibman, J. Anatomy of body water and electrolytes. *Am. J. Med.* 27:256, 1959.
7. Edelman, F. S., Olney, J. M., James, A. H., Brooks, L., and Moore, F. D. Body composition: Studies in the human being by the dilution principle. *Science* 115:447, 1952.
8. Hume, D. M., and Egdahl, R. H. The importance of the brain in the endocrine response to injury. *Ann. Surg.* 150:697, 1959.
9. Irvine, R. O. H., and Dow, J. W. Potassium depletion: Effects on intracellular pH and electrolyte distribution in skeletal and cardiac muscle. *Australas. Ann. Med.* 17:206, 1968.
10. Karnovsky, M. J. The ultrastructural basis of transcapillary exchanges. *J. Gen. Physiol.* 52:645, 1968.
11. Kleeman, C. R. In Maxwell, M. H., and Kleeman, C. R. (Eds.). *Clinical Disorders of Fluid and Electrolyte Metabolism* (2nd ed.). New York: McGraw-Hill, 1972.
12. Kruhoffer, P. Inulin as an indicator for the extracellular space. *Acta Physiol. Scand.* 11:16, 1946.
13. Leaf, A. Regulation of intracellular fluid volume and disease. *Am. J. Med.* 49:291, 1970.
14. Lindheimer, M. D., Lalone, R. C., and Levinsky, N. G. Evidence that an acute increase in G.F.R. has little effect on sodium excretion in the dog unless extracellular volume is expanded. *J. Clin. Invest.* 46:256, 1967.
15. Longerbeam, J. K., Lillehei, R. C., Scott, W. R., and Rosenberg, J. C. Visceral factors in shock. *J.A.M.A.* 181:172, 1962.
16. Bunag, R. D., Vander, H. J., Kaneko, Y., and McCubbin, J. W. In Page, I. H., and McCubbin, J. W. (Eds.), *Renal Hypertension.* Chicago: Year Book, 1968.
17. McKenzie, J. K., Lee, M. R., and Cook, W. F. Effect of hemorrhage on arterial plasma renin activity in the rabbit. *Circ. Res.* 19:269, 1966.
18. Mellander, S., and Lewis, D. H. Effect of hemorrhagic shock on the reactivity of resistance and capacitance vessels and on capillary filtration transfer in cat skeletal muscle. *Circ. Res.* 13:105, 1963.
19. Metcoff, J., Buchman, H., Jacobson, M., Richter, H., Bloomenthal, E. D., and Zacharias, M. Losses and physiological replacements for water and electrolytes after extensive burns in children. *N. Engl. J. Med.* 265:101, 1961.
20. Moore, F. D. Determination of total body water and solids with isotopes. *Science* 104:157, 1946.
21. Moore, F. D., Oleson, K. H., McMurrey, J. D., Parker, H. V., Ball, M. R., and Boyden, C. M. *The Body Cell Mass and Its Supporting Environment.* Philadelphia: Saunders, 1963.
22. Mueller, C. B., Surtshin, A., Carlin,

M. R., and White, H. L. Glomerular and tubular influences on sodium and water excretion. *Am. J. Physiol.* 165:411, 1951.

23. Nickerson, M., and Sutter, M. C. Angiotensin in shock. *Can. Med. Assoc. J.* 90:325, 1964.

24. Passmore, J. C., and Baker, C. H. Intrarenal blood flow distribution in irreversible hemorrhagic shock in dogs. *J. Trauma* 13:1066, 1973.

25. Raber, J. W., Taylor, I. M., Weller, J. M., and Hasting, A. B. Rate of potassium exchange in the human erythrocyte. *J. Gen. Physiol.* 33:691, 1950.

26. Rocchio, M. A., and Randall, H. T. Wound kinetics: Water and electrolyte changes from zero to sixty days in clean wounds. *Am. J. Surg.* 121:460, 1971.

27. Rothe, C. F., Schwendenmann, F. C., and Selkurt, E. E. Neurogenic control of skeletal muscle vascular resistance in hemorrhagic shock. *Am. J. Physiol.* 204:925, 1963.

28. Scornik, O. A., and Paladini, A. C. Angiotensin blood levels in hemorrhagic hypotension and other related conditions. *Am. J. Physiol.* 206:553, 1964.

29. Shaldon, S., Dolle, W., Guevare, L., Iber, F. L., and Sherlock, S. Effect of Pitressin on the splanchnic circulation in man. *Circulation* 24:797, 1961.

30. Steele, J. M., Berger, E. Y., Dunning, M. F., and Brodie, B. B. Total body water in man. *Am. J. Physiol.* 162:313, 1955.

31. Swan, R. C., and Pitts, R. F. Neutralization of infused acid by nephrectomized dogs. *J. Clin. Invest.* 34:205, 1955.

32. Vander, J. Control of renin release. *Physiol. Rev.* 47:559, 1967.

33. Vandongen, R., Peart, W. S., and Boyd, G. W. Adrenergic stimulation of renin secretion in the isolated perfused rat kidney. *Circ. Res.* 32:291, 1973.

34. Walker, W. F., Zileli, M. S., Reuter, F. W., Shoemaker, W. C., Friend, D., and More, F. D. Adrenal medullary secretion in hemorrhagic shock. *Am. J. Physiol.* 197:773, 1959.

4

Metabolism
·
Harold A. Harper

METABOLIC EFFECTS OF TRAUMA AND STRESS

Periods of trauma and stress are generally characterized by variable degrees of starvation. Consequently, as a means to understand the metabolic changes that occur in these states it is useful to summarize the important nutritional effects of starvation.

Carbohydrate as glycogen and glucose is stored in man in only very limited quantities (Table 4-1). Indeed, after 12 to 18 hours of fasting the liver becomes almost totally depleted of glycogen, and even under ideal conditions of storage, as after a high-carbohydrate meal, the total energy available as carbohydrate in storage form does not much exceed 1400 Calories, an amount enough for only a 12- to 24-hour supply to the brain. As a substitute for the limited direct sources of glucose, other substances are called upon to produce glucose through gluconeogenesis. Protein is the principal substrate for gluconeogenesis since most of the amino acids making up the protein molecule may, after deamination, be converted to glucose. The glycerol moiety of triglycerides, but not the fatty acids, derived mostly from

the lipid of adipose tissue, is also a source of glucose. The liver, and to some extent the kidney, is the organ in which gluconeogenesis is accomplished. Gluconeogenesis begins almost immediately after a meal so that tissue protein reserves, mainly from utilization of skeletal muscle, are drawn upon rapidly. It should be noted that there does not appear to be a significant amount of labile storage protein available. Consequently protein is mobilized almost entirely at the expense of structural functioning tissue.

A high priority on the use of glucose for energy is so characteristic of certain tissues that glucose can be regarded as virtually an obligatory metabolite for these tissues. Foremost among them is the brain. It utilizes daily 100 to 150 gm of glucose which under aerobic circumstances it can metabolize completely to carbon dioxide and water. Some other tissues also have a high requirement for glucose. Examples are erythrocytes, bone marrow, peripheral nerve, and renal medulla. Very important is the fact that tissues essential to wound healing, such as fibroblasts and phagocytes, are also utilizing glucose predominantly, metabolizing it anaerobically to

TABLE 4-1. *Storage of Carbohydrate in Normal Adult Man*

Liver glycogen	6.0% =	108 gm
Muscle glycogen	0.7% =	245 gm
Extracellular glucose	0.1% =	10 gm
Total: 363 gm × 4		= 1452 Cal

lactate and carbon dioxide. The other tissues of the body can also utilize fatty acids, or the products of their metabolism (ketones), as fuel, and they do so to an increasing degree, even to the point of exclusive use, when carbohydrate availability declines, as occurs in fasting. Examples of such tissues are heart and skeletal muscle and renal cortex.

During brief periods of fasting in normal man, 100 to 150 gm of glucose is sufficient to provide maximal protein-sparing action as evidenced by a reduction in gluconeogenesis from amino acids determined by measurement of the output of total nitrogen (mainly urea) in the urine. The requirement for calories is, to an increasing degree, met by breakdown of lipid from adipose tissue stores. Glucose, provided by gluconeogenesis, is diverted to tissues preferentially requiring this metabolite. Thus, whereas as much as 75 gm of protein per day (12 gm urinary nitrogen) may be excreted at the start of a total fast, adaptation to fasting, including a shift to mobilization of lipid for energy, produces a fall in protein breakdown to 20 to 25 gm per day or less. This protein-sparing action is a major aspect of the response to fasting. If protein losses equal to those that occur during the first few days of the fast were to continue, protein reserves (mainly muscle) would quickly decline. There is evidence that man cannot survive a loss of protein exceeding one-third to one-half of normal [8]. It is important to recall that muscle weakness, an inevitable result of protein depletion, extends also to the muscles associated with respiration—the intercostals, the diaphragm, and the secondary muscles of respiration. Inefficient clearing of the tracheobronchial tree, atelectasis, local infection, and bronchopneumonia, as well as sys-

temic infection, follow. This train of events explains why, aside from acute vascular episodes, sepsis secondary to debilitation is the major cause of in-hospital death. The most common focus for infection is the pulmonary system; terminal bronchopneumonia is frequently listed in pathological summaries as a contributor to the fatal end result. In addition to these important aspects of protein metabolism in disease, protein depletion seriously impairs resistance to infection as well as interfering with the proper healing of wounds.

During starvation, ketone bodies produced in the liver from the oxidation of fatty acids substitute for glucose as a source of energy for the brain. Indeed, the major reason for the ability of the organism during prolonged starvation to spare protein and glucose is the capacity to convert to the use of ketones as the chief source of energy. As noted above, even the brain, which normally gets all of its energy from glucose, can substitute ketones for up to 70 percent of its energy requirement. Fatty acid oxidation with ketone production in the liver during starvation can substitute for the energy normally obtained by the liver from amino acid oxidation, thus further sparing protein breakdown.

Contrary to former concepts, it is now clear that ketogenesis is a normal and essential metabolic adaptive response to starvation, reflecting as it does the mobilization of endogenous fat stores. It is by the maximal utilization of these reserves that nitrogen losses can be reduced to minimal levels.

Insulin plays a key role in regulating the balance between lipogenesis and lipolysis. When the blood sugar levels are elevated, insulin output is increased and ketogenesis is decreased through inhibition of lipolysis. Under these circumstances, excess administration of glucose inhibits utilization of the large reserves of energy present in adipose tissue depot fat. When the metabolic situation is favorable to utilization of endogenous lipid, therefore, the practice of infusing excess amounts of glucose in an effort to supply exogenous calories seems questionable. Admittedly this is done to spare catabolism of body proteins. In the light of recent information it appears that therapeutic approaches to sparing of protein should be directed toward utilization of endogenous stores of fat in patients for whom this is appropriate.

In contrast to the metabolic events occurring in short periods of starvation and the metabolic adaptation to more prolonged periods, stress due to trauma, sepsis, or infectious disease greatly enhances breakdown of glycogen and protein. The usual concomitant inadequate intake of nutrients and calories exacerbates the severity of the deranged metabolic environment in such an eventuality.

Studies bearing on this clinically important problem have been reported by Kinney and his co-workers [4]. These investigators evaluated what they termed the *rate of metabolic expenditure* (RME) by measuring the utilization of oxygen and the production of carbon dioxide. While the RME was found not to be significantly abnormal in preoperative, early postoperative, and septic patients, it was notably elevated in patients with burns and other kinds of injury. In a postoperative group in whom the early nitrogen excretion was 7.1 gm per square meter per day, it later fell to 0.1 gm per square meter per day as a consequence of the metabolic adaptation described above. In contrast, the rate for a group of burned patients remained at 7.7 gm per square meter per day, and for patients sustaining other types of trauma, 8.3 gm per square meter per day. These excessive rates of loss of body protein are at least three times what is expected during simple prolonged starvation. It was also observed that the respiratory quotient (RQ) was 0.84, indicative of metabolism predominantly of carbohydrate [4]. Had normal adaptive mechanisms come into play, the RQ would have fallen closer to 0.7, characteristic of endogenous metabolism of lipid.

Severe injury seems to impair mechanisms that normally minimize breakdown of protein even though mobilization of fat might in itself be adequate for the energy needs of the body. Apparently sepsis, when superimposed on starvation, interferes with the mobilization of endogenous fat stores. It is significant that during states of sepsis, trauma, and disease diabetes-like sugar tolerance curves (so-called diabetes of injury) have been observed, suggesting that insulin resistance is present. Measurement of insulin levels in these states reveals an actual increase in insulin activity; in the presence of elevated blood glucose, during these abnormal metabolic circumstances more insulin may be required to maintain normal blood glucose levels than is necessary in postabsorptive states or in those accompanying starvation not influenced by disease. The elevated insulin levels, by reducing lipolysis from adipose tissue, impair the acquisition of energy from this major endogenous source, and the consequent reduction in circulating fatty acids and ketones that could serve as fuel for the tissues creates a demand for more glucose and amino acid to serve as sources of energy. Rapid destruction of body protein is the inevitable result.

Protein Catabolic Effect

Among the several metabolic responses to injury, the protein catabolic effect has probably been the most extensively studied. After major trauma the urinary nitrogen, as an index of protein catabolism, may increase from a normal level of 4.6 gm per day, or less, to 7 to 15 gm per day; after very extensive injury or trauma, daily excretion of nitrogen may rise as high as 20 gm. Fractures or major injuries complicated by infection enhance the breakdown of lean tissue, resulting in a daily urinary nitrogen excretion rate of as much as 30 gm. This is equivalent to a loss of 180 gm of protein that would be derived from about 1 kg (wet weight) of lean tissue, largely skeletal muscle.

Nitrogen losses in the burned patient may be extremely serious. Where there is simply soft tissue trauma that progresses to uncomplicated convalescence and healing, the period of increased nitrogen excretion persists for only two to five days; after burns of even moderate severity, the nitrogen catabolic period is unduly prolonged. From a high level of excretion, which totals 25 to 30 gm of nitrogen per day, reached at seven days after the burn injury, negative nitrogen balance declines only slowly, sometimes not becoming positive until 20 to 40 days after the original injury.

In addition to the extensive and prolonged protein catabolic period after burning, losses of protein occur from the losses in the exudate, which is extremely rich in protein directly derived from plasma and interstitial fluid.

During the first 10 days after a severe burn a whole tissue loss of as much as 540 gm per day will occur when the mean nitrogen loss in the urine is 18 gm per day, a not unusual occurrence in major burning injuries. In one reported study burned patients lost 8.2 to 11.7 kg of lean body tissue during the protein catabolic period that followed the burn injury.

Potassium Balance

Potassium losses associated with trauma involving extensive tissue breakdown can be expected to be excessive since this element is normally concentrated intracellularly. Losses of potassium tend to occur very soon after injury. The first day after moderately severe trauma, 2.5 to 3.5 gm of potassium may be excreted. After a burn, a negative potassium balance of 2 to 5 gm per day occurs immediately. However, in contrast to the prolonged character of negative nitrogen balance, potassium losses usually decrease rapidly so that, if adequate amounts of potassium are provided, a positive balance of this element may be regained in three to six days.

NUTRITIONAL REQUIREMENTS RESULTING FROM STRESS, TRAUMA, AND INFECTION

Calories

Prompt weight loss is an inevitable feature of the immediate period after injury. The rate of loss is proportional to the severity of the injury. It is reasonable to assume that injury fosters large increases in metabolism and that, occurring as they do during a time of reduced caloric intake, they necessitate a greater use of the body's own tissues for fuel. Although body protein is being consumed more rapidly, this is not an important source of the extra energy. For example, when an amount of muscle tissue is sacrificed to account for a high daily nitrogen excretion of 20 gm, about 1 to 5 gm of glucose (by gluconeogenesis from amino acids) is produced. This accounts for only 500 Calories, and furthermore, such a rate of protein loss cannot be sustained very long. Preformed carbohydrate will supply no more than a total of about 300 Calories. Thus, it is the fat reserves in adipose tissues that must be counted on. In a normal man these reserves may produce as much as 100,000 to 150,000 Calories. The amount of stored fat in a given individual, therefore, bears a direct relationship to the length of time he can survive a total fast. At normal rates of consumption of energy the amount of stored fat in adipose tissues of previously healthy adults is adequate to supply energy for two to three months; loss of one-half or more of this total amount is not harmful.

In health, 25 to 30 Calories per kilogram per day are required for maintenance. In disease, this basal requirement may be markedly altered. Extra energy is necessary to support tissue repair during convalescence. Fever, by accelerating metabolism, increases energy demand by about 12 percent over the basal requirement for each degree centigrade by which the body temperature is above normal. Some authorities have suggested caloric needs of as high as 5000 to 6000 per day following a major injury such as an extensive burn. More recent studies have been conducted by indirect calorimetry using methods modified to be applicable to investigations on acutely injured patients [4]. These have permitted the establishment of ranges of resting metabolic expenditure of individuals according to size, sex, and age. The normal range was found to be ±10 percent of the classic figures given in standard tables for basal metabolic rates. Uncomplicated elective operations did not produce significant changes from preoperative values for the metabolic rate. Major skeletal injury resulted in increases of 10 to 30 percent for one to three weeks, followed by a decrease to 10 to 20 percent below normal. Infection in a major serous cavity may produce increases of 15 to 50 percent above normal; indeed, some elevation above normal will persist as long as inflammation is present notwithstanding the extensive tissue depletion and weight loss that have occurred. Most impressive is the hypermetabolism of extensive burns. Here the metabolic rate may remain at from 40 to 100 percent above normal for many weeks. Although there is little question that the metabolic rate increases after injury, it apparently does not increase to the heights previously suggested. In consequence, other reasons for the weight and nitrogen loss following injury must be sought.

In patients undergoing elective surgery, protein supplies an average of 15 percent of the total caloric expenditure, as it does in normal individuals. After major trauma and sepsis, protein supplies about 20 percent of the total expenditure of energy, which, itself, was increased about 20 percent over normal. However, in major burns with increase in energy expenditure about 60 percent greater than normal, protein supplied less than proportionate amounts of the total energy as compared to the other disease states studied even though the actual amounts of protein catabolized were significantly increased. This finding further supports the idea that the nitrogen loss is not simply a reflection of the use of protein to provide energy.

Consideration should also be given to the differences in water content of protein as contrasted with fat tissue. Fat may be thought of as essentially an anhydrous form of fuel containing 9 Calories per gram. Lean tissue yields only about 1 Calorie per gram because of its greater degree of hydration in the body, so that the 4 Calories contained per gram in dry protein yields only 1 Calorie per gram as the hydrated body protein is broken down.

Major injury or sepsis is associated with a relatively high proportion of lost lean tissue in the total mixture of energy-yielding substrates. Although lean tissue contributes perhaps but 15 to 20 percent of the total resting caloric output, it may be expected to yield as much as 60 to 70 percent by weight. This is the reason the extreme weight loss in major catabolic states is greater than would be expected merely from the need to provide sources of metabolic fuel from the tissues.

The oxidative metabolism of 1 kg of fat in the body produces slightly more than 1000 ml of water of oxidation; a similar amount of lean tissue when metabolized produces 250 ml of water of oxidation, which added to its contained water of hydration (referred to above) produces almost an additional liter of water. All of this "endogenous" water produced in severe trauma must be taken into account as a factor likely to contribute to overhydration of patients in the immediate period after trauma or injury, particularly if excess fluid is given either by mouth or as parenteral fluid.

Protein
It has been emphasized frequently that protein needs of sick or injured persons are often much increased—to as much as 200 to 300 gm per day in severe burns—as judged by measurement of nitrogen excretion in the urine as well as of direct losses of protein by exudation from the skin surfaces. Depletion of body protein leads to prolongation of convalescence, impaired healing of wounds, increased susceptibility to infection, muscle weakness, edema, anemia, impaired gastrointestinal motility, and the possibility of other postoperative complications.

However, there appears to be what is virtually an "obligatory" period of negative nitrogen balance associated with various disease states. The extent and duration of this protein catabolic period are related to the magnitude of the illness. In major trauma such as occurs with fractures or serious burns, particularly when complicated by infection, the protein catabolic event is most severe.

The metabolic response to injury produces physiological changes that are in large measure explainable by the anticipated response of the adrenal to stress. Increases in catabolism of protein and loss of potassium are examples of the expected metabolic result of hyperfunction of adrenal cortex.

Because of the apparently obligatory nature of nitrogen catabolism during the immediate post-traumatic period, it seems undesirable to attempt at that time to supply the very large protein and caloric intake necessary to equal the losses, even if it were practicable. There is no reliable evidence that the replenishing of muscle protein in the acutely traumatized patient can be accomplished by the giving of large quantities of protein orally or of amino acids parenterally.

Although, if possible, at least 100 gm of protein should be given to all sick or injured persons, caution should be exercised in proposing high-protein regimens for patients with impairment of hepatic or renal function. It is also important to provide enough fluid to support sufficient urinary output to permit the excretion of the nitrogenous end products of protein catabolism (principally urea). Patients with poor renal concentrating power must receive increased amounts of fluid to foster the excretion of adequate volumes of urine if retention of metabolic end products is to be avoided; the greater the amount of metabolic wastes to be eliminated (as in increased protein breakdown), the more the urine that must be produced, particularly as renal concentrating power declines. For example, a patient on a normal diet who is unable to form a urine more concentrated than 1.010 specific gravity must take enough fluid to permit a daily urine output of as much as 2100 ml per day if uremia is to be avoided; in contrast, the same load of metabolic wastes can be cleared with an output of as little as 700 ml of urine per day by a patient with maximal concentrating power—1.029 to 1.032 specific gravity.

After a variable period, usually only a few days following moderate stress, a protein anabolic period supervenes. During this time the body utilizes administered protein with much more efficiency if adequate calories are simultaneously available.

Many authorities have emphasized the difficulty of reversing protein breakdown, even after the protein catabolic period has passed, when provision of calories in larger than normal amounts is difficult. This is likely to be the situation if oral feeding is not possible or if consumption of nutrients in adequate amounts is hard to achieve.

Infusion of very large quantities of glucose may at certain periods during the patient's illness have little effect in reversing the catabolic events. As has been previously mentioned, there is now mounting evidence that high levels of blood glucose, as would occur during massive infusions of this sugar, provoke an increased output of insulin that acts to inhibit lipolysis from adipose tissue. Fatty acid mobilization is then reduced to rates insufficient to provide calories otherwise made available by oxidation of fatty acids and resultant production of energy-yielding ketones. A parenteral regimen using a relatively small amount of glucose, to minimize the insulin antilipolytic effect, together with amino acids, has been recommended. It is supported by the results of such therapy in a group of patients who during four days of conventional dextrose and water therapy (2 liters of 5% dextrose in water) had lost from 18 to 38 gm of protein. On amino acid infusion alone (90 gm per day), the same patients achieved a slight degree of positive nitrogen balance. There was some variation in nitrogen retention among the patients given glucose and amino acid mixtures. This would be expected as a manifestation of variations in the extent of insulin sensitivity related to the degree of sepsis or trauma, the previous nutritional state, and individual differences in glucose tolerance.

In the light of these observations the best intravenous regimen during partial starvation might be to provide necessary fluid as amino acid solutions together with such additional fluid as is necessary to supply electrolytes. Exclusion of carbohydrate should maximize lipid mobilization as a source of calories to spare protein. Two liters of isotonic (3%) amino acid solution provides 8.85 gm of nitrogen, approximately equivalent to that lost in skin, feces, and urine. It would appear that the ability of intravenously administered glucose to exert a protein-sparing action is the resultant of at least two factors: the desired effect of substituting exogenous glucose for that produced by gluconeogenesis from protein, and the undesirable effect on stimulation of insulin release with consequent inhibition of adipose tissue lipolysis. In most patients, particularly after the acute catabolic period induced by trauma and stress has passed, the first, favorable, effect predominates. Thus glucose administration does foster sparing of protein breakdown and tissue repair. However, if the insulin response so inhibits mobilization of fatty acids and ketone production that the caloric contribution from administered glucose is equivalent only to that obtainable from otherwise mobilizable endogenous lipid, the net sparing effect of the glucose is negated. Such an effect may conceivably be operative in states of severe caloric undernutrition—as in famine, when just enough carbohydrate is taken in the diet to inhibit the obtaining of additional calories from the already limited fat reserves. That the resulting critically inadequate supply of calories cannot prevent protein breakdown is evidenced by the occurrence of the classic signs of protein deficiency, particularly in children. These signs include muscle weakness, edema, and impaired physical and mental development.

Vitamins

When a normal individual is consuming an adequate balanced diet, all the required vitamins can be secured from dietary sources. But in abnormal states or when digestion or assimilation is impaired and the requirements for these nutrients are increased, supplementation must be considered. The recom-

mended daily allowances for normal persons for vitamins for which adequate information is available are given in Table 4-2. [6] It is very likely, however, that the recommended allowances will have to be increased in abnormal states. In these situations information is much less accurate with respect to appropriate vitamin requirements than is the case under normal circumstances of health.

The water-soluble vitamins of the vitamin B complex are directly involved as cofactors in important metabolic processes. Since these processes may be intensified as a result of the abnormal metabolic state incident to disease, it is desirable to increase the intake of these vitamins. The recommended therapeutic daily doses of the most important are as follows:

Thiamine (B_1)	5–10 mg
Riboflavin (B_2)	5–10 mg
Niacinamide	100 mg
Pantothenic acid	20 mg
Pyridoxine (B_6)	3 mg
Folic acid (folacin)	1.5 mg
Vitamin B_{12}	10 μg

Vitamin C (ascorbic acid) appears to have particular value in connection with disease processes accompanied by accelerated metabolism and stress. One of the best-demonstrated functions of vitamin C is its role in maintaining the normal intercellular material of cartilage, dentine, and bone, as well as in collagen synthesis. This relates the vitamin specifically to wound healing. Since there are large amounts of vitamin C in the adrenal cortex and the cortex is rapidly depleted of vitamin C when the adrenal gland is stimulated, as by stress, and since increased losses of vitamin C accompany infection and fever, special attention should be given to the intake of this vitamin in disease states characterized by trauma and stress. Therefore at least 500 mg per day of vitamin C should be provided as a therapeutic dose.

If supplementation with vitamins is necessary for only a short period until a normal diet

TABLE 4-2. *Recommended Daily Allowances of Certain Nutrients for Normal Persons*[a]

	Years	Weight (kg)	Weight (lb)	Height (cm)	Height (in)	Energy (kcal)[b]	Protein (gm)	Fat-Soluble Vitamins Vitamin A Activity (RE)[c]	Vitamin A Activity (IU)	Vita-min D (IU)	Vita-min E Activity[e] (IU)
Infants	0.0–0.5	6	14	60	24	kg × 117	kg × 2.2	420[d]	1400	400	4
	0.5–1.0	9	20	71	28	kg × 108	kg × 2.0	400	2000	400	5
Children	1–3	13	28	86	34	1300	23	400	2000	400	7
	4–6	20	44	110	44	1800	30	500	2500	400	9
	7–10	30	66	135	54	2400	36	700	3300	400	10
Males	11–14	44	97	158	63	2800	44	1000	5000	400	12
	15–18	61	134	172	69	3000	54	1000	5000	400	15
	19–22	67	147	172	69	3000	52	1000	5000	400	15
	23–50	70	154	172	69	2700	56	1000	5000		15
	51+	70	154	172	69	2400	56	1000	5000		15
Females	11–14	44	97	155	62	2400	44	800	4000	400	10
	15–18	54	119	162	65	2100	48	800	4000	400	11
	19–22	58	128	162	65	2100	46	800	4000	400	12
	23–50	58	128	162	65	2000	46	800	4000		12
	51+	58	128	162	65	1800	46	800	4000		12
Pregnant						+300	+30	1000	5000	400	15
Lactating						+500	+20	1200	6000	400	15

[a]The allowances are intended to provide for individual variations among most normal persons as they live in the United States under usual environmental stresses. Diets should be based on a variety of common foods in order to provide other nutrients for which human requirements have been less well defined. See text for more detailed discussion of allowances and of nutrients not tabulated.

[b]Kilojoule: (KJ) = 4.2 × kcal.

[c]Retinol equivalents.

[d]Assumed to be all as retinol in milk during the first six months of life. All subsequent intakes are assumed to be one-half as retinol and one-half as β-carotene when calculated from international units. As retinol equivalents, three-fourths are as retinol and one-fourth as β-carotene.

[e]Total vitamin E activity, estimated to be 80 percent as α-tocopherol and 20 percent other tocopherols.

82

Table 4-2 (continued).

	Water-Soluble Vitamins							Minerals					
	Ascorbic Acid (mg)	Folacin[f] (µg)	Niacin[g] (mg)	Riboflavin (mg)	Thiamine (mg)	Vitamin B6 (mg)	Vitamin B12 (µg)	Calcium (mg)	Phosphorus (mg)	Iodine (µg)	Iron (mg)	Magnesium (mg)	Zinc (mg)
Infants	35	50	5	0.4	0.3	0.3	0.3	360	240	35	10	60	3
	35	50	8	0.6	0.5	0.4	0.3	540	400	45	15	70	5
Children	40	100	9	0.8	0.7	0.6	1.0	800	800	60	15	150	10
	40	200	12	1.1	0.9	0.9	1.5	800	800	80	10	200	10
	40	300	16	1.2	1.2	1.2	2.0	800	800	110	10	250	10
Males	45	400	18	1.5	1.4	1.6	3.0	1200	1200	130	18	350	15
	45	400	20	1.8	1.5	1.8	3.0	1200	1200	150	18	400	15
	45	400	20	1.8	1.5	2.0	3.0	800	800	140	10	350	15
	45	400	18	1.6	1.4	2.0	3.0	800	800	130	10	350	15
	45	400	16	1.5	1.2	2.0	3.0	800	800	110	10	350	15
Females	45	400	16	1.3	1.2	1.6	3.0	1200	1200	115	18	300	15
	45	400	14	1.4	1.1	2.0	3.0	1200	1200	115	18	300	15
	45	400	14	1.4	1.1	2.0	3.0	800	800	100	18	300	15
	45	400	13	1.2	1.0	2.0	3.0	800	800	100	18	300	15
	45	400	12	1.1	1.0	2.0	3.0	800	800	80	10	300	15
Pregnant	60	800	+2	+0.3	+0.3	2.5	4.0	1200	1200	125	18+[h]	450	20
Lactating	60	600	+4	+0.5	+0.3	2.5	4.0	1200	1200	150	16	450	25

[f]The folacin allowances refer to dietary sources as determined by *Lactobacillus casei* assay. Pure forms of folacin may be effective in doses less than one-fourth of the RDA.

[g]Although allowances are expressed as niacin, it is recognized that on the average 1 mg of niacin is derived from each 60 mg of dietary tryptophan.

[h]This increased requirement cannot be met by ordinary diets; therefore, the use of supplemental iron is recommended.

Source: *Recommended Dietary Allowances* (8th rev. ed.). Food and Nutrition Board, National Research Council. Washington, D.C.: National Academy of Sciences, 1974.

can be taken, only thiamine, riboflavin, niacinamide, and ascorbic acid need be given. When these water-soluble vitamins are added to solutions to be given intravenously, large losses of the vitamins into the urine may occur. For this reason intramuscular or subcutaneous injection is preferred if the oral route cannot be used.

Vitamins A, D, and K are the fat-soluble vitamins generally considered important in human nutrition although a need for an exogenous source of vitamin D in adults is questionable since the small amounts required can be synthesized within the body. However, vitamins A and K do have generalized metabolic roles that are of continuing importance. A role of vitamin A in wound healing has been proposed; vitamin K is essential to the production of prothrombin by the liver and therefore in coagulation of the blood. Under normal circumstances vitamin A is present in adequate amounts in a balanced diet; the synthesis by intestinal bacteria of vitamin K assures its production in adequate amounts. But if fat digestion or absorption is impaired, as may occur in obstructive jaundice, biliary fistula, pancreatic disease, or any disease state extensively involving the gastrointestinal tract, these vitamins are not adequately absorbed from the intestine. For surgical patients a deficiency of vitamin K may be significant because of its effects on prothrombin production. When circumstances are such as to induce a vitamin K deficiency, it is important to administer vitamin K preoperatively by injection until the prothrombin level is at least 60 or 70 percent of normal. The dose of a water-soluble vitamin K preparation such as menadione sodium bisulfite (Hykinone) which is required is only 2 to 5 mg by intravenous or intramuscular injection.

MAINTENANCE OF NUTRITION IN THE SURGICAL PATIENT

Hyperalimentation

When the gastrointestinal tract cannot be used for nutritional purposes and only the intravenous route is available, supplying adequate nutrition is a formidable task. In fact, until recently it could safely be said that, except for brief periods, a totally intravenous regimen could not maintain patients in positive nitrogen balance and support growth and tissue repair. The principal problem during intravenous alimentation is to provide sufficient calories. The introduction of emulsions of fat intended for intravenous administration appeared to be a substantial contribution to the solution of this problem. However, their use was accompanied by untoward reactions in some patients, particularly after prolonged administration. Emulsions of fat for intravenous use are therefore not now generally available in the United States.

That the intravenous infusion of a fat-free amino acid and concentrated glucose solution could, under some circumstances, support normal growth and development has been conclusively shown by Dudrick and others [2]. The method used for total parenteral (IV) nutrition (hyperalimentation) is based on the infusion of glucose for calories and a protein hydrolysate as a source of nitrogen to provide for synthesis of protein. The hypertonic basal solution can be prepared in the hospital pharmacy by mixing routinely available solutions of glucose and 5% protein (e.g., fibrin or casein) hydrolysates. The details are as recommended by Dudrick et al. [1]:

A liter of solution providing 1000 Calories and 6 gm of nitrogen (equivalent to approximately 35 gm protein) is prepared by combining 860 ml of 5% fibrin hydrolysate (Aminosol*) in 5% glucose with 165 gm of U.S.P. anhydrous glucose. Sterilization must be accomplished by the use of a 0.22 micron membrane† since such a hypertonic glucose solution would suffer intense caramelization if autoclaved. This is the stock solution to which nutrients can be added. There are approximately 8 mEq Na, 14 mEq K, and traces of other mineral elements such as chloride, phosphate, magnesium, and calcium in the

---

*Abbott Laboratories, Chicago, Ill.
†Millprose, Bedford, Mass.

protein hydrolysate added. These values may vary slightly depending on the type of protein hydrolysate used (e.g., fibrin or casein digests).

An alternative method for preparing the basic stock solution consists in discarding 250 ml from a liter bottle of 5% protein hydrolysate in 5% glucose, then, using strict aseptic precautions, adding 350 ml of 50% glucose. The resultant 1100 ml of solution provides approximately 5.25 gm N (equivalent to 25 gm as protein), 212 gm glucose, 7 mEq Na, and 13 mEq K when fibrin hydrolysate is used. The caloric value is slightly less than 1 Calorie per milliliter.

Unless contraindicated, 50 mEq NaCl and 40 mEq KCl, using concentrated solutions of the electrolyte, should be added per liter of solution prepared by either procedure. Fortification with vitamins is most conveniently accomplished by addition, to one bottle of the daily infusate, of 10 ml of a commercially available multivitamin preparation of fat- and water-soluble vitamins.* Magnesium (4 to 8 mEq per day) may also be provided as magnesium sulfate. Vitamins B_{12} and K and folic acid if considered necessary, as may be the case during prolonged intravenous alimentation, may be given intramuscularly. If plasma analyses so suggest, calcium gluconate and potassium acid phosphate (KH_2PO_4) may also be supplied as necessary. Unless there has been a preexisting iron deficiency or extensive hemorrhage, or both, iron is probably not required. Transfusions of whole blood will supply iron, as will intramuscular injection of iron dextran if necessary. The trace mineral elements such as zinc, copper, manganese, cobalt, and iodine may be added if total nutrition by intravenous injection is prolonged beyond one month. Alternatively, 1 unit of plasma twice weekly will serve as a source of trace elements.

Table 4-3 summarizes the average nutrient composition of 2500 to 3000 ml of the solution, prepared as described above, for

*M.V.I., US Pharmaceutical Corporation, Tuckahoe, N.Y.

TABLE 4-3. *Average Composition of Adult Nutrient Solution*

Components	Amounts
Water	2500–3000 ml
Protein hydrolysate (amino acids)	100–130 gm
Nitrogen	12–18 gm
Carbohydrate (dextrose)	525–625 gm
Calories	2500–3000 Cal
Sodium	125–150 mEq
Potassium	75–120 mEq
Magnesium	4–8 mEq
Vitamin A	5000–10,000 USP units
Vitamin D	500–1000 USP units
Vitamin E	2.5–5.0 IU
Vitamin C	250–500 mg
Thiamine	25–50 mg
Riboflavin	5–10 mg
Pyridoxine	7.5–15.0 mg
Niacin	50–100 mg
Pantothenic acid	12.5–25.0 mg

Calcium and phosphorus are added to the solution, as indicated.
Iron is added to the solution, or given intramuscularly in depot form as iron dextran, or given as blood transfusion, as indicated.
Vitamin B_{12}, vitamin K, and folic acid are given intramuscularly or added for intravenous administration, as indicated.
Trace elements such as zinc, copper, manganese, cobalt, and iodine are added only after total intravenous therapy exceeds one month. Alternatively, 1 unit of plasma twice a week will provide required amounts of trace elements.

hyperalimentation of adults. Solutions intended for use in children requiring long-term nutrition exclusively by the IV route are prepared as for adults with only minor modifications.

Administration of the solution described above requires continuous infusion over the 24-hour day. The injection is made into a large-caliber vessel such as the superior vena cava, preferably by means of an indwelling catheter threaded carefully and with aseptic technique into the superior vena cava by way of the subclavian vein. For newborns or infants less than 10 pounds in weight the superior vena cava may be reached via the jugular vein. Initially only the normal amounts of fluid are given (2500 ml per day in adults; 125 ml per kilogram per day in infants). Then the volume infused is slowly increased over a period of several days as tolerated, with attention to avoiding overhydration. Measurement every other day of plasma electrolytes and of blood urea nitrogen and weekly of sugar should serve to monitor the safety of the infusion. Testing for urine sugar, collected at six-hour intervals during the infusion, is also recommended.

The rate of glucose utilization is between 0.5 gm per kilogram per hour in adults and 1.2 gm per kilogram per hour in infants, the average being 0.9 gm per kilogram per hour in an adult. These are the rates for normal individuals, but in seriously ill patients infusion rates may need to be lower; thus periodic adjustment in rate of administration of the nutrient solution may be required.

Giving glucose intravenously at a rate that permits less than 2 percent excretion of glucose in the urine avoids the danger of osmotic diuresis, with resulting dehydration and electrolyte imbalance. The normal pancreas will increase its output of insulin in response to the continuing infusion of glucose. If a diabetic patient is being treated, appropriate doses of insulin may be given subcutaneously every six hours or the total dose may be added to the intravenous fluid. Indeed, 5 to 25 units of crystalline insulin per 1000 Calories may be added routinely to the nutrient solution to improve utilization of glucose and promote nitrogen retention in elderly patients evidencing intolerance to glucose, or in patients with severe nutritional depletion.

Potassium in larger amounts than are used for maintenance is usually required in patients on hyperalimentation. A minimum dose would be 40 mEq of KCl per liter of infusate; more is required if there are substantial gastrointestinal fluid losses or extensive burns, with careful attention to the prevention of hyperkalemia. Although 50 mEq of sodium per 1000 Calories is a satisfactory intake in these patients, when the clinical state predisposes to retention of sodium, reduction of intake or even total elimination of sodium may be necessary at times.

Tubal Nutrition

Feeding by nasogastric tube may occasionally be called for to prevent serious malnutrition—for example, in severe anoxia, coma, obstructive lesions of the esophagus, and fractures of the jaw, and after severe burns. When liquid formulas are used, very small polyethylene nasogastric tubes (e.g., K-30) which may be left in place for many days are suitable. They may even be used for supplemental feedings in patients who can ingest some of their meals in the usual manner (such as burned patients who are unable to eat adequate quantities of protein).

In preparing formulas for tube feeding, one should probably avoid simple sugars, such as dextrose, and too much fat, such as cream, since both tend to cause diarrhea in tube-fed patients. The preferred source of carbohydrate is a dextrinized starch, such as Dexin or Dextri-Maltose. A simple formula for feeding by gastric tube is as follows:

Homogenized milk	2200 ml
Half-and-half (cream and milk)	600 ml
Eggs	6
Dextri-Maltose	7 tbsp

(In a total volume of 3000 ml this mixture contains 120 gm protein and 3000 calories.)

Homogenized milk alone is often the simplest substance to use at the beginning of a tube feeding regimen. It contains 3.5 gm of protein and about 70 Calories per 100 ml. During the first few days after an operation, the initial rate of feeding should not exceed 50 ml per hour. Thereafter the rate may be increased gradually in accordance with the patient's tolerance until a maximum of 150 to 200 ml every two hours is reached, usually about one week later. If at this time the patient is tolerating the feedings well, the homogenized milk may be fortified with 50 gm of a powdered protein hydrolysate and 30 gm of Dextri-Maltose or Dexin. If it is well tolerated, the carbohydrate may be gradually increased over a three-day period to 60 gm per liter. This final formula contributes 160 gm of protein and about 2500 Calories in 2400 ml. Vitamins may be added to the formula as a concentrated solution similar in composition to that already suggested for a therapeutic regimen.

The formulas and rates of administration described above may also be used for jejunostomy feedings.

A more concentrated tube feeding mixture is possible with the aid of a pump to maintain the flow of the mixture. A sample formula utilizing commercially available pureed infant foods is as follows:

	Protein (gm)	Calories
3½ oz strained beef	14.6	103
4½ oz beets	1.5	51
3 raw eggs	18.0	225
Homogenized milk (640 ml)	23.3	466
Totals	57.4	845

(Other meats and vegetables can be used to vary the formula.)

Precautions in Tube Feedings

1. If given rapidly by gravity drop or by injection into the gastric tube, the formula should first be warmed to body temperature.

2. Do not give over 200 ml at a time.

3. Use special care to prevent aspiration in unconscious patients.

4. Supply sufficient water in addition to the formula to permit excretion of nitrogenous end products. This is a particularly important point if the formula is high in protein.

5. When stopping or starting a feeding, or whenever the question of gastric retention arises, aspirate the gastric tube and wash it out with water.

6. Avoid constipation and fecal impaction in debilitated patients, if necessary by introducing 30 ml of milk of magnesia into the tube.

The Normal Diet

Parenteral and tube feedings should be discontinued as soon as possible in favor of a full normal diet taken by mouth. Foods should be palatable and attractively prepared as a stimulus to appetite. The physician should not overlook his responsibilities in this matter since a properly compounded nutritional prescription can be just as important to his patient's welfare as the drugs he may order.

The daily diet for the convalescent adult patient should contain 3000 to 5000 Calories and 100 to 150 gm of protein. It is not sufficient merely to place these nutrients on a tray within the patient's reach; one must make certain that the entire nutritional prescription is actually consumed.

It is often difficult for surgical patients to eat large amounts of high-protein foods such as muscle meats. Intermittent feedings may have to be given but must be carefully spaced so as not to spoil the patient's appetite for regular meals. Fruit juices and broths are of little value as supplementary nutrients because they contribute practically nothing toward remedying protein and caloric deficits, the major dietary faults in need of correction; in fact, these liquid supplements may actually dull the appetite and thus indirectly impair nutrition.

A simple supplementary drink may be prepared by stirring 50 gm of skimmed milk powder into 200 ml of water. This supplies 17 gm of protein and 26 gm of carbohydrate, more than is available in 1 pint of milk but in only half the volume. Six glasses will supply over 100 gm of protein of excellent nutritional quality. Other valuable protein supplements are ice cream, cottage cheese, and eggs.

REFERENCES

1. Dudrick, S. J., Wilmore, D. W., Steiger, E., Vars, H. M., and Rhoads, J. E. The

Use of Carbohydrates and Proteolysates for Long-Term Parenteral Feeding. In Fox, C. L., Jr., and Nahas, G. G. (Eds.), *Body Fluid Replacement in the Surgical Patient.* New York: Grune & Stratton, 1970. P. 301.

2. Dudrick, S. J., Wilmore, D. W., Vars, H. M., and Rhoads, J. E.   Long-term total parenteral nutrition with growth development, and positive nitrogen balance. *Surgery* 64:132, 1968.

3. Food and Nutrition Board, National Research Council. *Recommended Dietary Allowances* (8th rev. ed.). Washington, D.C.: National Academy of Sciences, 1974.

4. Kinney, J. M., Long, C. L., and Duke, J. H., Jr.   Energy Demands in the Surgical Patient. In Fox, C. L., Jr., and Nahas, G. G. (Eds.), *Body Fluid Replacement in the Surgical Patient.* New York: Grune & Stratton, 1970. P. 296.

5. Morgan, A., Filler, R. M., and Moore, F. D.   Surgical nutrition. *Med. Clin. North Am.* 54:1367, 1970.

6. Pollack, H., and Halpern, S. L.   *Therapeutic Nutrition.* Publication No. 234. Food and Nutrition Board, National Research Council. Washington, D.C.: National Academy of Sciences, 1952.

7. Stephens, R. V., and Randall, H. T.   Use of a concentrated, balanced, liquid elemental diet for nutritional management of catabolic states. *Ann. Surg.* 170:642, 1969.

8. Studley, H. O.   Percent of weight loss: A basic indicator of surgical risk. *J.A.M.A.* 106:458, 1936.

5

Blood and Blood Components
John M. Bowman

In many situations associated with trauma and with reconstructive surgery, administration of blood or a specific blood component is essential and is lifesaving. However, transfusion carries certain risks and should never be undertaken lightly. The hazards are relatively infrequent but when they arise they may be serious. This chapter begins with an outline of transfusion hazards and proceeds to a brief consideration of blood and its components, with indications for their use. No attempt will be made to describe their application in specific situations (burn shock, etc.), since that is discussed in detail elsewhere.

TRANSFUSION HAZARDS

The Hemolytic Transfusion Reaction

A rare but potentially lethal hazard, the hemolytic transfusion reaction, arises following the transfusion of blood or red cells containing an antigen against which the recipient has an antibody. Fatal transfusion reactions are nearly always caused by transfusions of ABO incompatible blood (group A blood to an O or B patient, group B blood to an O or A patient, etc.). Anti-A and anti-B are so-called naturally occurring isohemagglutinins. Both are invariably present in group O individuals; anti-B alone in group A and anti-A alone in group B people.

Anti-A and anti-B bind complement. When ABO incompatible blood is transfused, the binding of complement by the antibody to the antigen in the red cell membrane causes prompt and severe intravascular hemolysis. Hemoglobin is released into the plasma.

Other blood group system antibodies such as those in the Rh system are rarely if ever "naturally occurring." They develop only in people negative for the antigen following exposure to the antigen. The most familiar example is Rh immunization of an Rh-negative person after either an Rh-positive transfusion or an Rh-positive pregnancy. Rh antibody does not bind complement. Hemolysis in this situation is for the most part extravascular. Antibody-coated red cells are sequestered in the spleen and destroyed by phagocytosis. Although free hemoglobin appears in the plasma following extravascular hemolysis, levels are not as high as those following intravascular hemolysis.

Symptoms resulting from a transfusion of ABO incompatible blood appear within minutes of commencement of the transfusion. Initially, the patient, if conscious, complains of pain or burning along the vein into which the blood is being transfused. His face becomes flushed. He frequently speaks of a throbbing headache and then develops lumbar pain and a severe constricting pain in the chest. These symptoms are not seen in patients suffering from extravascular hemolysis although fever may develop.

Signs accompanying severe intravascular hemolysis are hypotension, shock, mental confusion, hemoglobinemia, hemoglobinuria, jaundice, abnormal bleeding, oliguria, and, in the most severe cases, anuria. The signs and symptoms described are almost all masked by general anesthesia or narcotics such as morphine. In the anesthetized or narcotized patient the only visible signs which may alert one to the possibility of a hemolytic transfusion reaction are persistent hypotension, despite apparently adequate blood replacement, and abnormal bleeding.

Some of the signs and symptoms accompanying a hemolytic transfusion reaction may be the effects of the release of vasoactive substances such as histamine. However, a major factor is the development of disseminated intravascular coagulation (DIC) brought about by the release of thromboplastic substances following intravascular hemolysis. DIC is characterized by thrombocytopenia, falling factor V, VIII, and IX levels, low levels of fibrinogen, presence of fibrin split products in the circulation, and presence of bizarre distorted and fragmented red cells. Again these signs, so frequent after intravascular hemolysis, are almost never seen following non-complement-medicated extravascular hemolysis. On rare occasions, if the non-complement-fixing antibody is present in exceedingly high titer (e.g., a severely Rh-isoimmunized pregnant woman), a por-

tion of the hemolysis induced may be intravascular and produce the signs and symptoms just described.

Animal experiments have shown that many of the signs and symptoms produced by intravascular hemolysis may be prevented by prior heparinization, direct evidence that DIC is a major factor in the dangerous effects of hemolytic transfusion reactions.

The major lethal hazard is renal failure. Renal failure is not an invariable result of intravascular hemolysis. It occurs only when hemoglobinemia is present. The three factors contributing to renal damage leading to anuria are direct renal toxicity of hemoglobin, interference with renal blood flow due to hypotension, and blocking of renal blood vessels by fibrin.

Management of Suspected Incompatible Blood Transfusion

PREVENTION. Careful attention to the standard precautions essential when ordering and transfusing blood is the most important factor in preventing the hemolytic transfusion reaction. Modern crossmatch facilities have stringent safeguards and back-checking techniques which make laboratory crossmatch mistakes extremely rare. A hemolytic transfusion reaction misadventure is almost always a patient misidentification error at the hospital ward, operating room, or emergency room level. Blood from the wrong patient is placed in the crossmatch blood specimen tube. In other words, correctly matched blood is given to the wrong patient. Such "human factor" mistakes can be prevented only by meticulous care in the ordering of blood, proper identification of the patient by name and hospital number when the crossmatch sample is being drawn, and again proper identification of the patient prior to administration of crossmatched blood.

Since the severity of the transfusion reaction and the likelihood of renal failure are directly related to the amount of incompatible blood transfused, an important precaution is to observe the patient for five minutes after commencement of the transfusion. If untoward symptoms develop (burning along the vein, etc.), immediate discontinuation of the transfusion will make the development of a severe hemolytic reaction much less likely. Unfortunately such observation is of no value in the anesthetized or narcotized patient.

TREATMENT. Once an acute hemolytic transfusion reaction is suspected, preservation and maintenance of renal function is all-important. There is experimental evidence that both alkalinization of the urine and inducing diuresis, which dilutes the toxic products of hemolysis (primarily hemoglobin), will reduce the risk of renal damage. A rapid infusion of 100 ml of 20% mannitol followed by 45 mEq of sodium bicarbonate added to 200 ml of 5% dextrose should be given. Fluids sufficient to keep urine flowing at a rate of 1 to 3 ml per minute are administered intravenously. A diuretic (furosemide, 80 to 120 mg for an adult) should be given with the parenteral fluids. If urine flow drops below 50 ml per hour, the mannitol should be repeated in two hours. If satisfactory urine flow cannot be maintained, renal damage (tubular necrosis) must be presumed to have occurred. Immediate treatment of a suspected hemolytic reaction is essential since a delay of an hour or two may allow irreversible renal damage to develop.

The management of the renal damage oliguria-anuria phase of the hemolytic transfusion reaction is beyond the scope of this chapter, as is the management of disseminated intravascular coagulation. Expert renal and hematological consultants with fully developed coagulation laboratory and renal dialysis facilities must be available to help in such situations. Fluid restriction is essential, since at this stage pulmonary and cerebral edema are ever present hazards. In one study of patients with renal damage following hemolytic transfusion reactions death was uncommon when fluid intake was kept below 2000 ml per day whereas 75 percent of those given more than 3500 ml daily died.

Infections Transmitted by Blood

Serum Hepatitis

At present the major problem associated with blood transfusion is the risk of serum hepatitis (hepatitis B). Serum hepatitis is common in addicts, who frequently may donate blood to commercial blood banks in order to receive money to support their habit. The incidence of post-transfusion hepatitis is much higher in patients transfused with blood obtained from commercial banks than in patients given blood from voluntary blood banks. The voluntary donor has an altruistic, not a financial, reason for donating blood.

With the discovery of the Australia antigen (hepatitis-associated antigen, hepatitis B antigen (HB_sAg) by Blumberg and the demonstration that administration of HB_sAg-positive blood carried a very high risk of serum hepatitis, a valuable tool for identifying serum hepatitis virus–containing donations became available. Electron microscopy reveals that the antigen consists of three particles: a 20 nm diameter spherical particle (most common), a 20 nm diameter tubular form, and a rarer, more complex, 40 nm sphere (the Dane particle). The 20 nm forms are not virus but probably represent virus coat. The central core of the Dane particle may be the virus itself.

HB_sAg testing of all blood and blood component donations prior to administration is now compulsory in North America and many other parts of the world. Using radioimmunoassay (RIA) techniques one can determine that about 1 percent of units donated to commercial blood banks are HB_sAg positive. When these units are excluded, about 1 unit out of 100 transfused will be contaminated with the virus. If a traumatized or burned patient receives 10 units of blood or plasma, he runs a

10 percent risk of exposure to hepatitis B virus. HB_s Ag-positive units detected by RIA make up 0.07 to 0.15 percent of voluntary donations (i.e., those to Red Cross and other voluntary blood banks). Use of blood provided by these agencies is 7 to 15 times less likely to cause serum hepatitis.

Although serum hepatitis is often quite mild (two-thirds of cases are asymptomatic), it may be very severe in the debilitated or the elderly. The mortality in symptomatic patients varies from 5 to 10 percent. A certain number of patients with asymptomatic serum hepatitis will have long-continued low-grade liver damage culminating in cirrhosis of the liver. The physician ordering whole blood, packed red cells, plasma, or components such as platelets, factor VIII, factor IX, and fibrinogen, all of which may contain the virus, must balance the risk of serum hepatitis against the expected benefits of the blood or blood components which will accrue to his patient.

Cytomegalovirus Infection

Certain completely healthy donors may carry cytomegalovirus in their blood. Following multiple blood transfusions an infectious mononucleosis–like syndrome has been described, particularly in, but not confined to, open heart surgery patients. This syndrome has been shown to be due to cytomegalovirus. Although relatively benign, it can be distinctly unpleasant.

Malaria and Syphilis

Both malaria and syphilis can be transmitted by contaminated blood. In a properly functioning blood bank with adequate medical and laboratory screening of donors, transmission of these two infections in donor blood should not occur.

Isoimmunization

Prior to the discovery of the Rh blood group system in 1940, transfusion of ABO compatible blood was associated with a 10 percent Rh immunization rate with its legacy

of subsequent transfusion reactions and erythroblastosis fetalis. Since the institution of the use of Rh(D) compatible blood for transfusions, Rh immunization should never occur as a result of blood transfusion.

One must not forget that transfused blood is compatible with the recipient's blood only insofar as the ABO system and one antigen (D) of the Rh blood group system are concerned. It is incompatible for many other blood group antigens. Although most are poor antigens, rarely producing specific antibodies, and the antibodies, once developed, are usually not strong, this is not an invariable rule. Kell and Kp^a in the Kell system and c in the Rh system are quite antigenic, and the antibody, once developed, is capable of causing a severe transfusion reaction or fatal erythroblastosis fetalis.

About 1 percent of transfused patients will develop "atypical" antibodies (antibodies other than anti-D of the Rh system). Although it is frequently easy to find compatible blood for such patients, in some cases it may be extremely difficult. Transfusions of emergency group O unmatched blood to patients with atypical antibodies may be associated with a hemolytic transfusion reaction.

The physician should weigh the risk of "atypical" isoimmunization against the expected benefits of the proposed transfusion. This precaution is particularly important in the young girl or the woman in her childbearing years since, as already noted, "atypical" isoimmunization can cause erythroblastosis fetalis.

Pyrogenic Transfusion Reactions

The three transfusion hazards described, although serious, are relatively rare. The fourth, development of fever during or following blood transfusion, is rather common; of 54,877 patients given 126,426 transfusions, 2.34 percent developed chills and fever. Pyrogenic transfusion reactions are usually caused by white cell agglutinins produced as a result of previous blood or blood component transfusions. Patients transfused in the past are therefore more likely to have a pyrogenic transfusion reaction. The antibodies are HLA antibodies. At the time of transfusion, if the leukocytes contain an HLA antigen to which the patient has produced an antibody, the antibody destroys the donor leukocytes, with release of pyrogens.

Although pyrogenic reactions are not usually serious, they may be exceedingly unpleasant. If powerful leukoagglutinins are present, severe chills, cyanosis, hypotension, and transient leukopenia may occur.

Allergic Transfusion Reactions

Almost as common as the pyrogenic reaction is the allergic transfusion reaction, reported in 2.1 percent of 54,877 patients transfused with 126,426 units of blood. Most allergic reactions are mild, consisting of urticaria or erythema with itching, but occasionally a severe anaphylactic reaction may occur, with bronchospasm, laryngeal edema, hypotension, and collapse.

Although some of these reactions may be due to specific anti-Gm antibodies, it is now quite certain that the majority if not all are related to the immune globulin IgA. Rare individuals, otherwise healthy, have no circulating IgA. They may, without known exposure to blood or blood products, produce "class-specific" anti-IgA. Following injection of as little as 10 ml they may develop an allergic reaction in the form of acute anaphylaxis.

More commonly individuals with one type of IgA produce "limited specificity" antibodies to another subgroup of IgA. Usually reaction following infusion of blood or a blood component containing the offending subgroup of IgA is mild, consisting of urticaria or erythema. However, sometimes "limited specificity" anti-IgA reactions are anaphylactic in nature.

Commercial immunoglobulins, although predominantly IgG, all have traces of IgA. On rare occasions intramuscular injections of immunoglobulins have produced severe

reactions in patients with circulating anti-IgA.

Since it is impossible to remove IgA from whole blood or plasma components, individuals with severe allergic transfusion reactions should be given only washed red cells. If a colloid blood volume expander is required, 5% albumin or dextran should be used. If it is absolutely necessary to give whole blood or plasma to such a patient, pretreatment with oral prednisone for 24 hours prior to administration is helpful in reducing the likelihood of an anaphylactic reaction. Less severe allergic reactions may be ameliorated by administration of an antihistamine such as diphenhydramine or promethazine before the transfusion.

Reaginic Antibodies

Care should be taken in transfusing the highly allergic individual since occasionally allergens in the donor's plasma may produce an acute allergic reaction. Conversely, and rarely, a patient transfused with blood or plasma from a very allergic individual, by passive transfer of the donor's reagins, will become temporarily allergic to the same allergens as the donor. For this reason extremely allergic people should not be accepted as blood donors. A well-recognized related problem is that of the patient receiving penicillin who develops an acute penicillin reaction following administration of blood from a donor allergic to penicillin.

Acute anaphylaxis as a result of blood transfusion requires prompt treatment. Parenteral epinephrine, in divided doses, intravenous corticosteroids, and parenteral antihistamines may all be helpful. In the most severe cases, with hypotension, vasopressor agents may also be required.

Transfusion Overload

Transfusion of blood or plasma in too large a volume or too rapidly may throw the patient into irreversible heart failure. This hazard is a particular problem in the very elderly or in the patient with severe nonhemorrhagic anemia. The writer has observed one such tragedy in a 9-year-old with congenital spherocytosis and a hemoglobin of 4 gm per 100 ml. In preparation for splenectomy the injudicious transfusion of too large a volume of blood too rapidly led to fatal irreversible heart failure. In this situation a partial exchange transfusion without increasing blood volume is a much safer method of raising hemoglobin levels.

In the patient in hemorrhagic or burn shock who requires large volumes of blood or colloids, careful monitoring of central venous pressure is helpful in determining the adequacy of blood or plasma replacement and avoiding the risk of overtransfusion, with overload, heart failure, and pulmonary edema.

Cold Blood

Rapid infusion of large volumes of refrigerated blood (temperature 4°C) has been reported to cause cardiac arrest. The risk of such an occurrence develops only if volumes infused are greater than 50 ml per minute. Paradoxically, the writer has noted no adverse effects when newborn infants are exchange-transfused with blood that has been removed from 4°C for only a few minutes; 20 ml aliquots were infused and removed at 30 to 45 second intervals up to a total blood volume of 500 ml in 35 to 50 minutes. However, the temperature of the donor blood at the time of infusion into these infants' circulations was in the neighborhood of 15°C, and the babies were being warmed by radiant heat.

If blood warming is required prior to transfusion, the water bath or heating device used must not allow overheating of the blood since temperatures higher than 47° to 50°C will produce acute hemolysis.

Citrate and Potassium Toxicity

The dating period for citrated blood is 21 days if properly stored at 4°C. However, with storage, potassium leaks out of the red cells into the plasma. After 10 days' storage,

plasma potassium levels average 15 mEq per liter, and by the end of the 21-day storage period levels average 30 mEq per liter. Moderate volumes of such blood given to a patient with reasonable kidney function will not produce a dangerous rise in serum potassium. But large volumes, particularly when given to patients with renal problems of a chronic or acute nature, may be associated with dangerously high serum potassium levels.

It must also be remembered that stored blood is citrated with no ionized calcium and that administration of large volumes of blood will be associated with a drop in ionized calcium. Calcium and potassium ion have reciprocal effects on myocardial irritability. Thus high circulating serum potassium and low ionized calcium levels make the hazard of ventricular fibrillation a real one.

When large volumes of blood are required, most of the units should be reasonably fresh (not more than three or four days old). If more than 2 units (1 liter) are given, 10 ml of 10% calcium gluconate should be infused slowly with each subsequent 1000 ml of blood.

Air Embolism

Air embolism is a major hazard if blood drawn into glass bottles is infused under pressure. The introduction of plastic donor unit equipment has completely eradicated this hazard. If blood drawn into glass units has to be infused under pressure, the unit must be observed continuously and the pressure released before the unit has emptied completely.

Blood Debris

Aggregates of leukocytes, platelets, and fibrin up to 200 μm in diameter form in blood during storage. In citrated blood, aggregates start forming by 24 hours and become marked by 8 to 10 days. In blood drawn in heparin, aggregates appear within two hours and are quite marked at the end of eight hours. These aggregates are not removed by passage through the standard 200-μm nylon mesh filter which is part of each blood administration set.

Some patients, following transfusions of large volumes of blood, become hypoxic. An important cause of the hypoxic state appears to be the blocking of pulmonary capillaries by the 200 μm aggregates present in stored blood. Although this hypoxic syndrome, called the *postperfusion lung syndrome*, is most often seen in patients undergoing cardiac bypass surgery, it is a well-established entity in post-trauma shocked patients. Its incidence and severity are related to the volume and length of storage of the blood transfused.

The risk of the postperfusion lung syndrome in patients requiring large volumes of blood may be reduced by using citrated blood which is as fresh as possible. When large volumes of blood stored for more than three or four days must be administered, it is wise to transfuse the blood through microfilters which are commercially available (Swank [Extra Corporeal Med. Spec., Inc., King of Prussia, Pa.] microemboli filter, Fenwal [Fenwal Laboratories, Deerfield, Ill.] microaggregate filter).

If for any reason large volumes of heparinized blood must be administered, the blood should be passed through a microfilter if it is more than five or six hours old.

Plasticizers

In order to render polyvinylchloride (PVC), the plastic used in making blood and blood component units, pliable, plasticizers must be added to it. They make up as much as 40 percent of the weight of each bag. The chief plasticizer in PVC bags is diethylhexylphthalate (DEHP). DEHP has been shown to appear in the lipid fraction of stored whole blood or plasma within 24 hours of storage. With continued storage it increases in amount.

Although oral ingestion of DEHP is not associated with adverse effects, its safety in stored blood remains to be determined. Experimentally, plasticizers in PVC tubing will arrest the beat of the isolated rat heart. It is suspected, but not yet proved, that postexchange transfusion necrotizing enterocolitis of the newborn may be due to the effect of DEHP on mesenteric vasculature.

There is no positive evidence that plasticizers in stored blood represent a major hazard, but they are blood contaminants which ideally should not be administered. Again, since plasticizers increase with storage, large-volume transfusions should consist of as fresh blood as possible.

Since plasticizers are concentrated in the lipid moiety of plasma, transfusion of packed red cells exposes the patient to much smaller amounts. Freezing plasma and storing it as such prevents leaching of DEHP from the plastic bag into the plasma.

Efforts are being made to find a more suitable plastic for blood and blood component storage. At present all units available commercially are made up of PVC plastic.

WHOLE BLOOD

The use of whole blood is unconditionally indicated only in the patient who is bleeding either from trauma or at surgery and when so much blood is lost that hypovolemic shock is likely. Blood pressure and pulse rate are helpful in assessing the need for transfusion and the degree of urgency in meeting this need. The loss of as much as 430 ml of blood within three or four minutes (the volume and time of a blood donation) usually causes little or no change in blood pressure or pulse rate. In many normal subjects withdrawal of as much as 1250 to 1300 ml in a 15- to 20-minute period (the amount of blood temporarily withdrawn at a double plasmapheresis) is associated with little or no drop in blood pressure and no specific symptoms provided the individual remains supine. If he sits up, blood pressure may then fall and syncope will follow. Loss of 1500 to 2000 ml (35 to 40 percent of the total blood volume) usually results in diminished cardiac output, tachycardia, pallor, syncope, and air hunger.

When 1000 ml of blood is lost, it takes 36 hours for the blood volume to be restored, and the replacement is initially entirely made up of plasma. Since replacement is slow, measurement of hemoglobin or hematocrit during or shortly after blood loss is not an accurate indication of the amount of blood lost, because the patient will still be hypovolemic. Irreversible hemorrhagic shock is entirely related to drop in blood volume. Assessment of blood loss and its adequate replacement is essential in the management of accidental or surgical trauma (see Chapter 10).

An emergency crossmatch takes about 45 minutes, and this time interval must be considered when blood is required for management of a traumatized individual. If unmatched group O emergency blood is administered, it must be remembered that this "universal donor" blood does contain anti-A and anti-B. If more than 3 or 4 units have been given, further crossmatched blood administered during the next few days should also be group O no matter what the blood group of the patient. He will now have sufficient anti-A and anti-B in his circulation so that administration of group A or B blood might be associated with a hemolytic transfusion reaction.

It should also be remembered (see Transfusion Hazards, above) that stored blood accumulates potassium and blood debris (aggregates). Further, as blood is stored, the level of red cell diphosphoglycerate (DPG), essential in allowing the release of oxygen from hemoglobin in the tissues, drops. Restoration of DPG levels in transfused stored blood takes many hours. If large volumes of blood have to be transfused, at least 50 percent of the blood should be reasonably fresh (not more than three or four days old). If large volumes of citrated blood are being administered, calcium replacement (see Citrate and Potassium Toxicity, above) is essential. Alternatively, when large volumes are to be given, citrated blood can be heparinized and recalcified just prior to transfusion.

Autologous Blood

In elective situations when blood is required for a patient who has an atypical antibody to a high-frequency blood group or who is a candidate for organ transplant, it should be understood that the safest blood for such an individual is his own blood. Provided he meets blood donor requirements, he may have blood donations taken and stored frozen for his own use at a future date.

In the patient with a high-frequency antibody or the one slated to receive an allograft, 4 units of his own blood 7 to 14 days old may be obtained by the so-called leapfrog technique. On day zero, unit A is withdrawn. On day seven, units B and C are withdrawn and unit A is given. On day 14, units D and E are removed and unit B is given. On day 21, F and G are removed and unit C is given. On day 28, at the time of operation, units D, E, F, and G are available.

This technique can be employed only if the patient's health and hemoglobin levels are adequate. Otherwise sedimented leukofiltered red cells (see Pyrogenic Transfusion Reactions, above) must be used.

PACKED RED CELLS

The sole indication for the use of whole blood is in the treatment of blood loss, either traumatic or surgical, severe enough to signal the risk of hemorrhagic shock. Barring this, reduced red cell mass in the presence of normal blood volume may be treated in many cases without transfusion, but by the use of iron, folic acid, etc. In nonhemorrhagic anemia with bone marrow unresponsiveness (following burns, for example) replacement of red cell mass is much more safely carried out by the administration of packed red cells. Improvement of hemoglobin levels may be attained with less increase in blood volume and therefore less risk of transfusion overload.

With modern transfusion equipment packed red cell units have the same dating as whole blood. Use of packed red cells also allows the retrieval of plasma from the donor unit. If whole blood is used exclusively, the blood bank will not have available to it fresh plasma, which either unchanged or in the form of one of its several components is an essential resource (see Plasma and Plasma Substitutes, and Bleeding Problems, below).

Since packed red cell transfusions are usually given for chronic anemia with a normal (or expanded) blood volume, rates of administration and volumes given should be monitored carefully. If the hemoglobin of the patient is between 5 and 8 gm per 100 ml, transfusion of 1 unit of 250 ml of packed red cells in one to two hours is safe. If the hemoglobin is below 5 gm per 100 ml, incipient heart failure is likely. Transfusion rates should not exceed 1 ml per kilogram per hour (70 ml per hour for a 70 kg man). With severe degrees of anemia, total volume at one transfusion should not exceed 200 ml. Modified exchange transfusion, raising the hemoglobin level without increasing total blood volume, is much safer. If available, monitoring of central venous pressure and regulating of the volume of blood transfused according to the venous pressure are valuable safeguards.

For elective surgical procedures, provision of half the blood required as packed red cells (up to 2 units) is perfectly safe and again conserves vital plasma for other uses. The units of red cells may be infused with normal saline solution.

PLASMA AND PLASMA SUBSTITUTES

Plasma removed from fresh blood and immediately frozen is a valuable resource. It can be administered unmodified after simple thawing or may be processed into plasma protein solution, albumin, and immune globulin, all of which are of value in the management of certain problems connected with reconstructive surgery, particularly in patients with nonhemorrhagic shock. Plasma extracted from outdated blood may also be processed

into albumin and immune globulin. Because of potassium levels and the possibility of bacterial contamination this type of plasma should not be administered unmodified. Pooled lyophilized plasma should not be used on account of the high risk of serum hepatitis.

Availability of sufficient plasma and plasma components to meet all patient requirements is possible only if a big proportion (35 to 75 percent) of all blood donations are used partially for this purpose. Therefore, in order to provide such large amounts of plasma, 35 to 75 percent of all blood transfusions must be in the form of packed red cells. If the physician or surgeon expects to have plasma and plasma components available to him, he must make certain that packed red cell transfusions replace whole blood transfusions wherever compatible with his patient's welfare.

Plasmapheresis of selected donors at weekly intervals is a highly effective means of producing large volumes of plasma. However, the method is relatively costly and is primarily reserved for the obtaining of specific plasma (Rh plasma, tetanus antitoxin plasma, etc.). Efficiently operated voluntary blood banks with adequate numbers of blood donors and proper widespread use of packed red cell transfusions should have a reasonable supply of fresh frozen plasma for use or for conversion to plasma components.

Fresh frozen plasma is the ideal colloid blood volume expander. As will be outlined in the section on bleeding problems, although it is still effective in the management of coagulation problems, because of the quantities required for this purpose it has been for the most part supplanted by concentrates (cryoprecipitate, lyophilized factors II, VII, IX, and X, etc.). Administration of fresh frozen plasma carries with it the risk of transmission of serum hepatitis. If plasma from a voluntary low-HB_sAg-incidence blood bank is available, the risk per unit is about 0.1 percent. If plasma from a commercial blood bank must be used, the 1.0 percent risk per unit may be too high when one considers that many units of plasma may be required for the treatment of nonhemorrhagic shock.

Two plasma components are available either commercially or through Red Cross blood transfusion services. Serum albumin, distributed in either 25% or 5% concentrations, is a very effective colloid blood volume expander. Plasma protein solution (trade name Plasmanate or Plasmaplex) is a 5% solution of plasma proteins, primarily albumin and alpha and beta globulins, the majority of the gamma globulins having been removed. Plasma protein solution is also an effective blood volume expander. Either 5% albumin or plasma protein solution may be used in the same volume as fresh plasma for the treatment of nonhemorrhagic shock. Both albumin and plasma protein are treated by heating to 60°C for 10 hours. This treatment destroys serum hepatitis virus—the major advantage of these two materials compared to fresh plasma. Both are considerably more expensive than fresh frozen plasma if fresh plasma is supplied by voluntary blood banks, and of course neither albumin nor plasma protein solution has any active coagulation factors or appreciable amounts of the gamma globulins. There is debatable evidence that the presence of the immune globulins in fresh plasma may confer some protection against infection in the burn patient treated with fresh plasma rather than with albumin or plasma protein solution. There is now substantial evidence that following major burns immunoglobulin levels, particularly IgG, drop and that phagocytic activity and ability to produce a primary immune response are depressed.

Dextrans

Even with the best efforts of the regional blood banks and the supply of plasma components, these natural colloid blood volume expanders may not be adequate to meet requirements, especially during disasters such as major fires and accidents. Much effort has been directed toward finding satisfactory plasma substitutes. The most suitable ones

are the dextrans. These are long chains of glucose units with variable degrees of branching. The dextrans ideally should have a narrow range of molecular weight between 70,000 and 100,000.

If large numbers of dextran molecules are of less than 70,000 molecular weight, they are rapidly excreted and their osmotic effectiveness in maintaining plasma volume is rapidly lost. Conversely, if many dextran molecules are of more than 100,000 molecular weight, red cell rouleaux formation and potential sludging of red cells in vivo become a problem. The three available dextran preparations are Rheomacrodex (mean m.w. 40,000), dextran 70 or Macrodex (mean m.w. 70,000) (Pharmacia, Uppsala, Sweden), and dextran 110 or Modified British Dextran (mean m.w. 110,000). Rheomacrodex produces little or no rouleaux formation and marked plasma volume expansion. However, because of rapid excretion its effect is gone within a few hours. Macrodex is intermediate. It produces little rouleaux and a somewhat longer plasma volume effect, which, however, disappears within 24 hours. Dextran 110 produces a volume expansion effect for a longer period than 24 hours but does induce rouleaux.

Dextran is a reasonably satisfactory plasma substitute for the treatment of nonhemorrhagic shock, and for immediate treatment of hemorrhagic shock while blood is being made available. Large volumes of dextran appear to be fairly safe. Nevertheless, the volume used should not exceed the patient's estimated plasma volume. Under ordinary circumstances dextran administration should be limited to 1 liter per day.

Rouleaux formation following dextran administration may make subsequent crossmatching for blood transfusion difficult. Therefore, the crossmatch sample should be obtained prior to commencement of dextran infusion. If a crossmatch sample must be drawn from a patient who is receiving dextran, the crossmatch laboratory should be notified to this effect.

Dextran rarely produces allergic reactions. However, large volumes of dextran (in excess of 1500 ml) interfere with platelet function; the higher the molecular weight of the dextran, the greater this effect. Prolongation of bleeding time persists from three to nine hours after administration of dextran. Risk of bleeding following dextran administration is low unless volumes administered exceed the patient's plasma volume (greater than 2500 ml).

Burn Shock

Burn shock is dealt with in detail in Chapter 10 and will be mentioned only briefly here. It must be emphasized that in severe burns plasma and fluid loss is rapid and extreme. Although there is evidence that burn shock can be treated successfully in its initial stages with noncolloid-containing solutions such as saline or Ringer's lactate, the volumes required to maintain a reasonably normal circulating blood volume are enormous. For example, if blood volume is being maintained by administration of electrolyte solutions alone, for every liter of plasma and fluid lost from the circulation 2.0 to 2.5 liters of fluid must be given. Massive edema follows. With severe burns hemolysis of red cells is always a factor. In an adult as much as 350 ml may be destroyed in the 48 hours after burning. The result is a 15 to 20 percent drop in hemoglobin level—for example, from 15 to 12 gm per 100 ml. This drop in hemoglobin is by itself not clinically significant provided blood volume is maintained. Therefore, although blood or red cell transfusions will be required in the later stages of management of the severely burned patient, they are not needed in the early management of burn shock.

BLEEDING PROBLEMS

The reconstructive surgeon will sometimes be called upon to treat patients with congenital or acquired coagulation defects that will complicate their surgical condition. Also, the primary disorder that he is to treat may be accompanied by loss of coagulation factors and a tendency to bleed. The help of a qualified hematologist should be enlisted when such problems arise. Blood components which are available for the treatment of bleeding problems are platelet concentrates and plasma coagulation factors.

Platelet Concentrates

The majority of the platelets in a unit of blood are found, following centrifugation, in the buffy coat. Blood used for platelet preparations must be fresh. After centrifugation the plasma and buffy coat are expressed into a satellite bag. If the platelets are not intended for immediate use, they may be stored in the plasma for about 48 hours. There is still controversy regarding the optimal method of storage. At present it appears that platelets are best kept at room temperature (22°C). After 48 hours' storage about 50 percent are still viable. Repeated gentle agitation of the platelet-rich plasma during storage is essential in order to prevent platelet aggregation and loss of viability. Prior to use the plasma is centrifuged and the supernatant removed, leaving a 5- to 10-ml button of platelet concentrate.

Platelets are very fragile, agglutinating and breaking down in vitro quickly. Whole blood, after 12 to 24 hours' storage at 4°C, contains few residual functional platelets. The technique of administering platelet concentrates is important in order to preserve as many of them as possible. The concentrates should be drawn into a plastic syringe through a large-bore needle (16-gauge); each empty unit should have 4 or 5 ml of isotonic saline solution added, and this should also be drawn into the syringe. They then should be given intravenously through a large needle or catheter. Gentle handling of platelets at all times is necessary if the patient is to reap any benefit from their administration.

Bleeding due to thrombocytopenia is not likely unless the platelet count drops below 30,000 to 40,000 per cubic millimeter. Indeed, in some conditions such as idiopathic thrombocytopenia and acute leukemia, bleeding may not occur until the platelet count drops well below 20,000 per cubic millimeter. Thrombocytopenia invariably accompanies severe hemorrhage requiring massive blood replacement. It is also commonly found in the badly burned patient.

Platelet estimations should be done at regular intervals on traumatized or burned patients. If the platelet count falls below 40,000 per cubic millimeter, platelets should be given. One unit of platelet concentrate will, on the average, increase the circulating platelet count of an adult by at least 5000 per cubic millimeter. Since a circulating platelet count of 30,000 per cubic millimeter is usually sufficient to stop bleeding, no more than 6 units of platelet concentrate need be given at one time. A single unit of platelet concentrate is adequate for infants up to 10 kg body weight, 2 units for children under 4 years old, and 3 to 4 units for children of school age. Although the half-life of the transfused platelet is said to be four days, in actual practice platelet counts usually drop back to preinfusion levels within two or three days unless spontaneous recovery from the thrombocytopenic state is occurring. For this reason repeated platelet transfusions may be necessary.

Since platelet concentrates always contain some donor red cells, it is wise to transfuse platelets from a donor who is ABO and Rh compatible with the recipient. This is a particularly important precaution if the patient is a girl or woman in the childbearing years, since very small amounts of red cells (0.1 ml) are capable of producing Rh isoimmunization.

Following repeated platelet transfusions many patients develop potent platelet isoantibodies. Platelet concentrates from unselected donors are rapidly destroyed. In these cases platelets from siblings or parents are less likely to contain the offending platelet antigen to which the patient has become isoimmunized. Platelet typing, although possible, is not widely available.

Plasma Coagulation Factors

Factors VIII and IX

Congenital plasma coagulation defects, if present, compound the problems of the surgeon. Hemophilia A and hemophilia B (Christmas disease), found only in males because of their X chromosome pattern of inheritance, are the principal disorders. Minor trauma in these individuals may be associated with severe bleeding. In the past major surgery could not be carried out on hemophiliacs. Hemophilia A is due to a lack of functional factor VIII, and hemophilia B is caused by lack of factor IX. Both factors are present in fresh plasma. Factor IX is quite stable but factor VIII is not, disappearing rapidly from plasma unless it is stored at temperatures below $-30°C$.

In the past it was exceedingly difficult to raise levels of these coagulation factors to hemostatic levels because of the huge volumes of plasma required. Now an easily prepared factor VIII concentrate has completely revolutionized the management of hemophilia A. When fresh plasma is frozen immediately and then thawed slowly at $4°C$, much of the functional factor VIII remains as a precipitate (cryoprecipitate). The thawed plasma is expressed, and the cryoprecipitate remaining in a volume of 5 to 10 ml represents about 50 percent of the factor VIII in the unit of blood. In order to raise factor VIII levels to 15 to 30 percent of normal (a hemostatic level except following major surgery), 6 to 12 units of cryoprecipitate daily will be required. In the presence of dangerous bleeding and particularly if major surgery is needed, doses of 10 to 20 units of cryoprecipitate every 12 hours may be necessary for 8 to 10 days in order to keep the factor VIII level always above 30 percent and to arrest or prevent hemorrhage. In such circumstances it is not unusual for a hemophiliac to require several hundred units of cryoprecipitate. Provision of adequate cryoprecipitate strains the resources of every blood bank; 25 to 35 percent of all blood donations must be used for cryoprecipitate production in order to keep up with the requirements.

Unfortunately, there is no easily prepared factor IX concentrate for treatment of hemophilia B, and the usual course is to administer plasma. Since factor IX is much more stable than factor VIII, the plasma need not be fresh or frozen. Recently, lyophilized commercial factor IX concentrates have become available which are effective. They also contain factors II, VII, and X. Commercial lyophilized factor VIII concentrates are likewise now obtainable. Both materials are expensive, and the factor IX concentrate carries with it the risk of transmission of serum hepatitis.

Extremely potent bovine and porcine factor VIII concentrates are available. They are effective for only 7 to 10 days because of the development of antibodies in the recipient which destroy the animal factor VIII. Indeed, some hemophiliacs will develop antihuman factor VIII antibodies, rendering further factor VIII administration of little or no value.

Fibrinogen

Fibrinogenemic states may be congenital or acquired. It is surprising how infrequently dangerous bleeding occurs in congenital afibrinogenemia. Acquired hypofibrinogenemia is usually associated with consumption coagulopathy (DIC), in which other coagulation factor defects are present.

Human fibrinogen is readily available in freeze-dried form. At one time it was administered in acquired coagulation defects associated with low fibrinogen levels. Since addition of further fibrinogen to patients simply increases the amount of intravascular coagulation, fibrinogen is not of value and should *not* be given. At present there is little or no indication for administration of fibrinogen. Since hepatitis virus appears to be concentrated in fibrinogen, commercial fibrinogen preparations carry with them the risk of producing serum hepatitis.

Disseminated Intravascular Coagulation (DIC)

DIC is a dangerous condition already referred to as a complication of hemolytic transfusion reactions. It may, however, complicate situations that confront the reconstructive surgeon. The development of DIC in patients with septic shock or burn shock or sepsis following severe burns must always be considered. For further discussion see Chapter 10.

IMMUNOLOGICAL PROBLEMS

Congenital immunological defects are rare and will not often complicate the management of the patient requiring reconstructive surgery. Sex-linked agammaglobulinemia (Bruton's type) associated with very low IgG levels and normal cellular immunity is benefited by regular injections of immune globulin. Other defects such as the Wiskott-Aldrich syndrome and the Swiss type of agammaglobulinemia are not similarly benefited since the defect is not confined to IgG, involving defects or absence of other immune globulins or defects in cellular immunity (thymus-derived lymphocyte defects). Some success has been reported with the treatment of these immunological defects with bone marrow from siblings with identical HLA groups.

Acquired immunological defects may occur following trauma particularly after severe burns (see Plasma and Plasma Substitutes, above). There is some evidence that administration of immune globulin to burn patients improves their chances of survival.

III

*The External Environment:
Its Violation and the
Breakdown of Body Defenses*

INTRODUCTION

Thus far we have dealt with aspects and factors that are inevitable or normal; genetic and embryological factors and maintenance of Claude Bernard's "milieu intérieur."

Part III presents those aspects of the hostile external environment that so often break down normal body defenses. Such a hostile environment leads to tissue damage, which frequently brings the reconstructive surgeon's special skills and training into the picture in an attempt to stop the damage or to modify the ravage that has been wrought upon the organism. When the body is no longer able to withstand the onslaught of the hostile external environment, breakdown of defenses may make itself apparent in various ways, from the small pimple in response to a microorganism to the total collapse of all defense mechanisms manifesting itself as the body in shock.

Chapters 6 through 10 are addressed to the most common aspects of external hostile factors which bring the reconstructive surgeon to the patient. In keeping with the spirit of the book, they discuss how the body reacts and what the end result is, but minimize or completely stay away from treatment, since this is not intended to be a "how-to" book.

6

Microorganisms and Sepsis
Charles F. T. Snelling

DEFINITIONS

An *abscess* is a cavity lined by a wall or pyogenic membrane containing pus; it may be sterile or infected. Pathogenesis of an abscess derives from inoculation followed by proliferation of microorganisms. These are most commonly *Staphylococcus aureus* but may also be *Streptococcus* or gram-negative organisms which cause tissue necrosis with polymorphonuclear leukocyte infiltration. Many of the organisms are killed, thereby releasing proteolytic enzymes, which in turn cause softening of the necrotic tissue with pus formation. Pus thus consists of necrotic material, tissue debris, leukocytes, edema fluid, fibrin, and microorganisms, both living and dead. The wall or pyogenic membrane is initially made up of edematous tissue infiltrated with polymorphs; then it becomes organized into granulation tissue. This description is of an *acute abscess*, which may drain spontaneously or be drained surgically and then go on to heal by scar tissue formation. If infection persists, a chronic abscess is formed, with the wall containing macrophages, plasma cells, and lymphocytes as well as polymorphs. *Staphylococcus aureus* produces such a lesion by virtue of alpha toxin, which causes local tissue necrosis. The body's acute inflammatory response produces the rest of the features.

The drainage channel from an abscess to the skin surface or into a hollow viscus is referred to as a *sinus*. If the abscess is superficial, with destruction of overlying epithelium, the lesion is an *ulcer*.

Impetigo is an intraepithelial abscess. *Gangrenous impetigo* (sometimes associated with chronic ulcerative colitis) is a confluence of multiple intraepithelial abscesses, with necrosis of skin and ulcer formation. A *furuncle* is an intradermal abscess and occurs commonly in a sebaceous gland, hair follicle, or sweat gland. If an abscess extends into subcutaneous tissue, it is a *carbuncle*. Because skin is attached to underlying fascia by fibrous septa, the cavity is compartmentalized and multiple separate draining sinuses are thus formed. *Suppurative hidradenitis* starts as an infection of the apocrine sweat glands of the axilla, perineum, areola of the nipple, groin, and perianal regions. Both an acute and a chronic form exist; the latter can spread into subcutaneous tissue and fascia forming a carbuncle-like lesion.

Cellulitis is an acute inflammation of subcutaneous tissue extending along tissue planes. It is diffuse, with an indistinct periphery, and is associated with swelling, pain, and redness. The usual cause is group A streptococci, and the tendency to poor localization is due to the enzymes hyaluronidase and streptokinase produced by these organisms. Abscesses may form later in the course of the inflammation, but the pus is watery and blood-stained on account of the presence of the enzymes streptodornase and streptokinase. *Erysipelas* is cellulitis combined with lymphangitis. It occurs most often on the face and is characterized by redness, marked swelling, and pain, with a definite line of demarcation between affected and normal tissue. *Lymphangitis* is an inflammation of superficial lymphatic channels visible as red streaking in thin skin whereas *lymphadenitis* is inflammation of nodes draining an area of acute infection.

Bacteremia is the presence of microorganisms in the bloodstream. Such a condition does not necessarily cause systemic toxicity and therefore suggests rapid removal of organisms by a functioning reticuloendothelial system. In contrast, *septicemia* indicates the presence of bacteria and their toxins in the bloodstream accompanied by an intense systemic host reaction. Septicemia may follow direct invasion of the bloodstream by organisms, release of infected venous thromboemboli, or invasion of the lymphatic system from infected nodes. *Pyemia* or *metastatic infection* is the formation of multiple disseminated abscesses following septicemia.

TETANUS

Tetanus is an infectious disease caused by *Clostridium tetani*. Symptoms and signs are produced by the exotoxin tetanospasmin, which is released by the vegetative form of the organism and which, by blocking interneural and neuromuscular transmission, causes spasm of skeletal, diaphragmatic, and laryngeal musculature. Under strict anaerobic conditions *C. tetani* organisms assume the vegetative or growing form, appearing as slender gram-positive motile rods. At all other times they exist in the spore or inactive form resembling a drumstick on account of the terminally located spore. Spores are found in human and animal feces, soil, operating room and hospital air, house dust, and contaminated heroin. Spores may remain dormant in old traumatic wounds and can be reactivated by re-injury or subsequent operation. The vegetative form producing the toxin is sensitive to heat and antiseptics. The spore form, however, is resistant to antiseptics and requires heat exposure of 120°C for at least 10 minutes to be killed.

Infection with *C. tetani* commonly follows puncture wounds and crush injuries in which tissues are devitalized and contaminated with soil or feces. However, a wide variety of injuries including burns, septic abortion, and reoperation on old traumatic wounds can be complicated by tetanus. Neonatal tetanus (invasion via the umbilical cord) is also known to exist.

Diagnosis of tetanus is usually made clinically by a history of trauma a week or two previously since one may not be able to culture the organisms at the site of the original injury by the time clinical tetanus develops.

The toxin tetanospasmin is produced by the organisms at the site of injury, migrates along the motor nerves, and is fixed to motor end-plates. Fixation then occurs at interneural synapses in the spinal cord as well as synapses in cranial motor nuclei and in the brain itself. Tetanus may manifest itself locally at the site of injury or may first present as generalized tetanus. The toxin may be neutralized with antitoxin before it becomes fixed to the synapse. Thereafter toxin must be allowed to metabolize, and the patient is treated symptomatically with respiratory support and a quiet environment to decrease stimuli promoting spasm. The basic pathophysiology at the neuroneural or myoneural junction is probably interference with the release of acetylcholine [35].

There are two forms of tetanus. *Local tetanus* manifests itself as a persistent spasm of muscles close to the site of injury. Spasm may continue for several weeks or months and will then disappear without residual signs. *Cephalic tetanus* is a variety of localized tetanus that follows facial injuries and middle ear infections. It has a rapid onset affecting the cranial motor nerves, particularly VII, IX, X, and XII. This form can be rapidly fatal. *Generalized tetanus* may occasionally follow localized tetanus but in most cases it is the initial presenting form, appearing one to two weeks after injury. Trismus is a usual presenting symptom followed by restlessness, irritability, stiffness of the neck, and rigidity of abdominal and thoracic muscles. Tonic contractures and tetanic seizures occur. Pathological changes in striated muscle may include bleeding, loss of striation, rupture, and homogenization. In some instances there are no demonstrable morphological changes, as these are ordinarily directly proportional to the duration of the illness. Mortality of treated tetanus exceeds 60 percent. Differential diagnosis includes consideration of tetanus, heterologous serum sickness following the use of equine tetanus antitoxin, tetany following thyroid surgery, meningitis, encephalitis, rabies, and strychnine poisoning.

Tetanus prophylaxis is effective. United States Army experience has indicated that a full course of active immunization with tetanus toxoid can lead to virtual elimination of tetanus. Thus no service cases have been reported since the Korean War. There has been a steady decline in the incidence of tetanus in the United States from 400 or more cases per year in the 1950s to less than 200 cases per year in 1971 [14]. Tetanus toxoid is a formalized toxin adsorbed on aluminum hydroxide. A full course of active immunization consists of three 1 ml doses of toxoid administered at one month intervals, plus a booster dose one year after the third

dose, following which effective circulating levels of antitoxin will be present for five years. An adequate anamnestic response to a booster dose of tetanus toxoid can definitely occur 10 years after the last booster dose of toxoid and probably occurs after a longer interval following an adequate course of active immunization. Since for five years after a booster dose sufficient circulating antitoxin is present, a booster dose is thus not necessary at the time of injury within this period [14]. From 5 to 10 years following the last booster dose tetanus toxoid should be given at the time of injury. After 10 years one should be given toxoid plus human immune globulin for a tetanus-prone wound although a booster dose alone is adequate for a minor wound. Indiscriminate use of tetanus toxoid may occasionally produce complications such as glomerulonephritis, peripheral neuropathy, and generalized urticarial reactions [7]. Human tetanus immune globulin (TIG)— 250 units when used together with toxoid—must be given in a separate site from the toxoid; otherwise it will neutralize the toxoid. For a particularly dirty wound in a patient who has not been actively immunized one may also use 1.2 million units of benzathine penicillin G or oxytetracycline (1 to 2 gm daily for three weeks) since these antibiotics will interfere with the organism itself. In the event that human TIG is unavailable, one must use 1500 to 3000 units of equine antitetanic serum (ATS) after a suitable intracutaneous test dose. Many patients do not know their current tetanus immunization status and must be treated as being unimmunized.

CLOSTRIDIAL MYONECROSIS AND OTHER HISTOTOXIC INFECTIONS

Clostridial myonecrosis or gas gangrene is the most severe form of disease caused by a group of histotoxic clostridia. All clostridia are saprophytes and as such require dead or decaying tissue in order to function and reproduce. *C. perfringens (welchii)* type A, isolated in 80 percent of cases, *C. oedematiens (novyi)*, in 40 percent of cases, and *C. septicum*, in 20 percent of cases, are the true pathogens, are all *saccharolytic*, and produce lethal toxins [21]. *C. histolyticum, C. sporogenes (fallax)*, and *C. bifermentans (sordellii)* are proteolytic, produce foul-smelling gases, and are secondary putrefactive saprophytes. Most infections contain a mixture of these organisms, *C. perfringens* being the most common and serious.

Clostridia exist either in the resting (spore) form with a central or subterminal spore when the organism finds itself under adverse conditions or in the active or vegetative (nonspore) form when it is seen as gram-positive rods. Spore forms of *C. perfringens* are rarely demonstrated in wound exudate smears whereas the other clostridia often demonstrate spores. *C. perfringens* is nonmotile and encapsulated; all other clostridia are motile and nonencapsulated. All are obligate anaerobes and require devascularized tissue or other anaerobic culture medium to grow. The organisms cause disease by virtue of toxin production. *C. perfringens* produces several toxins, the most important being alpha toxin, a lecithinase which is dermonecrotizing, destroys cell membranes causing cell death, and alters capillary permeability. It also generates hemolysin, collagenase, hyaluronidase, and deoxyribonuclease. The other saccharolytic clostridia produce a variety of toxins including leukocidin, protease, and lipase as well as some of those listed for *C. perfringens*.

Initiation of disease requires contamination by organisms of an anaerobic avascular wound with a reduced oxidation-reduction potential. Clostridia are widespread in nature, being inhabitants of animal and human gastrointestinal tracts, soil, and manure. Spores are highly resistant to destruction by normal methods of sterilization and thus can be readily isolated in the hospital environment. The decreased oxidation-reduction potential is created in deep wounds with crushed, devitalized tissue. Contamination of

such wounds with foreign bodies or other organisms will help to engender these conditions.

Simple contamination of a wound with clostridia is common. In this event muscle is not involved and gas production is not a feature. The wound features greenish-black slough, thin brownish seropurulent discharge, and an odor of putrefaction. Aerobic organisms are often cultured concurrently. This condition is self-limiting but under optimum conditions for the pathogen can occasionally progress to anaerobic cellulitis. Bornstein et al. found clostridial contamination alone in 85 percent of 144 patients from whom clostridia were isolated, with gas gangrene and anaerobic cellulitis each present in less than 2 percent of cases [3].

Anaerobic cellulitis develops in devitalized tissue four to seven days after injury or abdominal surgery. Healthy viable tissue is not involved. The process may be localized (the so-called Welch abscess) or it may be quite diffuse. There are few systemic signs, local pain is minor, and there is no swelling. Gas formation is a striking and prominent feature. The gas extends along fascial planes, separating muscle groups without invading muscle. The wound is dirty and foul smelling and exudes a brown seropurulent discharge. The overlying skin may be edematous but not discolored. If gas is abundant, extensive, and easily demonstrable and there are no systemic effects, the patient does not have gas gangrene [36]. Histological examination of wound exudate will show both gram-positive rods and numerous inflammatory cells.

Clostridial myonecrosis or *gas gangrene* is distinguished by involvement of normal uninjured muscle. It can follow trauma, septic abortion, lower limb amputation in diabetics, and many abdominal operations, particularly bowel resections and biliary tract procedures. The incubation period is 12 hours to 3 days and occasionally longer. With a suitable environment the organisms convert to the vegetative form, proliferate, and produce lecithinase. This diffuses into normal muscle causing cellular death and thus provides additional suitable medium for invasion and proliferation of organisms. A vicious cycle is created, and the process spreads rapidly [11]. Systemic signs are severe: tachycardia, pale and sweaty skin, hypotension, agitation, and disorientation. The local lesion presents with swelling, tenderness, and a serosanguineous discharge having a putrid odor. Initially the skin is edematous, later it becomes red, and then bullae containing gas and fluid form. Eventually cyanosis and necrosis of skin occur. The underlying muscle is extensively involved far beyond the initial margins of the wound. This muscle does not bleed when cut and does not contract when stimulated. Gas formation is minimal and takes place within muscle, which becomes bright red or pink. Histologically the muscle shows loss of striation and nuclei. The wound exudate shows gram-positive rods but no inflammatory cells. To differentiate anaerobic cellulitis from myonecrosis the following criterion is used: In cellulitis systemic signs are minimal, with marked local gas formation and an inflammatory cell infiltrate, whereas in myonecrosis the reverse is true.

Anaerobic streptococcal myonecrosis can be confused with gas gangrene clinically, but histologically there are gram-positive cocci in muscle and connective tissue. Apart from an elevated temperature and flushed dry skin, systemic signs are minimal. Gas formation is moderate, and there is serosanguineous discharge with severe local pain. The insidious onset over three to four days, pyrexia, and a demonstration of gram-positive cocci in the wound exudate differentiate this condition from anaerobic cellulitis and myonecrosis [21].

Therapy of established gas gangrene is primarily surgical, with hyperbaric oxygen, antibiotics, and antisera as valuable adjuncts. Surgical treatment used to consist in removal of all necrotic muscle and tissue. In the past this often meant amputation or mutilating excision. Recent reports suggest that preliminary opening of the wound followed by re-

peated treatments with hyperbaric oxygen permits less extensive surgical excisions to be effective treatment [30].

A course of hyperbaric oxygen therapy is 100% oxygen at 3 atmospheres of pressure for two hours, repeated three times on day 1 and twice on days 2 and 3 for a total of seven doses [30]. The rationale of hyperbaric oxygen therapy and its mode of action is not clear, but saturation of the normal tissue at the border between living and necrotic tissue with oxygen would appear to produce tissue oxygen levels sufficient to last long enough to inhibit clostridia from invading later. Obviously very high tissue levels of oxygen must be obtained since the alpha toxin invades living muscle and kills it prior to invasion of the clostridia [17].

Antibiotics in high doses may kill organisms not removed surgically although this result too is difficult to explain with the relative avascularity of the infected tissues. Presumably high antibiotic tissue levels are built up prior to invasion of the alpha toxin in order to have effective residual amounts. Recommended doses of antibiotics include penicillin (12 million units per day), erythromycin (4 gm daily), or cephalothin (12 gm daily) for two weeks [36].

Passive immunotherapy is employed. Horse serum containing 10,000 units *C. perfringens*, 10,000 units *C. oedematiens*, and 5000 units *C. septicum* antitoxin is commercially available. After suitable skin testing it is administered intramuscularly, intravenously, and directly into the site of infection for a total of 75,000 units. Injections into the vicinity of the wound are often made. In sheep experiments it was found that antitoxin must be given within nine hours of wounding and inoculation to be effective [5].

Active immunization has been experimentally evaluated [4]. Because of the short incubation period for gas gangrene, active immunization would be effective only with a prior course of active immunization combined with appropriate boosters since effective circulating antitoxin levels would be necessary at all times. There would be too short a latent interval to rely on an anamnestic response to a booster dose as is successfully done in tetanus prophylaxis.

PROGRESSIVE BACTERIAL SYNERGISTIC GANGRENE

Progressive bacterial synergistic gangrene is a chronic superficial necrosis of skin and subcutaneous tissue often starting in an abdominal operative wound. The lesion is characterized by three zones of skin color change, an outer erythematous ring surrounding a middle cyanotic zone and a central core of black necrosis. Brewer and Meleney first described the condition in detail (although earlier case reports appear in the literature); hence the name *Meleney's synergistic gangrene* [6]. Meleney has attempted to elucidate the etiology and pathogenesis [23, 24].

Careful bacteriological studies have demonstrated that a microaerophilic nonhemolytic streptococcus and *Staphylococcus aureus* are both cultured from the lesion. The streptococcus is recovered from the peripheral erythematous zone and even beyond, and both organisms are found in the necrotic central area. Meleney could duplicate this lesion in dogs and guinea pigs only when both organisms were injected *together* whereas injecting the organisms separately would not produce the lesion [23]. Lyall and Stuart produced a similar lesion in guinea pigs with *Proteus* and microaerophilic nonhemolytic streptococcus [19].

Most frequently synergistic gangrene follows abdominal surgery or trivial trauma and occurs around colostomy or ileostomy openings. In the case of abdominal wounds retention sutures have often been used. Ten days to two weeks postoperatively, after the wound has been healing satisfactorily, there is onset of intense pain and erythema, swelling, and tenderness at the operative site. The erythematous zone spreads, central cyanosis develops, and finally gangrene is present. If allowed to progress, the condition can gradually involve extensive areas of the trunk and limbs. Once the necrotic areas have separated, there may be reepithelialization from deeper undamaged epidermal appendages, but generally skin grafting will be required. Systemic signs are minor until the condition progresses to cause general debilitation. Diagnosis is made on the basis of careful bacteriological studies, including cultures from the outer zone which demonstrate microaerophilic nonhemolytic streptococcus. Demonstration of this organism plus *Staphylococcus aureus* or a gram-negative organism from the central necrotic area is pathognomonic. Differential diagnosis includes consideration of necrotizing fasciitis, chronic burrowing ulcer, and synergistic necrotizing cellulitis as well as noninfectious causes of cutaneous gangrene. Death can result if the process is allowed to go on unchecked. In the past, treatment consisted of wide excision beyond the advancing edge of the process, but now appropriate antibiotic therapy combined with a more modest excision is effective [26].

NECROTIZING FASCIITIS

Necrotizing fasciitis is a clinical condition characterized by progressive necrosis of subcutaneous tissue and superficial fascia with extensive undermining of the overlying skin. Skin changes can vary from cellulitis with or without blister formation to complete necrosis. The skin is separated from the underlying fascia quite widely from the original portal of injury. In the original description of this condition under the term *hemolytic streptococcus gangrene* [22], group A streptococcus was the only organism isolated. However, *Staphylococcus aureus* [37] and gram-negative aerobes [29] have subsequently been cultured from the patients.

Whether hemolytic streptococcus gangrene and necrotizing fasciitis are separate entities or the same disease is a matter of great dispute in the literature. It would appear that both terms—as well as *hospital gangrene, necrotizing erysipelas, suppurative fasciitis*, and *Fournier's gangrene*—describe essentially the same disease process.

The infection occurs in the extremities, perineum, and trunk following cuts, scratches, needle punctures, splinter wounds, insect bites, and surgery to the abdominal and thoracic cavities as well as incision and drainage of infected lymph nodes. Occasionally no initiating injury is identified. Debilitated patients, diabetics, and patients with rheumatoid arthritis who have had long courses of steroid therapy are often affected.

The process starts rapidly, 24 to 72 hours after surgery or injury. Moderately elevated temperature is accompanied by a tachycardia out of proportion to the fever. Hemolytic anemia and shock due to intravascular fluid loss into the extracellular space can occur. At first the skin has an appearance suggestive of cellulitis, with redness, swelling, and edema. Later the skin becomes anesthetic and cyanotic, and a blister forms. Group A streptococci may be isolated from the fluid aspirated from the blister. Probing below the surface demonstrates wide undermining of the skin with separation from the fascia overlying the muscle bundles. The subcutaneous fat is edematous, and a thin serosanguineous turbid fluid exudes. The fascia is gray and necrotic and separates easily from the deep fascia. Muscle is not involved. The overlying skin finally becomes necrotic after thrombosis of the small perforating vessels occurs.

The pathogenesis of subcutaneous fat and fascial necrosis may be a hypersensitivity reaction of the Arthus or Shwartzman type as suggested by Meleney [24]. McCafferty and Lyons suggest that the collagen of fascia is particularly vulnerable to a proteolytic serum lysin factor activated by streptococcal fibrinolysin. Beathard and Guckian [2] have elucidated the work of Cromartie et al. [10], who demonstrated that the pathological picture of this condition can be reproduced experimentally with group A streptococcus cell wall extracts. Hyaluronidase produced by group A streptococci facilitates the rapid spread of the involvement when the organism is established. However, if other gram-positive and gram-

negative organisms can produce the same clinical picture, further investigation of the organisms and host is necessary to determine the pathogenesis. Anaerobic organisms have not been cultured.

Treatment includes surgical incision and exposure of all areas of involvement combined with the appropriate antibiotics. Supportive measures such as fluid and blood replacement are required. Beathard [2] suggests 20 million units of penicillin per 24 hours. A few cases have been treated with cortisone, although many patients suffering from this disease have already received long-term steroid therapy. Once the infection has been eliminated, the wound usually requires skin grafting.

SYNERGISTIC NECROTIZING CELLULITIS

In 1972 Stone and Martin described 63 cases of a disease characterized by extensive necrosis of fascia and muscle with or without less extensive necrosis of overlying fat and skin usually involving the perineum or adjacent thigh (79 percent of cases) [33]. Bacteriologically this entity is typified by a mixed flora of aerobic gram-negative rods (98 percent of cases) and anaerobic bacteria (80 percent of cases) with *Bacteroides* in 30 percent and anaerobic streptococci in 57 percent. In presentation it resembles necrotizing fasciitis, and its mixed flora suggests progressive synergistic gangrene, but neither of these involves muscle.

The disease is often associated with diabetes (61 percent of cases). The lesion starts as an ulcer which drains reddish brown foul-smelling fluid, so-called dishwater pus. There may be gas formation, with crepitation and a minor degree of skin necrosis. The course is chronic. Systemically there will be moderate pyrexia (100° to 102°F) and signs of generalized toxicity. Overall mortality is 76 percent, with a poorer prognosis in patients treated by simple incision and drainage than in those treated by wide excision which may necessitate hip disarticulation. Colostomy may also be necessary.

MELENEY'S ULCER (CHRONIC UNDERMINING ULCER)

Meleney [25, 27] described *chronic undermining* or *burrowing ulcer*, a discrete clinical entity caused by microaerophilic hemolytic streptococcus. It can begin in an operative wound following gastrointestinal or genital tract surgery, after incision and drainage of an infected lymph node, or in a traumatic wound. The organism is a member of the normal human oral, bowel, and vaginal flora and colonizes the wound, which presents initially as an ulcer. There is progressive liquefaction of fat, and undermining and thinning of adjacent skin take place. Secondary ulcers develop to create intervening thin skin bridges which may break down or become circumferentially epithelialized. If the condition is allowed to progress unchecked for several months, invasion occurs along fascial planes between muscle masses and along lymphatics, and finally erosion of large blood vessels can occur. Muscle necrosis is not a feature. The base of the ulcer is covered with grayish friable granulation tissue. Local symptoms vary from minor to severe pain with occasional peaks of temperature. The condition is a chronic progressive debilitating process, nonfatal itself but producing potentially lethal complications such as hemorrhage.

Therapy prior to the development of antibiotics included opening the wound and applying zinc peroxide topically to create an aerobic environment. Penicillin has reduced the tissue destruction and the need for extensive surgical resection [18]. Failure to request anaerobic cultures, however, may lead to delay in making the correct diagnosis and initiating effective therapy.

RABIES

Rabies is a viral disease endemic in wild and domestic animals and transmitted to man usually through animal bites and scratches, causing central nervous system damage and disease. Skunks, foxes, cats, dogs, bats, raccoons, and farm animals are most commonly affected. The incidence of rabies in the United States reported for all animals has declined from over 8000 cases in 1953 to 3276 cases in 1970. From one to three human cases per year have occurred in the United States in the past decade [1].

Virus is present in the saliva of the infected animal up to 10 days preceding clinical disease while the incubation period in man varies from one to three months, with extremes of nine days to eight months being reported. As a rule, for transmission to take place open cuts, abrasions, or bites to human skin must be contaminated with saliva of the animal although inhalation of virus has produced human disease [8]. An unprovoked attack by any animal must be considered a serious sign whereas a provoked attack by a domestic animal would necessitate a 10-day observation of the animal to determine whether rabies develops.

In human disease the initial prodromal stage, lasting up to four days, is characterized by wound symptoms such as numbness, tenderness, tingling, and inflammation, general symptoms such as malaise, nausea, headaches, and dysphagia, and changes in personality. This is followed by the excitement stage, marked by restlessness, nervousness, high fever, and intense muscle spasm associated with pain, thirst, and dehydration. The patient's saliva is infected, there is frothing at the mouth, and the patient becomes comatose, with Cheyne-Stokes breathing, convulsions, and finally complete respiratory paralysis leading to death. Mortality is virtually 100 percent [1].

Prevention is the most effective cure. Formerly it was routine practice to leave animal bite wounds open. Currently, if the patient presents within 6 to 12 hours for treatment, thorough cleansing of the wounds including application of quaternary ammonium compounds, debridement, and primary closure are acceptable practice [34]. The use of immunotherapy depends on the availability and condition of the attacking animal and the severity of the injury. As the animal is often unavailable, immunotherapy must be used speculatively. The diagnosis of rabies is made on examination of the animal's brain for Negri bodies. If the animal appears normal at the time of injury, it must be observed for 10 days to rule out rabies. If rabies is suspected, the animal is killed and its head is packed in ice and sent to the appropriate health department where the brain is examined for Negri bodies or used in fluorescent antibody tests. The salivary glands of the animal are also used in performing tests.

Active immunization with vaccine and passive immunization with horse serum are available. The safest and most commonly used vaccine is the duck embryo vaccine (DEV), prepared from a killed virus grown in duck embryo. The side-effects of this vaccine are infrequent and minor. The Semple's vaccine, made from a phenol-killed virus grown in rabbit brain tissue, has a high incidence of neurological side-effects. A new tissue culture vaccine grown in hamster kidney is currently under evaluation [1]. The dose of either vaccine is 2 ml of 5% tissue emulsion given subcutaneously for 14 to 21 consecutive days with a booster dose 10 and 30 days after the last daily dose. Side-effects include a mild local reaction, serum sickness, and allergic encephalomyelitis. The incidence of neurological side-effects with duck embryo vaccine is 1 in 25,000 cases and with the Semple's vaccine 1 in 4000 cases [28]. Passive immunization is with horse serum, the dose being 40 IU per kilogram of body weight as a single dose, with 46 percent of patients developing serum sickness and anaphylactic shock [15, 31]. A human immune globulin (HRIG), under evaluation but not generally available, causes only occasional febrile reactions [31].

The guidelines for the use of immunotherapy in rabies are clearly laid out by Cox [9]. If clinical rabies is present in the attacking animal, active immunization is started immediately and a full course given. If the animal is normal and can be observed for 10 days, the course of treatment depends on the severity of the injury. For scratches and minor bites no treatment is initiated unless the animal develops rabies during the 10-day observation period, at which time immunization is begun. For severe injuries a course of vaccination is started, but if the animal remains healthy at the end of 10 days the course of vaccination is not completed. If the animal cannot be found or followed and rabies is considered a possibility, a full course of vaccination is carried out. For severe multiple injuries in all categories one dose of rabies antiserum is also given early in addition to the course of active immunization.

HAND INFECTIONS

Hand infections are essentially abscesses or cellulitis due usually to common pyogenic bacteria. They have gained special significance because of the varied and complex anatomical characteristics of the hand which uniquely influence their presentation. In recent reviews [13, 32] gram-positive organisms alone caused 67 to 95 percent of infections, with *Staphylococcus aureus* accounting for 75 percent of these and group A streptococci most of the remainder. Gram-negative organisms alone caused 5 percent, *Klebsiella*, *Enterobacter*, and *Escherichia coli* being the most common. Mixed infections were present in 30 percent of cases [13]. A wound inflicted by human teeth in the region of the metacarpophalangeal (MP) and proximal interphalangeal (PIP) joint is an exception as anaerobic streptococcus (peptostreptococci), *Bacteroides*, and other oral anaerobes may be introduced directly into the joint and cause persistent indolent refractory infection.

Swelling of the dorsum of the hand may be due to cellulitis or abscess or be a secondary lymphadematous manifestation of a volar infection such as a palmar or web space infection. Before treating dorsal swelling as the primary and only infection, one must examine the rest of the hand, as all of the palmar lymphatics drain to the dorsum, which is looser and swells readily.

Fingernail infections include *acute paronychias* involving the lateral nail folds, *eponychia* involving the cuticle, and *subungual abscesses* involving the nail bed deep to the nail plate. All may be present at the same time. Chronic paronychias are often infected with *Candida albicans*.

Pulp space abscesses of the volar distal phalanges (felons or whitlows) are complicated by the presence of tethering fibrous bands extending from skin to bone which prevent skin movement. Infection causes swelling, but these nonelastic bands prevent expansion and lead to increased pulp pressure with the ultimate possibility of bone necrosis, or osteitis, with loss of the bulk of the fingertip. The epiphysis is usually preserved because its vascular supply is proximal to the distal phalanx. The diaphysis may regenerate if the periosteum remains intact and the general shape of the distal pulp is preserved. Pulp space infections of the proximal and middle phalanges may be mistaken for acute tenosynovitis but are more localized. Pulp space infections usually follow puncture wounds although they may be a complication of paronychia.

Acute suppurative tenosynovitis is an infection of the synovial sheaths of the digital flexor tendons. These extend distally to the insertion of the profundus tendon. The proximal extension is variable, but generally speaking the sheaths of the index, middle, and ring fingers are separate and originate at the MP joints, while the thumb sheath is continuous with the radial bursa of the wrist, and the small finger sheath is continuous with the ulnar bursa. Since the radial and ulnar bursae often communicate, the thumb and small finger as well as the wrist can be involved. Acute tenosynovitis usually follows a puncture wound directly into the sheath but can be secondary to a pulp space infection, osteomyelitis of a phalanx, or a palmar space infection. The classic signs of Kanavel [16] are the flexed position of the digit, fusiform swelling of the whole digit, severe pain on extension, and tenderness over the entire tendon sheath. Treatment philosophy is divided between conservative (systemic or intrathecal instillation of antibiotics [20]) and surgical incision and drainage. Failure to recognize and treat can leave a stiff thickened finger often with destruction of the flexor tendon.

Subfascial palmar infections close to the webs are *web space infections* and present with both palmar and dorsal swelling of the web and separation of the adjacent digits. Web space infections require drainage through both volar and dorsal separate incisions at least 1 cm proximal to the web. More proximal infections are referred to as *collar-button abscesses* because of the coexistence of infection both superficial and deep to the palmar fascia. The collar-button abscess requires incision of the palmar fascia and drainage of the subfascial pocket in addition to the superficial subdermal locus.

Palmar space infections involve the potential spaces deep to the profundus flexor tendons at the level of the carpal and metacarpal bones between the thenar and hypothenar muscle masses. A septum joining the synovium of the middle finger tendons to the third metacarpal divides the thenar space laterally from the midpalmar space medially. These infections are recognized by a localized palmar swelling if only one space is affected or a diffuse swelling if both are involved. In some cases marked dorsal swelling of the hand is the most striking presenting feature and can lead to misplaced drainage incisions. Palmar space infections can follow puncture wounds or be extensions from acute purulent tenosynovitis or osteomyelitis of the metacarpals.

Wounds of the MP and PIP joint region due only to fights are often contaminated with oral anaerobic organisms. These wounds should be left open until the likelihood of infection has been ruled out.

OSTEOMYELITIS

Acute hematogenous osteomyelitis occurs primarily in the metaphysis of long bones of the lower limbs in children, is due to *Staphylococcus aureus*, and is seldom seen in standard plastic surgical practice while osteomyelitis as a complication of compound fractures of the tibia, mandible, and hand is rather likely to be seen. Proliferation of microorganisms produces acute inflammation with edema. This compromises blood supply, on account of the rigidity of bone, leading to further necrosis, which fuels the infection. The necrotic bone fragment, termed a *sequestrum*, is enveloped by subperiosteal new bone formation, the so-called involucrum. Following osteoclastic action the sequestrum is isolated from living tissue and must be spontaneously or surgically removed before healing can occur. Tibial fractures complicated by osteomyelitis are often associated with inadequate or unstable skin coverage that must be corrected before definite treatment can be carried out. Fractures of the mandible which secondarily develop osteomyelitis often reveal carious teeth with apical abscesses. Personal preference appears to dictate the indications for removal of teeth as part of the definitive fracture care [12]. Osteomyelitis of phalanges is usually a complication of delayed or inadequate debridement and inadequate soft tissue coverage.

REFERENCES

1. *Annual Summary—Rabies 1970.* Centre for Disease Control, Zoonoses Surveillance. Washington: U.S. Department of Health, Education and Welfare, Public Health Service, Health Sciences and Mental Health Administration, October 1971.
2. Beathard, G. A., and Guckian, J. C. Necrotizing fasciitis due to group A beta-hemolytic streptococci. *Arch. Intern. Med.* 120:63, 1967.
3. Bornstein, D. L., Weinberg, A. N., and Swartz, M. N. Anaerobic infection: Review of current experience. *Medicine* (Baltimore) 43:207, 1964.
4. Boyd, N. A., Thomson, R. O., and Walker, P. D. The prevention of experimental *Clostridium novyi* and *Cl. perfringens* gas gangrene in high velocity missile wounds by active immunization. *J. Med. Microbiol.* 5:467, 1972.
5. Boyd, N. A., Walker, P. D., and Thomson, R. O. The prevention of experimental *Clostridium novyi* gas gangrene in high velocity missile wounds by passive immunization. *J. Med. Microbiol.* 5:459, 1972.
6. Brewer, G. E., and Meleney, F. L. Progressive gangrenous infection of the skin and subcutaneous tissues following operation for acute perforative appendicitis: A study in symbiosis. *Ann. Surg.* 84:438, 1926.
7. Christensen, P. Side Reactions to Tetanus Toxoid. In *Report*, Third International Conference on Tetanus, São Paulo, Brazil, 1970.
8. Constantine, D. G. Rabies transmission by non-bite route. *Public Health Rep.* 77:287, 1962.
9. Cox, H. R. Rabies: Laboratory diagnosis and post exposure treatment. *Am. J. Clin. Pathol.* 57:794, 1972.
10. Cromartie, W. J., Schwab, J. H., and Craddock, J. G. The effect of a toxic cellular component of group A streptococci on connective tissue. *Am. J. Pathol.* 37:79, 1960.
11. De Haven, K. E., and Evarts, C. M. The continuing problem of gas gangrene. *J. Trauma* 11:983, 1971.
12. Donahue, W. B., and Abelardo, L. M. Osteomyelitis of the jaw. *Can. Med. Assoc. J.* 103:748, 1970.
13. Eaton, R. G., and Butsch, D. P. Antibiotic guidelines for hand infections. *Surg. Gynecol. Obstet.* 130:119, 1970.
14. Furste, W., and Wheeler, W. L. Tetanus: A team disease. *Curr. Probl. Surg.* October 1972. P. 1.
15. Hattwick, M. A., Rubin, R. H., Music, S., Sikes, R. K., Smith, J. S., and Gregg, M. B. Post exposure rabies prophy-

laxis with human rabies immune globulin. *J.A.M.A.* 227:407, 1974.

16. Kanavel, A. B. *Infections of the Hand* (6th ed.). Philadelphia: Lea & Febiger, 1933. P. 60.

17. Lambertsen, C. Oxygen in the therapy of gas gangrene. *J. Trauma* 12:825, 1972.

18. Leacock, A. A case of chronic undermining ulceration treated with penicillin. *Br. Med. J.* 2:765, 1945.

19. Lyall, A., and Stuart, R. D. Progressive postoperative gangrene of the skin: Observations of aetiology and treatment in two cases. *Glasgow Med. J.* 29:1, 1948.

20. MacDougall, E. P. Acute suppurative tenosynovitis. *Can. J. Surg.* 11:41, 1968.

21. MacLennan, J. D. The histotoxic clostridial infections of man. *Bacteriol. Rev.* 26:177, 1962.

22. Meleney, F. L. Hemolytic streptococcus gangrene. *Arch. Surg.* 9:317, 1924.

23. Meleney, F. L. Bacterial synergism in disease processes with a confirmation of the synergistic bacterial etiology of a certain type of progressive gangrene of the abdominal wall. *Ann. Surg.* 94:961, 1931.

24. Meleney, F. L. A differential diagnosis between certain types of infectious gangrene of the skin with particular reference to haemolytic streptococcus gangrene and bacterial synergistic gangrene. *Surg. Gynecol. Obstet.* 56:847, 1933.

25. Meleney, F. L. Zinc peroxide in the treatment of microaerophilic and anaerobic infections with special reference to a group of chronic ulcerative burrowing non gangrenous lesions of the abdominal wall apparently due to a microaerophilic haemolytic streptococcus. *Ann. Surg.* 101:997, 1935.

26. Meleney, F. L., Friedman, S. T., and Harvey, H. D. The treatment of progressive bacterial synergistic gangrene with penicillin. *Surgery* 18:423, 1945.

27. Meleney, F. L., and Johnson, B. A. Further laboratory and clinical experiences in the treatment of chronic undermining burrowing ulcers with zinc peroxide. *Surgery* 1:169, 1937.

28. Mozar, H. N., Finnigan, F. B., Petzold, H., Spitler, L. E., Emmons, R. W., and Rothenberg, B. Myelopathy after duck embryo rabies vaccine. *J.A.M.A.* 224:1605, 1973.

29. Rea, W. J., and Wyrick, W. J., Jr. Necrotizing fasciitis. *Ann. Surg.* 172:957, 1970.

30. Roding, B., Groeneveld, P. H. A., and Boerema, I. Ten years' experience in the treatment of gas gangrene with hyperbaric oxygen. *Surg. Gynecol. Obstet.* 134:579, 1972.

31. Rubin, R. H., Sikes, R. K., and Gregg, M. B. Human rabies immune globulin, clinical trials and effects on serum anti-gamma globulins. *J.A.M.A.* 224:871, 1973.

32. Sneddon, J. *The Care of Hand Infections.* London: Edward Arnold, 1970.

33. Stone, H. H., and Martin, J. D. Synergistic necrotizing cellulitis. *Ann. Surg.* 175:702, 1972.

34. Thompson, H. G. Small animal bites: The role of primary closure. *J. Trauma* 13:20, 1973.

35. Weinstein, L. Tetanus. *N. Engl. J. Med.* 289:1293, 1973.

36. Weinstein, L., and Barza, M. A. Gas gangrene. *N. Engl. J. Med.* 289:1129, 1973.

37. Wilson, B. Necrotizing fasciitis. *Am. Surg.* 18:416, 1952.

7

Antimicrobial Therapy

Allan R. Ronald

Discovery of antimicrobial agents, drugs able to destroy the invading pathogen and remain largely innocuous for the host, has been one of the most dramatic accomplishments of modern medicine. Together with improvements in sanitation and immunization, chemotherapy has greatly reduced the scourge of life-threatening communicable diseases and brought about a significant shift in the types of etiological agents responsible for infection. Organisms indigenous to man now cause the vast majority of infections requiring antimicrobial therapy. Also, these organisms have the ability to acquire resistance to antimicrobial therapy, and this is a continuing challenge. The initial enthusiasm for antimicrobial "coverage" of the patient has now been replaced by concern about the consequences of the antimicrobial action on the ecology of the host and the danger of substituting more resistant pathogens in the vacuum created by the eradication of normal flora. The decision to use an antimicrobial agent and its selection require a rational approach and an adherence to basic microbiological and pharmacological principles. In order to assure that

an appropriate decision has been made, the surgeon prescribing antimicrobials must have the knowledge to answer certain questions:

1. Is an infection present? If so, what is the most likely etiological agent? Symptoms or signs suggesting infection, including fever, local inflammation, and exudation, can be mimicked by a number of disease processes. Objective evidence to diagnose infection with laboratory confirmation should be obtained in most instances in which antimicrobial use is indicated. In soft tissue infections, if no exudate is apparent, an injection of 0.5 ml of saline solution into the infected area followed by aspiration of tissue fluid will frequently reveal the organism on culture. Microscopical examination of infected material can be carried out immediately and often provides guidelines as to the kind of infection present. The Gram stain in particular should be considered an integral part of the initial clinical evaluation. This permits organisms to be grouped into categories by the stain reaction and also confirms the accuracy of the final culture report. The clinical

presentations of many infections together with the Gram stain allow an accurate etiological "guess" to be made, and with the knowledge of the predictable susceptibility of many microorganisms to chemotherapeutic agents a rational plan of therapy can be formulated.

2. What is the most appropriate antimicrobial agent? How should it be administered, and in what dose? The laboratory fulfills a significant role in guiding the physician's choice of therapy with certain limitations. Only pure cultures of presumed pathogens should be tested. Inocula, media, antimicrobial content, and interpretation must be standardized and controlled if reproducible meaningful results are to be obtained [8]. The disk agar diffusion method is most widely used because of its cost and technical simplicity. If carried out correctly, it satisfactorily differentiates susceptible from resistant organisms. Although other, more complex techniques involving antimicrobial dilution in agar or broth give more precise answers, these techniques are no less subject to error.

Bactericidal drugs should be used in patients with impaired host defenses and in those with life-threatening infection. However, in the great majority of infections antimicrobials are necessary only to retard the proliferation of microorganisms and allow normal mechanisms to eradicate the pathogens. In these instances bacteriostatic drugs may be as effective as bactericidal agents. Parenteral therapy is mandatory in all patients with serious infection. Intravenous therapy is usually preferable particularly if the patient is hypotensive, has a bleeding diathesis, or has infection located in sites where antimicrobial penetration may be difficult. The ideal dosage of an antimicrobial agent is the least amount of drug to achieve the desired effect while producing no untoward reactions. Fortunately, most recommended dosage schedules ensure optimal therapeutic effect, and increases in dosage are seldom indicated.

3. What is the risk of the agents to be prescribed? The patient's history of drug allergies should be ascertained before therapy is begun. Toxic reactions to antimicrobials are numerous and are usually related either to excessive dosage or to impairment of drug metabolism or excretion. Hepatic function and renal excretion are important to consider in choosing an antimicrobial agent. Direct toxicity of antimicrobials usually manifests itself as specific toxic effects on organ systems. Hypersensitivity reactions may follow the use of any drug but are most frequent with penicillins and sulfonamides. The most serious of these are anaphylactoid reactions, which usually occur within 30 minutes after administration of the offending agent. Treatment must be prompt and vigorous. Delayed reactions including fever, skin rashes, and cholestatic hepatitis are rarely life-threatening and can usually be controlled by discontinuing the responsible drug. Changes in the ecology of the patient's flora have only recently been recognized as an important untoward effect of antimicrobial agents. With suppression of normal inhabitants of the skin, overgrowth with *Candida albicans* or *Staphylococcus aureus* can occur. This is particularly common in the hospital environment.

CLASSIFICATION

Antimicrobial agents can be grouped by their chemical structure, by their mechanism of action, and by the kinds of microorganisms affected. Unfortunately, the introduction of many new antimicrobial agents during the past 20 years has made any classification unwieldy. In order to deal effectively with this large number of agents we will consider them within the following seven groups: (1) the penicillins, (2) the cephalosporins, (3) the macrolide antibiotics and lincomycin-clindamycin, (4) the aminoglycosides, (5) the sulfonamides, (6) the tetracyclines, and (7) chloramphenicol.

THE PENICILLINS

The basic structure of all penicillins is a β-lactam thiazolidine configuration. The mode of action is through inhibition of the synthesis of the cell wall mucopeptide. This structure is unique to bacteria and not present in mammalian cells. Therefore the penicillins can be administered in very high quantities with minimal dose-related toxicity.

The isolation of the nucleus of the penicillin molecule, 6-aminopenicillanic acid, permitted the synthesis of a potentially endless series of penicillins. Many of these analogues have useful clinical applications. Three groups are distinguishable on the basis of their antibacterial spectrum: penicillinase-susceptible, penicillinase-resistant, and gram-negative spectrum penicillins.

Penicillinase-Susceptible Penicillins

Penicillin G (benzylpenicillin) is the most widely used penicillin. It is susceptible to degradation by acid solution and is variably absorbed from the gastrointestinal tract. Phenoxymethyl penicillin (penicillin V) is acid stable and preferable to penicillin G for oral administration. Penicillin G remains the drug of choice for parenteral administration. However, it has a very short half-life of 30 minutes, and to prolong this, penicillin G has been compounded with several salts. Procaine penicillin G is less irritating, can be administered intramuscularly every 12 hours, and provides adequate levels for most susceptible organisms. Following intramuscular injection benzathine penicillin G provides a very low but measurable concentration of penicillin for as long as three weeks.

The antibacterial spectrum of these penicillins includes most gram-positive organisms except penicillinase-producing *Staph. aureus* and some group D streptococci (*Streptococcus faecalis*).

Penicillinase-Resistant Penicillins

The emergence of staphylococci with the ability to enzymatically inactivate penicillin led to epidemic staphylococcal disease. The discovery of penicillins highly resistant to cleavage by penicillinase was a major advance. A number of clinically useful antistaphylococcal drugs are now available. The only indication for their use is infection caused by penicillinase-producing *Staph. aureus*. Methicillin, the first antistaphylococcal penicillinase-resistant penicillin, is not absorbed orally. It is also the least potent and least stable of the penicillinase-resistant penicillins. Oxacillin, cloxacillin, nafcillin, and dicloxacillin are all antistaphylococcal penicillins with little to choose between them. Cloxacillin and dicloxacillin are reliably absorbed after oral administration and one of these should be chosen as the oral agent of choice in treating penicillinase-producing staphylococci.

Although methicillin-resistant strains of staphylococci have become a serious problem in many parts of the world, they are still rarely isolated in the United States.

Gram-Negative Spectrum Penicillins

Ampicillin is a penicillinase-*susceptible* penicillin that is stable in gastric acid and includes in its spectrum gram-negative pathogens including *Hemophilus influenzae*, *Escherichia coli*, and many enteric pathogens. Group D streptococci (*S. faecalis*) are also more susceptible to ampicillin than they are to penicillin.

Carbenicillin widens the spectrum of ampicillin to include *Pseudomonas aeruginosa*. However, these organisms are only relatively sensitive to carbenicillin, and bactericidal serum levels can be achieved only with high-dose intravenous therapy (200 to 500 mg per kilogram per day).

Allergic reactions to penicillins occur in 1 to 10 percent of patients treated. At least two chemical determinants are involved in the sensitization phenomena. The most serious immediate allergic reactions are mediated by skin-sensitizing antibodies that are usually specific for the "minor determinants," including a mixture of metabolic products of penicillins [10].

Allergic reactions occur with any dose of penicillin, and the history of an allergy to one type of penicillin compound increases the risk to the patient of a reaction with any other penicillin. Although many patients will not necessarily have a repetition of an allergic event on subsequent exposure, a history of allergy to any of the penicillins is usually sufficient grounds to choose an alternative agent.

The virtual absence of dose-related toxicity has permitted the use of very large doses of penicillin for long periods of time in patients with normal renal function without significant side-effects.

CEPHALOSPORINS

The cephalosporin family has a basic structure similar to the penicillins with a dihydrothiazine-β-lactam ring configuration common to all cephalosporins. The mode of action is thought to be identical to that of the penicillins. Like the penicillins, a great many cephalosporin antimicrobials are being synthesized and marketed for clinical use. All the clinically available cephalosporins share a similar antibacterial spectrum. Cephalosporins are active against both gram-positive and gram-negative microorganisms including group A *Streptococcus pyogenes*, penicillin-resistant and penicillin-sensitive *Staph. aureus*, and most other gram-positive pathogens. In addition, most strains of *E. coli*, *Proteus mirabilis*, and *Klebsiella* species are susceptible to the cephalosporins. *P. aeruginosa*, group D streptococci, and anaerobic gram-negative rods (*Bacteroides fragilis*) are generally resistant.

The cephalosporins are the drugs of choice in only a few specific situations. In the acutely ill patient with sepsis of undefined etiology a cephalosporin combined with an aminoglycoside may be an appropriate initial choice until the bacterial etiology is known and sensitivities are determined. Patients with a history of penicillin allergy may usually be treated safely with a cephalosporin. Despite the β-lactam ring common to both families of drugs, cross-sensitivity between the agents is only occasionally observed. Finally, the cephalosporins may be indicated when antibacterial sensitivities suggest that they are the drugs of choice.

Four parenteral and three oral cephalosporins are currently available for use. Cephalothin and cephapirin are both rapidly excreted by the kidneys after parenteral administration. Cephaloridine and cefazolin are less rapidly excreted, and adequate levels persist for 8 to 12 hours after intravenous or intramuscular use. Cephaloglycin is available for oral use but is so poorly absorbed that only urinary levels are antibacterial. Cephalexin and cephradine are well absorbed, and very substantial blood levels are achieved.

Allergic reactions with the cephalosporins are relatively infrequent and usually take the form of cutaneous reactions. A recent study suggests that high-dose prolonged parenteral cephalosporin therapy can cause a systemic illness characterized by malaise, fatigue, and a "serum sickness-like syndrome" [12]. Cephaloridine and, to a lesser extent, cephalothin have been associated with renal insufficiency. Clinical experience with cephapirin and cefazolin has not yet documented any harmful effects on renal function. The wide spectrum of all the cephalosporins results in profound disturbances of normal flora, and overgrowth with resistant, potentially dangerous pathogens, particularly *P. aeruginosa* and *C. albicans,* may be a serious outcome of therapy.

ERYTHROMYCINS AND LINCOMYCINS

The erythromycins belong to the macrolide antibiotics, a group of drugs consisting of a lactone ring with attached deoxy sugars. A number of macrolide antimicrobials have been marketed (e.g., oleandomycin and trioleandomycin), but the erythromycins are the only ones with current clinical significance. Lincomycin and its analogue, clindamycin, are structurally not macrolides, but they otherwise resemble this group of compounds. The mechanism of action involves the binding of the compound to the 50S subunit of ribosomes with inhibition of polypeptide synthesis in the ribosomal complex.

Erythromycin absorption is enhanced by its combination with stearate or estolate. The antibacterial spectrum of erythromycins includes most gram-positive cocci. In addition, they are effective against *Mycoplasma pneumoniae*. Erythromycin-resistant *Staph. aureus* organisms have become a problem in some hospitals. Fortunately, they are rare outside the hospital environment.

The erythromycins infrequently cause allergic reactions. Erythromycin estolate is associated with idiosyncrasy characterized by a cholestatic jaundice which mimics acute cholecystitis. This reaction reverses when the drug is stopped. Erythromycin is also often the cause of epigastric distress, nausea, and vomiting. Although several preparations are available for parenteral use, pain on injection and phlebitis are so common that it is usually advisable to select other antimicrobial agents for parenteral use.

Lincomycin and clindamycin share the antibacterial spectrum of the erythromycin. In addition, they are effective against anaerobic gram-negative rods (*Bacteroides* species). Clindamycin has a definitive advantage in absorption and antimicrobial effectiveness over lincomycin and has essentially replaced it.

Clindamycin is well absorbed after oral administration even in the nonfasting state. A parenteral preparation can be given either intravenously or intramuscularly. Since cardiac arrhythmia may occur if the drug is given as a rapid infusion, it should be infused over at least 30 minutes.

Erythromycin is an effective alternate choice to penicillins in patients with gram-positive cutaneous infections. Clindamycin may be preferable to erythromycin in patients with recurrent staphylococcal infections and in patients with osteomyelitis if a penicillin is contraindicated or ineffective. Clindamycin is an effective drug in anaerobic infections originating from the gastrointestinal tract or the female genital tract.

Clindamycin occasionally causes a skin rash. A more serious side-effect is diarrhea, which occurs in about 10 percent of patients. This may lead to an acute severe, sometimes fatal, pseudomembranous colitis [13].

THE AMINOGLYCOSIDES AND POLYMYXINS

The aminoglycosides are a closely related group of antimicrobial agents effective against aerobic gram-negative organisms. Highly charged polar agents, they form stable salts and are usually marketed as the sulfate salt. Each drug is a complex of different sugars with amino groups. Streptomycin was the first antimicrobial agent with significant effect against gram-negative rods. Unfortunately, the rapid emergence of resistant organisms limited its usefulness, and, except for its value in combination with other agents in the treatment of tuberculosis, it is seldom indicated in current medical practice. Neomycin is sufficiently toxic on parenteral administration so that it is used only topically. Kanamycin and gentamicin are currently the most frequently prescribed parenteral aminoglycosides. They both have a broad range of activity against most aerobic gram-negative organisms, and gentamicin includes *P. aeruginosa* in its antibacterial spectrum.

Aminoglycosides have many features in common. None are absorbed to any extent after oral ingestion, and they must be administered parenterally to treat systemic infection. Bacterial death results from misreading of the genetic code with the production of defective progeny. All the aminoglycosides have two important toxic effects: (1) Damage can occur to renal tubular epithelium with an impairment in renal function. (2) The cochlear structure is susceptible to injury resulting in high-tone deafness or an impairment of balance. Hypersensitivity phenomena and skin rashes occur frequently with the aminoglycosides. During surgical procedures one must be cognizant of the curare-like effect of these drugs, which can be additive, with the anesthetic agents potentiating neuromuscular blockade.

The aminoglycosides are now the therapy of choice in serious aerobic gram-negative rod infections. This includes invasive pyelonephritis, cholangitis, burn wound sepsis, gram-negative pneumonia, and aerobic infection arising from gut flora. Although gentamicin is several times more potent than kanamycin, its therapeutic ratio is similar. However, for the patient in whom *P. aeruginosa* is a potential pathogen, gentamicin becomes the aminoglycoside of first choice.

Aminoglycosides are all primarily excreted by the kidney. In the presence of any degree of renal impairment there is accumulation with increased potential for toxicity. Although rough guidelines are available to modify either the dose given or the time interval between doses, direct measurement of serum antibiotic concentration is necessary to validate the correctness of the dosage schedule. In particular, in patients with changing renal function and severe infection, serum aminoglycoside determinations should be obtained daily.

All aminoglycosides have been used from time to time orally as agents to suppress aerobic gram-negative gut flora prior to operative procedures or in patients with hepatic coma.

The polymyxins are cationic detergents that interfere with bacterial metabolism by disorientation of the lipoprotein membrane. They are bactericidal. Their antibacterial spectrum is limited to gram-negative organisms, and prior to the introduction of gentamicin and carbenicillin they were the therapy of choice for *P. aeruginosa* infections. Because both neurotoxicity and nephrotoxicity occur, their use is limited to patients with *P. aeruginosa* resistant to carbenicillin and gentamicin.

THE SULFONAMIDES

The sulfonamides remain optimal therapy for most patients with urinary infection, despite 40 years of use, an antimicrobial spectrum limited primarily to aerobic gram-negative rods, and a bacteriostatic mechanism of action. Drug rashes and fever occur in 2 to 4 percent of patients. Granulocytopenia and erythema multiforme are less frequently seen. Although numerous soluble, rapidly excreted sulfonamides are on the market, there is little to choose between them.

A significant new therapeutic advance is a combination of a sulfonamide, sulfamethoxazole, with the pyrimidine analogue trimethoprim. Together they act synergistically to retard folic acid synthesis in the bacterial cell, the sulfonamide by competitively antagonizing the conversion of para-aminobenzoic acid to folic acid, and trimethoprim by blocking the enzyme dihydrofolate reductase [9]. This combination is bactericidal for most aerobic gram-negative rods except *P. aeruginosa*. Trimethoprim has remarkably little affinity for the corresponding mammalian enzyme, so its use is rarely associated with folic acid deficiency. At present the major therapeutic indication for this drug is persistent urinary infection refractory to more conventional therapy.

TETRACYCLINES

This group of antimicrobial agents was introduced into clinical medicine in 1948. The drugs were the first "broad-spectrum" antimicrobial agents in that they were effective against not only bacteria but also *Chlamydia*, *Rickettsia*, and *Mycoplasma*. The tetracyclines are derivatives of polycyclic naphthacenecarboxamide. They bind specifically to 30S ribosomes and prevent access of transfer RNA. Although a number of tetracyclines are now available, their properties are similar. They are essentially all bacteriostatic, inhibiting bacterial growth but not killing organisms in readily achievable concentrations.

Chlortetracycline, oxytetracycline, and tetracycline were initially available for both oral and parenteral use. Demethylchlortetracycline, methacycline, doxycycline, and minocycline are low-dose modifications of tetracyclines which can be given less frequently and still achieve satisfactory blood levels.

The antimicrobial spectrum of the tetracyclines includes both gram-positive and gram-negative bacteria. *P. aeruginosa* and most strains of *Proteus* are innately resistant. Over the years many organisms have developed resistance to the tetracyclines, and in the hospital setting many strains are now resistant.

The tetracyclines rarely cause allergic reactions. However, they all may produce gastrointestinal irritation with epigastric distress, vomiting, or diarrhea. Phlebitis often follows intravenous administration. Several tetracycline preparations have also been shown to cause a phototoxic reaction. More serious side-effects are seen in patients with renal impairment, who rapidly become more azotemic. The tetracyclines are also responsible for hepatic injury, particularly in pregnant patients. This appears to be dose related and rarely occurs in patients receiving less than 2 gm per day. Tetracyclines are chelated to a calcium orthophosphate complex and are deposited in the skeleton and teeth of the human fetus and infant. In the teeth the result is a brown discoloration. Because of these untoward effects, tetracyclines are not prescribed during pregnancy or the first eight years of life. The wide antibacterial spectrum of the tetracyclines can account for major changes in the host ecology during a course of therapy, leading to superinfections, especially with *C. albicans* and tetracycline-resistant staphylococci.

CHLORAMPHENICOL

Chloramphenicol has an antibacterial spectrum similar to that of the tetracyclines. Its mechanism of action is primarily on the 50S ribosome, preventing the binding of RNA.

Chloramphenicol is readily absorbed from the gastrointestinal tract and metabolized in the liver by glucuronyl transferase.

Allergic reactions are relatively uncommon with chloramphenicol. The most important and dramatic side-effect is bone marrow aplasia secondary to a presumed idiosyncrasy. Although this risk is small, it is usually fatal and has resulted in sharply circumscribed indications for chloramphenicol. Chloramphenicol should be used only if no alternative agent is effective, and repeated courses should be avoided. Many patients on chloramphenicol do develop anemia secondary to the direct toxic effects of chloramphenicol on the bone marrow. This transient suppression of bone marrow function recovers rapidly when the drug is stopped.

TOPICAL ANTIMICROBIALS

Topical antimicrobial therapy is widely used for superficial infection. Evidence of its efficacy in many clinical situations is sparse, and in at least one skin infection, streptococcal impetigo, systemic therapy is more effective than locally applied antibiotics [7]. The prophylactic value of topical antimicrobial therapy has been well documented in burns, and it is often used in other situations involving widespread skin injury. Antimicrobials applied topically can be potent cutaneous allergens. Administration of gentamicin over a large surface area for a prolonged time can lead to auditory toxicity.

ANTIMICROBIAL COMBINATIONS

Despite the popularity of antimicrobial mixtures in treating infection the combined use of two or more agents is indicated in only a few specific situations: under conditions of life-threatening sepsis of unknown etiology, in the presence of mixed infections, particularly those arising from gut flora, and in neutropenic patients. Multiple drugs are routinely used in tuberculosis to prevent the emergence of resistant *Microbacterium tuberculosis*, but this appears to be almost a unique example. True antibacterial synergy, or a state in which two drugs together are more effective than their combined action, is seldom of clinical significance. An exception is the synergy of streptomycin and penicillin in group D streptococcal infection. The disadvantages of combined therapy include increased cost, more frequent untoward reactions (particularly serious alterations of bacterial ecology with resulting superinfection), and antibacterial antagonism. Classically antagonism between two agents is said to occur when a bactericidal agent is combined with a bacteriostatic agent. Although this appears to be an uncommon event in clinical use, combination of bacteriostatic and bactericidal drugs should be avoided unless very specific indications exist for each.

ANTIMICROBIAL PROPHYLAXIS

Antimicrobial prophylaxis of infection during surgical procedures has been in vogue intermittently since the advent of antibiotics. Indiscriminate use with haphazard administration has resulted in an overall negative impression of their efficacy in preventing postoperative infection. However, recent demonstration of the host's response to bacterial infection during surgery has emphasized the importance of natural resistance to bacterial contamination of tissues [6]. The outcome of the interaction between the host and contaminating bacteria with regard to the occurrence of infection is decided within hours of tissue contamination, and experimental evidence suggests that this can be altered in favor of the host by the presence of antimicrobial activity in the tissue when contamination occurs [5]. Therapy need not be prolonged following the procedure unless major contamination of tissue has taken place. Patients with significant alteration in host resistance may benefit from this kind of selective, preventive antimicrobial therapy.

ANTISEPTICS AND DISINFECTANTS

The reduction of bacterial counts on the hands of the surgeon and the skin of the patient prior to operation is routinely accepted as essential to patient care. The phenolic hexachlorophene, despite its effectiveness against *Staph. aureus*, has fallen into disfavor because of its proved central nervous system toxicity following long-term use in neonates and its lack of effectiveness against most gram-negative rods. A two-minute 70% alcohol rinse following a scrub with soap or detergent is a well-established effective procedure. Povidone-iodine, an aqueous iodine preparation, is a satisfactory alternative for preoperative scrubbing. Chlorhexidine, in a 4% detergent solution, is a well-tolerated disinfectant with wide antibacterial activity against both gram-positive and gram-negative organisms. Residual activity persists and accumulates with repeated use. Allergic effects and toxicity have not been a problem to date [11].

GENERAL REFERENCES

1. Cluff, L. E., and Johnson, E. J. *Clinical Concepts of Infectious Diseases.* Baltimore: Williams & Wilkins, 1972.
2. Goodman, L. S., and Gilman, A. *The Pharmacological Basis of Therapeutics* (5th ed.). New York: Macmillan, 1975.
3. Hoeprich, P. D. *Hoeprich's Infectious Diseases: A Guide to the Understanding and Management of Infectious Processes.* New York: Harper & Row, 1972.
4. Top, F. H., and Wehrle, P. F. *Communicable and Infectious Diseases* (7th ed.). St. Louis: Mosby, 1972.

SPECIFIC REFERENCES

5. Burke, J. F. Effective period of antibiotic action in experimental incisions and dermal lesions. *Surgery* 50:161, 1961.
6. Burke, J. F. Preventive antibiotic management in surgery. *Annu. Rev. Med.* 24:289, 1973.
7. Dillon, H. C., Jr. The treatment of streptococcal skin infection. *J. Pediatr.* 76:676, 1970.
8. Ericsson, H. M., and Sherris, J. C. Antibiotic sensitivity testing. Report of an international collaborative study. *Acta Pathol. Microbiol. Scand.* S217:1–90, 1971.
9. Grunberg, E. The effect of trimethoprim on the activity of sulfonamides and antibiotics in experimental infections. *J. Infect. Dis.* S478:130, 1973.
10. Levine, B. B. Immunologic mecha-

nisms of penicillin allergy. A haptenic model system for the study of allergic diseases of man. *N. Engl. J. Med.* 27:1115, 1966.

11. Lowbury, E. J. L., and Lilly, H. A.   Use of 4% chlorhexidine detergent solution (Hibiscrub) and other methods of skin disinfection. *Br. Med. J.* 1:510, 1973.

12. Sanders, W. E., Jr., Johnson, J. E., III, and Taggart, J. G.   Adverse reactions to cephalothin and cephapirin. Uniform occurrence on prolonged intravenous administration of high doses. *N Engl. J. Med.* 290:424, 1974.

13. Tedesco, F. J., Barton, R. W., and Alpers, D. H.   Clindamycin-associated colitis. A prospective study. *Ann. Intern. Med.* 84:429, 1974.

8

Trauma by Physical Agents

Any agent which interacts with tissue in such a manner that the tissues are left injured is a candidate for discussion in this chapter. Thus a whole host of agents could potentially be considered along with the pathological conditions they leave in their path. A veritable textbook of pathology would result instead of a single chapter if one were to consider solar energy, invasion by microorganisms, mechanical trauma, and deprivation of tissues of blood supply, to mention a few.

Discussion is limited, therefore, to those agents of particular interest to the reconstructive surgeon: heat, cold, electricity, radiation, and chemicals—the latter being restricted to acids and alkali.

These agents have systemic effects on the body as well as local effects. Either type of effect may be a common effect (i.e., one that follows no matter which agent it is) or an effect due to the specific agent (i.e., characteristic of that agent). Similarly, effects may be considered on a histological versus a biochemical level and finally in a time relationship (i.e., early [acute], intermediate, or late [chronic]).

COMMON SYSTEMIC AND LOCAL EFFECTS

LARS M. VISTNES

SYSTEMIC EFFECTS

The systemic effects caused by the agents under discussion are in direct proportion to the magnitude of exposure of the organism to the agent. Thus, the burning of a finger on a hot stove, the exposure to the radiation needed to get a chest film, or the electrical spark from a small battery is not sufficient to cause an observable or measurable general effect. Contrariwise, no one would question the far-reaching and devastating general effects produced by massive radiation or by an extensive body burn. Common systemic effects of these agents or any other form of trauma are essentially those of the organism going into shock. There is increased activity of the sympathetic nervous system with release of circulating epinephrine and norepinephrine as well as a rapidly increased rate of release of adrenal corticosteroids. The latter have secondary effects at vascular regions remote from the area of trauma, besides affecting small vessel changes in the area of injury.

In addition to being responsible for rapidly induced defects in both the cellular and humoral immune response, the same adrenal corticosteroids have been implicated in the acute gastrointestinal ulcers that may occur in situations of physical stress (e.g., in burns: Curling's ulcers). The sympathetic overactivity with its accompanying general vasoconstriction reduces circulating blood volume (which is worsened by the loss of plasma into locally injured tissue). Jointly, these components result in reduced blood flow to the damaged area as well as the area surrounding it, with decreased nutrition, a change from aerobic to anaerobic metabolism (the product of which is lactic acid), and generalized acidosis. Most of the agents under discussion change the skin in such a way that its ability to act as a vapor barrier is altered by destroying a water-holding lipid in the stratum corneum [5]. With the subsequent increase in water loss, the vaporization process requires an energy expenditure drawn from endogenous source calories which is associated with a markedly increased metabolic rate. Massive problems in terms of protein and calorie balance then arise [10].

Similarly, because the damaged skin contains much of the body's collagen, which by virtue of the injury becomes denatured, protein metabolism is considerably altered as the body attempts to clear itself of protein debris [5].

Finally, there is inhibition of insulin production, leading to both inefficient glycogen mobilization and inefficient glucose utilization at the cellular level [5]. Although the detailed local wound situation will be dealt with later, it must be mentioned here because of its systemic implications that the injured

cells will leak potassium, allowing sodium to enter in exchange. Thus the wound becomes a repository for sodium drawn from the plasma, and the kidney is presented with a large load of potassium derived from the wound. This potassium must be excreted in the distal tubule in direct competition with hydrogen. As potassium is excreted, hydrogen must be retained, thus aggravating the metabolic acidosis already started by the reduced tissue perfusion.

All these processes, added to and augmented by the effects of local tissue damage to be discussed below, produce the clinical picture we know as shock. This is evidenced on a histological level as a reduction in velocity of flow of the formed elements of the blood, in both arterioles and venules, in uninjured tissue. The effect is noted as early as five to seven minutes following injury, along with a simultaneous reduction in lumen of the vessels, all indicative of early traumatic shock [2]. Brånemark theorizes that the local damage with its microvascular changes leads to simultaneous increase of permeability of intestinal capillaries. The latter causes absorption of endotoxins into the general circulation, which in turn leads to systemic microvascular disturbances, including further injury in the area of initial trauma. A vicious cycle is thus established, leading to ultimate shock [2]. (For further information on shock, see Chapter 10.)

Trauma to tissue by the etiological agents discussed (and by other means, including mechanical trauma) will cause damage to vascular endothelium and thereby give rise to increased permeability of the vessel wall. This results in the extravascular loss of the protein fractions of the serum. Smaller molecules (albumin and gamma globulin) will leave first, so that the relative intravascular fibrinogen concentration is increased. Circulating proteins from the area of injury, denatured by the injury, tend to precipitate on the surface of erythrocytes, thereby causing red blood cell aggregation and a tendency toward greater blood viscosity [13]. The latter, along with increase in plasma protein concentration, also occurs because water and electrolytes are lost into the massive wound more rapidly than are plasma proteins. Nevertheless, proteins too are lost from the plasma into the area of tissue damage, heavily contributing to the clinical shock seen in these injuries if massive and untreated. The combined loss from the intravascular compartment of fluid and proteins results in decreased circulating plasma volume [1]. The organism tries to compensate by drawing fluid from the extracellular spaces of undamaged areas, by vasoconstriction, especially of skin and gut, and by drawing fluid from the gut.

The object of treatment, not within the scope of this discussion is obviously to reverse all these tendencies and to replace what has already been lost. (See Chapter 9.)

LOCAL EFFECTS

Just as the body exhibited a systemic response to injury away from the area of injury, so there is also a marked local response. The tissues still alive modify their physiological responses in such a way that plasma and leukocytes can enter the injured tissue. This is known as *acute inflammation*, a process that continues as long as damage to the tissue continues [12]. Following removal of the agent producing damage, necrotic tissue and debris are removed by phagocytic cells, and healing may then take place.

If, on the other hand, the injury has been sufficiently severe to destroy tissue completely, there is no inflammatory response in the tissue destroyed, because inflammation by definition is "the reaction of vascular and supporting elements of a tissue to injury, resulting in the formation of a protein-rich exudate" [12]. In such a case, the inflammatory response is seen at the junction of viable and destroyed tissue [11].

Thus, the common effect of the agents being discussed is acute inflammation. The changes are related predominantly to the vascular response and to edema and exudation.

Normally, in uninjured tissue, there is free flow in all vessels with good mixing of blood from anastomosing vessels. Red cells are well segregated, and white cells do not adhere to the walls of the vessels [9]. The cellular elements occupy the center of the stream, with a peripheral plasma zone.

Upon injury, there is an initial and very short-lived vasoconstriction in the microvasculature, followed in short order by vasodilatation, which lasts as long as the injury continues [12]. Lewis postulated that this vascular response is caused by histamine liberated from damaged cells, or if not, that at least histamine is an important factor [8]. This hypothesis has held up through the years, although the nervous system is also felt to play some part [14].

With injury, as soon as vasodilatation occurs, blood flow slows down. The character of the stream changes by virtue of the fact that white cells move to the peripheral plasma zone. An increase in the total number of granulocytes is seen. All the formed elements of the blood tend to adhere to the vessel wall. In the small vessels, a combination of platelets and fibrin may form microthrombi, which adhere to the walls and either partly or completely occlude the lumen [2]. This phenomenon is enhanced because endothelial cells become swollen and covered with a sticky, gelatinous material [12]. The granulocytes that become trapped along this lining are disrupted, and the granules (histamine containing) are liberated and cause tissue destruction. Accordingly, there is endothelial wall disruption with leakage of plasma into the extravascular tissues [9]. If the disruption is sufficiently severe, there is also loss of red cells (microhemorrhage). Loss of plasma from the blood increases viscosity, which aggravates stasis, sometimes leading to complete thrombosis.

With endothelial wall damage and continued loss of plasma into the tissues, the feature most characteristic of acute inflammation appears: a fluid exudate with or without a cellular component. Unlike normal interstitial fluid, this exudate has a high fibrin content and a low specific gravity, and contained fibrinogen leads to easy clot formation [12].

In addition to allowing passage of plasma proteins and red cells, the damaged vessel wall permits passage of white cells, but whereas the passage of plasma occurs largely by virtue of differences in hydrostatic and osmotic pressures, and red cell passage by virtue of diapedesis, white cell passage takes place actively by ameboid action. The white cells are seen to push through the gaps between the damaged endothelial cells [3]. Following exit, the white cells move toward the area of tissue damage, another significant feature of an acute inflammatory response.

Probably as a result of the plasma leakage, the level of soluble proteins in damaged tissue rises, probably because the ability of injured tissue to synthesize protein is reduced. Similarly, there are significant increases in concentration of lysosomal enzymes in both skin and muscle, thought to be due to enzyme activation, on the cellular level one of the earliest responses to injury [7]. All these changes are reflected in corresponding changes in the lymph draining the injured area.

When the tissue damaged is skin, the grossly visible result of the foregoing microscopical pathophysiological changes is blister formation. Intercellular edema, along with separation of the junction between dermis and epidermis, is believed to be responsible for the blistering [4, 11]. The blister fluid itself is thought to be a transudate originating from the capillary network in the papillary dermis. Heat loss from skin thus injured is considerable. Evaporation of water from an unruptured blister is twice that from normal skin. When the blister has ruptured, the evaporation is increased 10-fold, a powerful argument against early deliberate rupture. Another argument is that epithelialization under the blister is more rapid. By the same token, a deeper injury resulting in a dry eschar showed a water loss nearly 20 times that of normal skin [6].

Common local reaction on a cellular level

to heat, cold, chemical, and electrical injuries is coagulative tissue necrosis [4]. Cellular changes in skin and its appendages include nuclear pyknosis with a perinuclear halo effect, disruption of sebaceous glands, and a condensation of sweat glands, particularly eccrine glands [11]. Necrotic collagen fibers are seen to fuse, and there is refractile eosinophilia. Ultrastructurally, swelling of endoplasmic reticulum, fragmentation of the cell membrane, necrosis of endothelial cells, and exposure of the basement membrane take place [4].

REFERENCES

1. Artz, C. P., and Moncrief, J. A. *The Treatment of Burns.* Philadelphia: Saunders, 1969.
2. Brånemark, P. I., Breine, U., Joshi, M., and Urbaschek, B. Microvascular pathophysiology of burned tissue. *Ann. N.Y. Acad. Sci.* 150:475, 1968.
3. Florey, H. W., and Grant, L. H. Leucocyte migration from small blood vessels stimulated with ultraviolet light: An electron microscope study. *J. Pathol. Bacteriol.* 82:13, 1961.
4. Foley, F. D. Pathology of cutaneous burns. *Surg. Clin. North Am.* 50:6, 1970.
5. Jelenko, C., III. Systemic response to burn injury: A survey of some current concepts. *J. Trauma* 10:10, 1970.
6. Lamke, L. O., and Liljedahl, S. O. Evaporative water loss from burns, grafts and donor sites. *Scand. J. Plast. Reconstr. Surg.* 5:17, 1971.
7. Lewis, G. P., Lowe, T. J., White, A. M., and Worthington, J. Biochemical changes in skin and muscle after thermal injury. *Br. J. Exp. Pathol.* 51:7, 1970.
8. Lewis, T. *The Blood Vessels of Human Skin and Their Response.* London: Shaw, 1927.
9. Schoen, R. E., Wells, C. H., and Kolmen, S. N. Viscometric and microcirculatory observations following flame injury. *J. Trauma* 11:7, 1971.
10. Thomson, A. E. Conjoint Burn Conference. University of Manitoba, Winnipeg, Canada, March 12, 1971. Unpublished.

11. Vistnes, L. M., and Hogg, G. A. The burn eschar: A histopathological study. *Plast. Reconstr. Surg.* 48:56, 1971.
12. Walter, J. B., and Israel, M. S. *General Pathology* (3rd ed.). London: Churchill, 1970.
13. Weatherley-White, R. C. A., Knize, D. M.,

Geisterfer, D. J., and Paton, B. C. Experimental studies in cold injury: V. Circulatory hemodynamics. *Surgery* 66:1, 1969.
14. Zweifach, B. W., Grant, L., and McClusky, R. T. *The Inflammatory Process.* New York: Academic, 1965.

COLD INJURIES

LARS M. VISTNES

SYSTEMIC EFFECT

The systemic effect of cold injury varies somewhat depending on the method of exposure. If an individual gets his feet wet in cold weather and walks to his shelter in below zero temperature, he is likely to get his feet frostbitten. Similarly, if he loses his gloves or gets them wet, he is likely to get his fingers frozen. The systemic effect of such an injury is no different from what has already been described as *common effects*. If, however, the entire person falls through the ice or even when dry is exposed to prolonged low temperatures, the situation is changed. Even though only his feet and hands may become frozen, the effects of which are still the same as before, certain systemic effects specific to the results of exposure of the entire organism to the cold are *added* to these effects. They are generally those of hypothermia, a complex series of events beyond the scope of the present chapter. The reader interested in pursuing the subject is referred to the hundreds of articles appearing each year in the literature, listed in *Index Medicus* under Cold and Hypothermia.

LOCAL EFFECTS

Changes specifically associated with cold injury in the exposed area are (1) hemodynamic changes and (2) changes in protein synthesis.

The hemodynamic alterations take place on the basis of physiological responses as well as being secondary to changes in vessel flow (rheologic). Before there is any actual injury, but as progressive cooling takes place, the rate of circulation through the tissue being cooled increases. Presumably a physiological attempt at temperature regulation [12], this compensatory "rewarming response" mechanism has never been explained to everyone's satisfaction. If the mechanism fails, however, the tissue has now lost its last protective measure, and tissue temperature falls rapidly until it is the same as that of its surroundings. As the temperature falls, there is a progressive parallel decrease in blood flow, until at the time of actual freezing the latter completely stops. Another explanation of events is that rapid vasoconstriction occurs in skin vessels on exposure to cold, with reduction in blood flow in order to diminish heat loss and conserve body temperature. This vasoconstriction is the result of a stimulus from the vasomotor center which initiates the direct and continuous stimulation to the vessels in response to two stimuli: (1) cooled blood reaching the center and (2) afferent impulses from the cooled area. The resulting decrease in blood flow in the cooled part makes a fall in temperature inevitable, and a vicious cycle is established [2, 3, 10]. The latter explanation seems more tenable as it embodies the principle often found in nature: sacrifice of the part in order to salvage the organism as a whole.

The factors already enumerated under general effects are in operation as well: alterations in plasma proteins, circulation of protein breakdown products, and erythrocyte aggregation enhanced by relative increase in fibrinogen concentration caused by loss of albumin [4, 12].

When the frozen part is rewarmed by the application of external heat, arterial flow returns rapidly and becomes stabilized at a rate actually greater than the preinjury flow. This return, however, is transient, because tissues damaged by freezing have been found to be excluded from circulation by vascular occlusion as early as 30 minutes after rewarming [12]. Clinically seen as a promising return of flow with a bright pink part having sensation at first, it is followed by sharp demarcation with dry gangrene of the most distal part as time progresses. Just as no two species of animals or plants have the same resistance to freezing, so different cells and tissues within the same organism differ in their resistance to low temperature [1]. The total effect of freezing temperatures is a combination of temperature, time, and space, a relationship Rinfret has termed the *thermal history* of the tissue involved [8].

Similarly, the rate of freezing as well as the rate of thawing will affect the eventual viability or destruction of the cells. With slow cooling, there is formation of large ice crystals in the intercellular spaces. As rate of freezing accelerates, ice crystals are also formed within the cell [6]. The extracellular ice formation causes minimal cell injury on a mechanical basis [7] whereas the intracellular formation is far more deleterious to cell survival, involving chromosomal injury [9].

Because of a gradient in vapor pressure created between cytoplasm and intercellular spaces by ice crystal formation, water migrates across the cell membrane, resulting in cell dehydration and intracellular electrolyte concentration. Many investigators regard the latter as a significant factor in ultimate cell death [13]. Slow thawing is more harmful to tissue than rapid thawing because it exposes the cells to concentrated electrolytes for a longer period of time. There is, in fact, indica-

tion that thawing may be more harmful than freezing [5].

These facts have a significant bearing both on the clinical management of frostbite and on the technique of cryosurgery, in which cold is used in deliberate tissue destruction. In the former, the recommendation of rapid rewarming becomes valid as well as the warning never to thaw a frozen part until the patient can be kept permanently warm. If a part were thawed as an emergency measure and refrozen during transportation to a permanent medical facility, greater damage would occur than if it were kept frozen. Similarly, this double freeze-thaw cycle and its added tissue damage is taken advantage of in cryosurgery [11, 13].

REFERENCES

1. Cameron, G. G., and Mehrotra, R. M. L. Differences in the response to injury in various tissues. *J. Pathol. Bacteriol.* 65:1, 1953.
2. Fuhram, F. A., and Crimson, J. M. Studies on gangrene following cold injury: I. A method for producing gangrene by means of controlled injury by cold. *J. Clin. Invest.* 26:229, 1947.
3. Jarrett, J. R., and Paletta, F. X. Cold injury. *Mo. Med.* 67:3, 1970.
4. Laiho, K., and Hirvonen, J. Reactions of the guinea pig's skin and adipose tissue to experimental frostbite. *Acta Pathol. Microbiol. Scand.* [A] 79:91, 1971.
5. Mazur, P. Physical and Chemical Basis of Injury in Single-Celled Microorganisms Subjected to Freezing and Thawing. In Merryman, H. T. (Ed.), *Cryobiology.* New York: Academic, 1966. P. 250.
6. Merryman, H. T. Mechanics of freezing in living cells and tissues. *Science* 124:124, 1956.
7. Merryman, H. T. Review of Biological Freezing. In Merryman, H. T. (Ed.), *Cryobiology.* New York: Academic, 1966. P. 48.
8. Rinfret, A. P. Thermal history. *Cryobiology* 2:171, 1966.
9. Sherman, J. K., and Kim, K. S.

Freeze-thaw induced ultrastructural alterations of chromosomes following intracellular ice formation. *Cryobiology* 3:367, 1967.

10. Sjostrom, B., Weatherley-White, R. C. A., and Paton, B. C. Experimental studies in cold injury: I. The individual response to a standard cold environment. *J. Surg. Res.* 4:12, 1964.

11. Vistnes, L. M., Harris, D. R., and

Fajardo, L. Evaluation of cryosurgery of basal cell carcinoma. *Plast. Reconstr. Surg.* 55:71, 1975.

12. Weatherley-White, R. C. A., Knize, D. M., Geisterfer, D. J., and Paton, B. C. Experimental studies in cold injury: V. Circulatory hemodynamics. *Surgery* 66:1, 1969.

13. Zacarian, S. A. *Cryosurgery of Skin Cancer.* Springfield, Ill.: Thomas, 1969.

ELECTRICAL INJURIES

LARS M. VISTNES AND RONALD P. GRUBER

SYSTEMIC EFFECTS

During Benjamin Franklin's numerous experiments to prove that lightning was a form of electricity, he suffered two severe electrical shocks resulting in unconsciousness. Such an instantaneous result on exposure to electricity makes this agent unique among the agents discussed here. In many instances, because of the peculiar nature of electricity, it is indeed difficult to separate local effects from systemic ones.

Ohm's law states that the current in any electrical system as measured in amperes (I) is related to the voltage (V) and resistance (R, measured in ohms), as follows: $I = V/R$. Resistance, voltage, and current always play a part in any electrical injury, and their relationship must not be forgotten. It is conveniently remembered as Ohm's triangle:

in which the function of any covered letter is expressed as the visual relationship between the remaining two: for example, $V = I \cdot R$ or $R = V/I$.

The severity of damage to an organism exposed to electricity depends on (1) duration of contact, (2) voltage, (3) type of contact (AC or DC), (4) resistance of body tissues, (5) pathway of the electricity through the body, and (6) grounding [11]. Duration and voltage are probably the main factors. Type of current is also important, however. AC (alternating current) is in effect an on-and-off electrical shock that occurs 120 times per second. It results in tetanization of the muscles causing the victim to freeze to the contact point, prolonging the duration of contact. Whereas AC tends to be dangerous at lower voltage, DC is more dangerous at the high voltages. The reason for this discrepancy has not been explained. Resistance in the body is obviously a major factor when the body is the conductor of current. Thus, a dry hand is much more resistant to the passage of electricity than a wet hand. Specific tissues have their own resistance, as follows (in decreasing order of resistance): (1) bone, (2) fat, tendon, and skin, (3) brain, (4) muscle, (5) mucous membrane, and (6) blood vessel and nerve. It is of interest that a tissue with low resistance (a good conductor) permits the rapid passage of electricity and therefore suffers little of the electrical effect locally. Tissues that conduct poorly (have high resistance) do suffer the consequences. For example, since bone is highly resistant, it is readily damaged by electrical current. Blood vessels and nerves, on the other hand, although offering little resistance and hence allowing rapid flow of electricity, are still *very sensitive* to electrical effects. Probably the explanation is that the body itself is a complex electrical system (the "man-instrument system") [3] with neuromuscular synapses, etc., which are easily upset. As it happens, the tissues that are designed to carry the normal action potentials with ease are also the ones that carry accidental bursts with least resistance. Such accidental conduction is achieved with less cellular (anatomical) damage than occurs in tissues with high resistance, but with greater physiological (functional) upset. Consequently, the tissues offering the least resistance are still most easily damaged functionally by electrical currents despite their low resistance, at first an apparent paradox.

The pathway taken by electricity through the body also determines the severity of the injury [2]. On a path from the left hand to the right hand, electricity is likely to pass through the heart, causing an arrhythmia and even cardiac arrest. Passing from the left hand to the right foot, the electricity may go through various viscera and injure them. The pathway is not predictable unless one part of the body is grounded, in which case the pathway is from point of contact to point of grounding via the tissues of least resistance.

Most electrical injuries will be found as damage to the extremities, even if the current has passed through the thorax or abdomen. The rare occurrence of damage to the thorax and abdomen is in large part due to the "current density" phenomenon. As electricity enters one of the extremities, it passes through a protoplasmic structure of relatively small diameter. As it reaches the thorax and abdomen, however, the current diffuses to encompass the entire diameter of the thorax and abdomen. The current density, therefore, decreases and its overall net effect is a dilution of electrical energy throughout the body. It is well to remember that when grounding is proper and resistance to electricity lower there may be no local tissue damage whatever and yet the setup may be fatal. For example, a man in a bathtub (well grounded)

who reaches for the electric switch may receive an electrical shock that is spread diffusely throughout his body and is therefore not of sufficient "concentration" to produce a local burn, but sufficient to produce ventricular fibrillation. A small child, on the other hand, who sucks on an electrical cord and is poorly grounded when he is on a rug does not have a diffuse spread of current throughout his body yet suffers a local injury to the lips.

Several properties of electricity produce an electrical injury. Arcing is a phenomenon peculiar to electricity. Ten thousand volts can produce an arc of several centimeters. Thus a potential victim does not need to touch the high-voltage wire to receive a shock. A construction worker who moves his crane to within several feet of a very high-voltage wire may still be electrocuted. Moreover, once the arc is established between the source of electricity and the contact (victim), it can be extended in length despite the victim's withdrawal from the high-voltage wire. It is also worth noting that electricity can pass along the flow of a liquid stream [8]. A young boy who urinates upon a high-voltage wire is likely to be shocked by the retrograde passage of electricity along the stream of urine to his penis. Lightning is a special form of electrical injury that is frequently fatal. Electrical injury to a person struck by lightning has been noted to be so severe that the belt buckle was melted and the electricity exploded through the ends of the feet, shattering his shoes.

Death due to electrical contact is often from ventricular fibrillation when voltage is low and from respiratory paralysis at high voltage. The minimum voltage that is still dangerous to life is 25 volts, 60 cycles per second [6]. Although no fatalities have been reported with this voltage (fatalities have been recorded above 40 volts [60 cycles]), a voltage of greater than 25 is considered potentially lethal.

When the victim survives, there is frequently renal damage, due primarily to (1) myoglobin precipitation within the tubules,

(2) shock, which in itself can cause acute tubular necrosis, or (3) direct damage to the kidney from the passage of electrical current through that organ [9]. The myoglobin precipitation within the kidney tubules is directly attributable to the fact that following muscle destruction by electricity myoglobin is released into the bloodstream. It is then precipitated within the kidney tubules in the presence of acidosis. Hemoglobin and other substances may also be precipitated within the kidney tubules, again particularly in the presence of acidosis. Some pigment, mostly myoglobin, is excreted in the urine.

Central nervous system (CNS) complications are infrequent and transient. The skull probably prevents severe CNS injuries. Permanent damage to the cord or brain is unusual. Transitory effects include paralysis and sensory losses. Even the immediate coma that follows a severe electrical shock often subsides in three to five days. Some of these effects are secondary to vascular damage to the brain and spinal cord. The pathological changes seen at autopsy are the result of permanent damage and are often said to be similar to those found in multiple sclerosis. Personality changes and permanent psychotic changes have been reported as a result of electrical injury.

Visceral changes are infrequent for the reasons stated previously. However, when they occur, they often go undetected. Fractured vertebrae are not uncommon. They result from severe muscular contraction of the body including episthotonos. Cardiac problems may be seen as well, including nonspecific ST-T wave abnormalities and cardiac arrhythmias. Cases of delayed onset of myocardial infarction due to electrical damage in preexisting myocardial disease have been reported.

The pathophysiology of electrical injuries can best be explained by the Joule effect: Electrical energy is converted to heat, and it is the heat that causes the primary damage to the tissues. The formula for this conversion is $C = KI^2RT$, where C equals calories, K is a constant, I is the current, R is resistance, and T equals time. Otherwise stated, $C = KV^2T/R$, where V represents the voltage. That is, the heat produced by electrical injuries is directly proportional to the square of the voltage, directly proportional to the duration of contact, and inversely proportional to the resistance. Most investigators today believe that the trauma from electrical injuries is the result of this conversion from electrical energy to heat.

Nerve damage, however, may not be directly due to heat injury alone. Ugland demonstrated that several changes may be produced in nerves by an electrical current that results in temperatures of 40°C or less [16]. This temperature by itself would not have any heat effects. Some of the changes seen in such electrically damaged nerves are (1) increased stimulus threshold, (2) decreased amplitude of response to supramaximal stimuli, and (3) decreased conduction velocity. The fibers that conduct most rapidly are most vulnerable. Histologically, examination of damaged nerves revealed fragmentation of the axons with fusion of the nuclei in the sheath of Schwann [4].

Serial angiographic studies have demonstrated peculiar vascular lesions related to electric injury [12]. There is a progressive occlusion of the vessels over three months. Histologically, arteritis was seen in the excised specimens, suggesting (although not proving) that the current itself produces a specific injury to vessels. In contrast to these studies, a prior study by Jaffe et al. indicated that the damage caused by an electrical current applied to the femoral vessels of animals is similar to that following dry heat applied to the same type of vessel [5]. Moreover, the damage to the vessel wall was seen only when electrical damage was severe enough to cause coagulation of the blood. It was concluded that heat damage as a result of electrical current was prevented by intact circulation and that when the heat from the electricity was sufficient to cause coagulation the continuous flow of blood was no longer able to prevent damage to the vessels. Jaffe also noted that the media was the most sensitive part of the vessel wall to electrical current. As a result of the current, fusiform aneurysms often occurred. This fact helps explain the frequently seen delayed hemorrhage of blood vessels following electrical injuries.

LOCAL EFFECTS

Three types of local surface injuries are seen: (1) an entry-exit wound, (2) an arc burn, and (3) a flame burn. The entry wound is usually where the individual makes contact; the exit wound is often in another extremity where the electricity discharges to the grounding source. The arc burn is due to the arcing of electricity from the source to the skin and may reach a temperature of 3000° to 20,000°C [1]. More often, it is in the neighborhood of 2500°C. The burn from the arc is generally more severe to the skin than that from direct contact to the source. Interestingly, however, arcing does not tend to cause muscular tetanization or the locking phenomenon as seen with lower-voltage injuries that are not associated with an arc. The flame burn is secondary to the arc burn igniting clothing. Finally, there is a "current mark," usually an insignificant wound seen adjacent to the entry wound. It is due simply to the local arcing of electricity from one portion of skin to another.

A low-voltage contact wound exhibits (1) a central charred point, (2) a gray or white surrounding area, and (3) a periphery of blood-red coagulation necrosis [13]. All three of these regions represent full-thickness loss of tissue. The wound resulting from the arc injury is a blackened epidermis—with almost a charred color to the surface of the skin. One occasionally sees subcutaneous emphysema after very severe electrical injuries. Its cause is unclear, but presumably it is due to the sudden release of heat within the tissues.

The hand is frequently involved in electrical burn cases—as much as 75 percent of the time. A characteristic finding from an electrical burn to the hand is a "clawhand" [14]. This injury is a direct result of arcing across a volar aspect of the wrist causing a severe flexion contracture.

Electrical burns to the lip are a special problem [15]. The pathophysiology of an electrical lip burn is not completely understood. Electrical resistance of the well-vascularized lip is low, and one might expect that a local injury should not occur but rather that electricity should pass through the body causing a more pronounced systemic effect such as ventricular fibrillation. Actually, fibrillation has occurred, and in some series approximately 5 percent of oral contacts with a live electrical wire resulted in death [10]. Nevertheless, a local injury is generally the rule perhaps because the individual is poorly grounded. Kazanjian and Converse hypothesized that an arcing occurs across the lip and is the prime cause of the burn near the commissure [7].

Some electrical burns are iatrogenically induced. The Bovie, if incorrectly placed beneath the patient during surgery, will cause arcing of electricity across the buttocks, resulting in a second- if not third-degree burn. This occurs quite frequently and is simply due to poor contact to the electrode. Rarely, a malfunction of a surgical diathermy can inadvertently apply a large amount of electricity to the tissues of the patient and has been known to produce complete necrosis of a lower extremity [6].

REFERENCES

1. Baxter, C. R. Present concepts in the management of major electrical injury. *Surg. Clin. North Am.* 50:1401, 1970.
2. Brown, K. L., and Moritz, A. R. Electrical injuries. *J. Trauma* 4:608, 1964.
3. Cromwell, L., Weibell, F. J., Pfeiffer, E. A., and Usselman, L. B. *Biomedical Instrumentation and Measurements.* Englewood Cliffs, N.J.: Prentice-Hall, 1973.
4. Fischer, H. Pathological effects and sequelae of electrical accidents. *J. Occup. Med.* 7:564, 1965.
5. Jaffe, R. H., Willis, D., and Bachem, A

The effect of electric currents on the arteries. *Arch. Pathol.* 7:244, 1929.

6. Jellinek, S. The pathological changes produced in those rendered unconscious by electric shock and the treatment of such cases. *Arch. Radiol. Electrobiol.* 27:316, 1923.

7. Kazanjian, V. H., and Converse, J. M. *The Surgical Treatment of Facial Injuries.* Baltimore: Williams & Wilkins, 1959.

8. Krizek, T. J., and Ariyan, S. Severe acute radiation injuries of the hands. *Plast. Reconstr. Surg.* 51:14, 1973.

9. Malbec, E. F., and Quaife, J. V. Plastic surgery in radiation burns. *Plast. Reconstr. Surg.* 20:232, 1957.

10. Occonomopoulos, C. T. Electrical burns in infancy and early childhood. *Am. J. Dis. Child.* 103:35, 1962.

11. Peterson, R. A. Electrical Burns. In Grabb, W. C., and Smith, J. W. (Eds.), *Plastic Surgery* (2nd ed.). Boston: Little, Brown, 1973. P. 653.

12. Ponten, B., Erikson, U., Johansson, S. H., and Olding, L. New observations on tissue changes along the pathway of the current in an electrical injury. *Scand. J. Plast. Reconstr. Surg.* 4:75, 1970.

13. Skoog, T. Electrical injuries. *J. Trauma* 10:816, 1970.

14. Taylor, P. H., Pugsley, L. Q., and Vogel, E. H. The intriguing electrical burn. *J. Trauma* 2:309, 1962.

15. Thomson, H. G., Juckes, A. W., and Farmer, A. W. Electrical burns to the mouth in children. *Plast. Reconstr. Surg.* 35:466, 1965.

16. Ugland, O. M. Electrical burns, a clinical and experimental study with special reference to peripheral nerve injury. *Scand. J. Plast. Reconstr. Surg.* Suppl. 2, 1967. P. 74.

RADIATION INJURIES

RONALD P. GRUBER AND LARS M. VISTNES

Acute radiation injuries present an uncommon but important problem to the reconstructive surgeon. An understanding of elementary physics is a prerequisite for appreciation of the burn that results from an acute radiation injury. Table 8-1 indicates the various types of radiation one is likely to encounter and the depth of penetration the radiation can attain. Radiation is basically either electromagnetic or particulate [2]. Electromagnetic radiation is comprised of those forms of radiation from the electromagnetic spectrum, which include ultraviolet light. Particulate radiation involves particle radiation, such as alpha or beta particles.

Beta radiation is essentially energetic electrons. They have a penetration of only a few millimeters. Alpha radiation is radiation of helium nuclei which penetrates no more than 40 microns (the thickness of a piece of paper).

Neutrons are a form of particulate radiation with deep penetration. Among the forms of electromagnetic radiation are x-rays and gamma rays, which also penetrate deeply. The shorter the wavelength, the greater the depth of penetration. When the radiologist speaks of "soft x-rays," he is referring to longer-wavelength x-rays (deep penetration).

The amount of radiation one receives is expressed in rads. A rad is the absorbing dose, defined as 100 ergs per gram of absorbing medium. It should be emphasized that this form of measurement is in energy per *volume* of tissue. Therefore, the total body exposure following 1000 rads to the tonsillar area is not nearly as large as that following 1000 rads to the side of the neck.

The actual mechanism of damage by radiation is unclear [6]. It is hypothesized that bombardment by electrons, protons, and neutrons is associated with energy release in

TABLE 8-1. *Depth of Penetration by Various Types of Ionizing Radiation*

Type	Depth of Penetration
Electromagnetic	
1. X-ray	Deep
2. X-ray (gamma)	Deep
Particulate	
1. Alpha (helium nucleus)	40 microns
2. Beta (electron)	Few millimeters
3. Neutron	Deep

the cell. Electromagnetic waves such as x-rays accelerate either an electron or a proton within the cell that they hit, thereby causing energy release. This energy release results in ionization of water, which in turn is associated with the release of hydrogen peroxide and chemical radicals that interfere with normal enzymes. The release of histamine-type chemicals has also been postulated. It is well known that the lethal effects of such radiation are particularly intense in proliferating cells, especially those in prophase. This fact is compatible with the recently discovered sensitivity of DNA to ionizing radiation. Most important, the ionizing effect from either particulate or electromagnetic radiation is cumulative over the lifetime of the individual. Finally, the shorter the wavelength of radiation, the longer the interval prior to the onset of signs and symptoms.

SYSTEMIC EFFECTS

To better understand the effects of radiation, a brief discussion of the acute radiation syndrome is useful. A patient who has recently been exposed to acute radiation of the hand must be evaluated for total body irradiation and the possibility that he has systemic involvement from the radiation. Total body irradiation of the human body in sufficient dosage causes death by one of two mechanisms: injury to the hematopoietic system or injury to the gastrointestinal system.

The hematopoietic system is the most sensitive tissue to radiation. Damage to it results in leukopenia and, consequently, infection. The mucous membrane of the gastrointestinal tract is also sensitive to radiation, with resulting gastrointestinal hemorrhage. Table 8-2 lists five syndromes associated with acute radiation injury. Dose estimates are based on a midline total body dose exposure (not a surface dose exposure). In group I, for example, patients receiving a total dose of 150 rads are relatively asymptomatic. At 400 rads (total body dose), hematopoietic complications, including sepsis, are manifest. With 400 to 600 rads, a more severe hematopoietic syndrome ensues. It is at the latter dosage that the lethal dose, median (LD_{50}) in man is said to occur, with death in 30 days. With an exposure of 600 to 1500 rads, gastrointestinal symptoms prevail before hematopoietic symptoms can become manifest. With more than 5000 rads, cardiovascular and cerebral symptoms are severe from immediate damage to the cells. Death is imminent and not preventable.

In general, it is difficult to tell what quantity of radiation the patient has been exposed to. A great deal depends on the nature of the radiation, the duration of exposure, and knowledge of parts of the body that have been exposed. Only a careful dosimetric study can help evaluate the approximate midline total body exposure dose. As a rule, a serial absolute lymphocyte count will help predict the severity of the acute radiation illness. There is a direct correlation between the severity of lymphocytopenia and the severity of illness.

The pathological condition of an acute radiation burn is usually nonspecific. There is an obliterative endarteritis associated with progressive fibrosis and obliteration of blood vessels. It has been unclear whether the effect of cell necrosis is related to primary damage to the cells or represents secondary damage from the vascular lesion. What is important to recognize is that the pathology of the radiation effect is cumulative over a lifetime. Also,

TABLE 8-2. *Five Entities Associated with Radiation Injury*

Group No.	Clinical Manifestations	Dose Estimate (rads)	Predominant Organ System Involved
I	Mostly asymptomatic; occasional prodromal symptoms	<150	
II	Mild form of acute radiation syndrome; transient prodromal nausea and vomiting; mild laboratory and clinical evidence of hematopoietic derangement	<400	Hematopoietic
III	A serious course; hematopoietic complications severe, and some evidence of gastroenteric damage present in upper portion of group	400–600	Hematopoietic
IV	An accelerated version of acute radiation syndrome; gastroenteric complications dominating clinical picture; severity of hematopoietic complications related to survival time after exposure	600–1500	Gastrointestinal
V	A fulminating course with marked cardiovascular and/or central nervous system impairment	>5000	Cardiovascular-cerebral

the shorter the wavelengths, the longer the latency before the onset of objective findings.

The treatment of acute radiation injury is nonspecific; that is, there are no specific antidotes. If it has been determined that the patient is still radioactive, however, precautions must be taken to protect others from being contaminated. Bowel sterilization for acute radiation syndrome when the patient is leukopenic is helpful to prevent sepsis. Blood and platelets are replaced as necessary and as indicated by serial hematocrit and platelet counts. Procedures such as marrow transplantation are experimental at this time.

Complications include leukemia, sterility, and cancer of the involved organ or digit [7]. With respect to the hand, one of the more common cancers is osteosarcoma. Nevertheless, it is felt that amputation should not be undertaken on the basis of probable consequent cancer. The incidence, although not definitely known, is low enough so that prophylactic amputation is not indicated [4]. A critical dose of radiation may be required to induce a carcinoma. In the case of radon, for example, the cancer is not seen below 100 rads. However, the incidence of cancer seems to decrease when exposure has been greater than 12,000 rads.

LOCAL EFFECTS

The local lesion seen as a result of acute radiation injury occurs following careless handling of radioactive material, prolonged exposure during fluoroscopy, or improper irradiation [1]. Physicians, dentists, and technical personnel are particularly prone to injury in the first two categories. The lesion manifests itself initially as incomplete destruction of the epithelium, known as moist desquamation. Eventually it is replaced by a radiation scar and finally by an ulcer.

Figure 8-1 shows the hands of a man exposed two weeks previously to 38 curies of iridium. He inadvertently manipulated a piece of iridium with his fingers for an unknown duration of time. His radiation badge read 250 rads of exposure. The badge was worn at waist level. One week after the exposure the patient decided to inform his physician. It was obvious at the time that he did not suffer from acute radiation syndrome as he

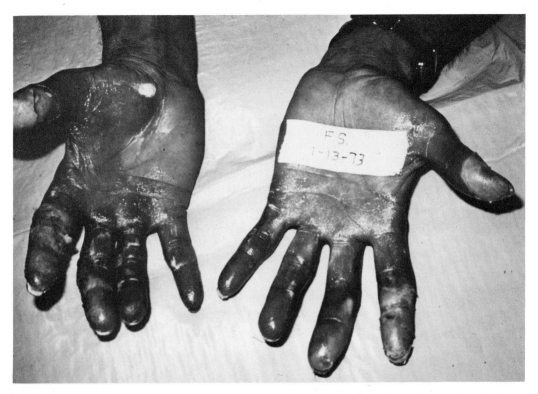

FIGURE 8-1.   *Two weeks following manipulation of a piece of iridium for unknown length of time (38 curies). See text for complete history.*

did not develop nausea, vomiting, and signs of hematopoietic damage prior to the first week. The problem was one of an acute local radiation injury. Dosimetric studies indicated that the patient's fingers were exposed to 30,000 rads at the skin surface assuming he had a one minute exposure to the iridium. It must be kept in mind, however, that this is a calculated skin exposure dose to a radiation which is primarily beta ray and some gamma ray. The badge reading of 250 rads was a midline reading but at the surface. Dosimetric calculation indicated the midline total body exposure dose to be 70 to 100 rads. The amount of radiation to the tendons beneath the skin and to the bone was calculated to be considerably less. When these films were taken of the patient's hand, the radiation burn was two weeks old and the patient had considerable pain in his fingers. The skin of the

tips of the index fingers and thumbs required split-thickness grafts at first and eventually amputation because of the progressive obliterative endarteritis. Figure 8-2 emphasizes the fact that, although the clinical signs and symptoms occurring shortly after a radiation injury may subside, they may reappear with the passage of time. The cutaneous and subcutaneous pathological changes progress at a rate faster than that expected of aging tissues [3]. This case points out how difficult it is to predict the ultimate outcome of the lesion. A great deal depends upon exact dosimetric study, the type of radiation, and the individual's susceptibility to radiation.

Radiation may cause a local tissue injury years after the actual injury. It occurs in three main forms: (1) chronic radiodermatitis, (2) osteoradionecrosis, and (3) malignancy. A chronic radiodermatitis may occur following

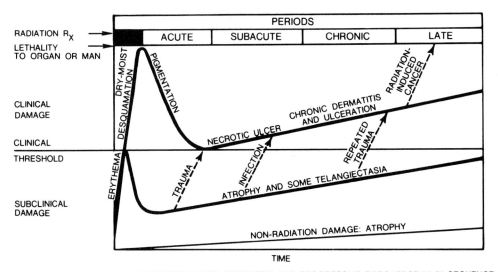

FIGURE 8-2. *Effects of radiation on skin. The lower line illustrates the effect of an erythematous dose level with rapid recovery and minimal changes. However, trauma or infection may unmask latent radiation change. The top line shows the probable damage from a large dose of irradiation in which a moist desquamation occurs and in which atrophy and pigmentation are immediately evident. A necrotic ulcer may occur as a result of minimal trauma. Radiation-induced cancer may follow in time. (From P. Rubin and G. W. Casarett,* Clinical Radiation Pathology. *Philadelphia: Saunders, 1968. Reprinted by permission.)*

prolonged repeat low-dose radiation exposure. It is manifested by (1) atrophy of the skin, (2) fissures in the skin, (3) telangiectasis, and, if severe enough, (4) ulcerated lesions. This condition is often seen after radiation to the face for acne or to the neck for radiation treatment for thyroid disease. Osteoradionecrosis is manifested by pain of the involved bone, a draining sinus to the bone, or, more rarely, a pathological fracture. Often the maxillofacial bones are involved where a large dose of roentgen rays was given to treat a malignancy. Malignancy follows radiation injury particularly if there is a long-standing history of radiodermatitis with ulceration. For this reason, a persistent ulcer should be examined by biopsy for malignancy. The most common skin malignancy following radiation injury is squamous cell carcinoma; next comes basal cell carcinoma and third,

sarcoma. The latency between time of radiation and onset of malignancy is 5 to 10 years but often 20 to 30 years.

The histopathology of the radiodermatitis consists in (1) hyperkeratosis, (2) parakeratosis, (3) atrophy, and (4) loss of rete pegs in the epidermis.

In the dermis, one sees (1) a thickening or fibrosis of the intima of the arterioles, (2) thrombosis and tortuosity of the vessels, (3) chronic inflammatory response, (4) atrophy of dermal appendages, and (5) dysplastic fibroblasts.

Treatment for radiodermatitis depends on the severity of the lesion. For atrophy and minor ulcerations, bland ointments and dressing changes suffice. Hyperkeratosis can be treated by excision. Some surgeons employ electrodesiccation. To prevent aggravation of existing lesions, protection from further radiation injury is mandatory. For example, ointments such as those containing benzophenones can be used to protect the skin from solar radiation. Ulcerative lesions require excision and grafting. Depending on the location, ulcer reconstruction with flaps may be necessary. Because the tissue underlying the ulcer is also abnormal and contains abnormal vessels that retract poorly, postoperative bleeding is a problem. For this reason skin grafting may be postponed one to two days following excision of the ulcer.

Osteoradionecrosis is treated by excision of the necrotic bone. Often, bone graft or a prosthesis is used to replace the excised specimen. The treatment of skin tumors secondary to radiation injury is much like that of any other type of skin cancer with two exceptions: (1) The cell tumors are less likely to result in local lymph node metastases, perhaps because the dermal fibrosis often seen in these lesions inhibits metastases; therefore, a prophylactic of lymph node excision may not be necessary. (2) If lymph nodes are enlarged, the condition may be due to a granulomatous lymphadenitis caused by the ulcerative radiodermatitis. However, one is obliged to perform a lymph node dissection under these circumstances, since the possibility of metastatic squamous cell carcinoma cannot be ruled out otherwise.

REFERENCES

1. Cramer, L. M., Waite, J. H., Edgecomb, J. H., Powell, C. C., Tuohy, J. H., Van Scott, E. J., and Smith, R. R.   Burn following accidental exposure to high energy radiation. *Ann. Surg.* 149:286, 1959.
2. Hartwell, S. W., Jr.   Radiation Injury. In Grabb, W. C., and Smith, J. W. (Eds.), *Plastic Surgery* (2nd ed.). Boston: Little, Brown, 1973. P. 646.
3. Jellinek, S.   The pathological changes produced in those rendered unconscious by electric shock and the treatment of such cases. *Arch. Radiol. Electrobiol.* 27:316, 1923.
4. Krizek, T. J., and Ariyan, S.   Severe acute radiation injuries of the hands. *Plast. Reconstr. Surg.* 51:14, 1973.
5. Malbec, E. F., and Quaife, J. V.   Plastic surgery in radiation burns. *Plast. Reconstr. Surg.* 20:232, 1957.
6. Peterson, R. A.   Electrical Burns in Plastic Surgery. In Grabb, W. C., and Smith, J. W. (Eds.), *Plastic Surgery* (2nd ed.). Boston: Little, Brown, 1973. P. 653.
7. Robinson, D. W., and Masters, F. W.   Surgery for radiation injury. *Arch. Surg.* 80:946, 1960.

CHEMICAL INJURIES

RONALD P. GRUBER

Chemical burns, while infrequent as compared to thermal burns, are a difficult therapeutic challenge. Most are the result of accidental exposure, and many, if not most, are due to industrial accidents.

THE AGENTS

Common agents involved include KOH, NaOH, and ammonia among the alkalies, and H_2SO_4, HCl, and HNO_3 from the acids. In addition, hydrofluoric acid must be mentioned; it is one of the strongest inorganic acids known, used in the semiconductor industry and as a component of rust-removing agents. War contributes to a large percentage of chemical burns, particularly the white phosphorus injury. (Insecticides and rat poisons are also known to contain white phosphorus.) Mustard gas can result in a burn because of its alkalization effect, and tear gas has a weak acidic effect and can cause a second-degree burn [2].

Trichloroacetic acid is often used by dermatologists in the destruction of skin lesions. Phenol (carbolic acid) is used for chemical "skin peeling" but has been known to produce severe chemical burns [1], either accidentally by patients or iatrogenically. It was utilized by Lister as one of the first antiseptics in surgery. When used in chemical peeling, it is also capable of producing local anesthesia. Croton oil, originally used as a cathartic, is often combined with phenol to potentiate its effect. In significant concentration and duration croton oil too can cause vesiculation of the skin [7].

Chemical burns are not unlike local thermal burns in appearance. The burn area is generally smaller than that of a thermal burn, and consequently the mortality is less. The lesion is usually very painful. When first seen, it may appear as no more than the erythema of a first-degree thermal burn or the bullae of a second-degree burn. But in a matter of hours or days it may manifest itself as a full-thickness skin loss.

As with the other agents discussed, the overall morbidity and mortality of chemical burns are directly related to the area of the burn, as well as the patient's age and general health at the time of injury.

SYSTEMIC EFFECTS

A persistent chemical burn involving a significant enough surface area may, by continual necrosis of large amounts of tissue and pH aberrations, result in shock. This is particularly the case with agents such as hydrofluoric acid. The latter may also cause hypocalcemia and, if the burn is severe, alterations in clotting mechanisms.

Phosphorus can bring about liver and renal damage, with nephrotoxicity being the primary cause of death. The cause of the renal damage is unknown. Although increased serum glutamic-pyruvic transaminase (SGPT) levels are seen, the liver damage is not severe enough for death to ensue, as occurs following phosphorus ingestion. Sudden early death can come even after as little as a 10 to 15 percent phosphorus burn surface area [5]. Serum calcium is decreased, serum phosphorus is increased, and occasional cardiac arrhythmias can be produced experimentally. ST-T wave abnormalities and prolonged QT intervals may be noted. It is not

yet clear whether it is the decreased calcium or the increased phosphorus level that causes a sudden lethal arrhythmia, although pilot studies suggest that giving calcium intravenously does not improve survival chances. Moreover, excision of the eschar at one hour does not prevent calcium and phosphorus shifts and consequent arrhythmias [9]. Ben-Hur and Appelbaum suggested that early death may also be related to the potassium intoxication which is secondary to acute renal failure [4]. Sodium and potassium levels are similar to those following acute renal failure.

Although copper sulfate ($CuSO_4$) neutralizes H_3PO_4, it may cause symptoms and signs of copper toxicity (vomiting, diarrhea, hepatic necrosis, and cardiorespiratory collapse). Because it is a competitive inhibitor of glucose 6-phosphate, an enzyme of the pentose cycle of the red blood cells, $CuSO_4$ may also cause hemolysis, hematuria, and consequent renal failure.

The systemic effect of phenol includes CNS signs such as seizures, but increased neuromuscular transmission and muscle tremor are seen too. In the late stages, depression and coma ensue. Cardiac toxicity, nephrotoxicity, and an unexplained antipyretic effect have also been noted. In the usual dose employed for chemical peeling, these systemic findings are not likely to occur, and no serum phenol level is detectable. Ayres, however, reported serum levels up to 50 mg per 100 ml when large areas are covered by phenol every two to three days [3]. Under these circumstances, transient urinary signs such as granular casts were seen.

Another general effect of chemical burns that often goes unsuspected is the inhalation of fumes such as HCl or ammonia. Such inhalation of fumes results in a severe tracheobronchitis.

LOCAL EFFECTS

The pathophysiology of a chemical burn is usually more complicated than one realizes. The chemical burn, particularly that caused by alkali, is a *persistent* burn. The alkali (such as KOH, NaOH, and ammonia) combines with a fat producing a soap and an exothermic response [2]. This agent also has a hygroscopic action resulting in cellular dehydration and protein precipitation. When inadequate treatment is rendered, alkali in the eschar retains uncombined alkali and, therefore, the burn continues for several days. It may persist in spite of the fact that the patient remains asymptomatic.

Acids (such as HCl, H_2SO_4, HNO_3, phenol, and trichloroacetic acid) induce an exothermic reaction, sudden tissue dehydration, and protein precipitation. Hydrofluoric acid, in addition to the above, causes liquefaction and calcification.

Although the treatment of chemical burns is beyond the scope of this section, the chemical reaction of the various chemicals is of importance in terms of the pathophysiology. All acids are neutralized by bicarbonate whereas most alkalies are neutralized by acetic acid solutions (0.5% to 5.0%) or ammonium chloride (5.0%). *The heat generated from these reactions, however, is itself a cause of local tissue damage*; therefore, the primary treatment of chemical burns is copious irrigation with saline solution [11]. It must be begun immediately if it is to be effective. To some extent, there is a slight latency in the onset of the corrosive effect of potassium hydroxide and sodium hydroxide which apparently is due to the general protective qualities of skin surface oil and keratin. Formerly, 30 to 60 minutes of irrigation was deemed satisfactory. Recent studies by Bromberg et al., in which wounds were irrigated from six hours to six days, indicated that up to 24 hours may be necessary to completely irrigate a wound and eschar of remaining acid or alkali [6].

The importance of hydrotherapy has been confirmed experimentally [8]. Standard burns were made on the backs of mice using either 50% HCl or 36% NaOH. At varying intervals of time after the burn, treatment consisting of a 10-minute brief washing or an eight-hour shower was employed. Hydrotherapy by an eight-hour shower decreased the gross and microscopic severity of the burn. If the subcutaneous pH of HCl and NaOH burn wounds is plotted as a function of time, it is found that NaOH causes a much more severe deviation of the pH from normal than does HCl and that, as is unlike the case with HCl, the pH does not approach near normal levels for as much as 6 to 12 hours. If a burn wound received a brief washing, the pH could immediately be returned to more normal levels although it never approached the preburn level. However, a brief washing could not alter the pH of the NaOH burn older than one hour or the HCl burn older than 15 minutes; hence the emphasis on early irrigation of burn wounds.

Hydrofluoric acid has an even longer-lasting necrosing effect than other chemicals. In addition to producing a burn as an acid, it releases free fluoride ion that causes necrosis of tissues and decalcification of bones by trapping calcium to form insoluble calcium fluoride. Because calcium binds so well to the fluoride ion, 10% calcium gluconate is used to neutralize the effect of hydrofluoric acid. Treatment is by intradermal or subcutaneous injection directly into the burned tissues [10]. Hypercalcemia does not seem to be a problem despite massive doses of calcium gluconate.

Phenol causes a white pellicle of precipitated protein. It is best made soluble and hence washed from the skin by combining it with 50% alcohol or glycerine and even water.

White phosphorus burns have a peculiar pathophysiology in that, unlike other chemical burns, they are the only ones in which the *thermal* component is the major factor in producing the burn. Phosphorus ignites spontaneously upon drying and exposure to air where it is oxidized to P_2O_5 and other anhydrates of phosphoric acid. During the process of oxidation heat is liberated. In addition to the heat effect, the acid produced is capable of tissue destruction. If $CuSO_4$ is added to phosphorus, as is often done to treat phosphorus burns, and if bicarbonate is also added, the resultant reaction tends to have a neutralization effect:

$$H_3PO_4 + NaHCO_3 + CuSO_4 \rightarrow$$
$$CuCO_3 + Na_2HPO_4 + CuPO_3$$

White phosphorus melted by body temperature penetrates the skin, causing a blue-green color. It produces coagulation necrosis as a result of its heat-generating capacity. It can be extinguished by water but re-ignites when dry; therefore, when debrided from the wound in the operating room, it should be placed carefully in water so that it does not re-ignite or explode.

The complications of chemical burns are similar to those of thermal burns, including contraction, susceptibility to breakdown of tissues, and trophic ulceration. If the eyes are involved, corneal ulceration, iritis, and increased intraocular pressures may follow. Cataract formation is a frequent consequence in 10 percent of cases. Because of the severity of the burn, white phosphorus in particular can result in joint contracture, chondritis of the ear, and panophthalmitis—the latter requiring enucleation in some instances.

REFERENCES

1. Abraham, A. J. A case of carbolic acid gangrene of the thumb. *Br. J. Plast. Surg.* 25:282, 1972.
2. Artz, C. P., and Moncrief, J. A. *The Treatment of Burns.* Philadelphia: Saunders, 1969.
3. Ayres, S. Superficial Chemosurgery. In Epstein, E. (Ed.), *Skin Surgery* (2nd ed.). Philadelphia: Lea & Febiger, 1962.
4. Ben-Hur, N., and Appelbaum, J. Biochemistry, histophathology and treatment of phosphorus burns. *Isr. J. Med. Sci.* 9:40, 1973.
5. Bowen, T. Z., Whelan, T. J., and Nelson, T. G. Sudden deaths after phosphorus burns. *Ann. Surg.* 174:779, 1971.
6. Bromberg, B. E., Song, I. C., and Walden, R. H. Hydrotherapy of chemical burns. *Plast. Reconstr. Surg.* 35:85, 1965.
7. Brown, K. L., and Moritz, A. R. Electrical injuries. *J. Trauma* 4:608, 1964.
8. Gruber, R. P., Vistnes, L. M., and Laub, D. R. The effect of hydrotherapy on the clinical course and pH of experimental cutaneous chemical burns. *Plast. Reconstr. Surg.* 55:200, 1975.
9. Harrison, S. T. Lightning burns. *Br. J. Plast. Surg.* 8:154, 1955.
10. Iverson, R. E., Laub, D. R., and Madison, M. S. Hydrofluoric acid burns. *Plast. Reconstr. Surg.* 48:107, 1971.
11. Wolfert, F. G., DeMeester, T., Knorr, N., and Edgerton, M. T. Surgical management of cutaneous lye burns. *Surg. Gynecol. Obstet.* 131:873, 1970.

9

Thermal Burns

TISSUE RESPONSE TO HEAT

LARS M. VISTNES

SYSTEMIC EFFECTS

It is becoming increasingly clear that a person who sustains a burn is a victim of trauma just as surely as if he had received a crushing injury in a car accident [3]. Thus, the circumstances outlined under Common Systemic and Local Effects on page 129 are induced, but in addition, certain circumstances related to the postburn status are set in motion. Most of these are on a local level and will be dealt with later, but the same local circumstances induce or amplify the systemic changes already enumerated.

The only notable situation in which heat as a specific agent results in systemic effects peculiar only to heat is in the so-called pulmonary burn. As defined by Stone et al., this is a condition in which two of the following three criteria are satisfied: (1) burn in an enclosed space, (2) singed nasal vibrissae or soot in the mouth, (3) burns about the face [4].

Because animal studies in which thermistors have been placed at various levels in the respiratory tract to detect the temperature of inhaled hot steam have shown rapid heat dissipation, it has been concluded that the heat does not produce damage; rather, the observed complications arise from inhalation of the noxious products of combustion which in turn irritate the mucosa of the bronchial tree [1]. This irritation is manifested clinically by the typical wheezing, rales, and rhonchi of pneumonia, and systemically by changes in otherwise stable blood gas values. Thus, decreased PO_2 values commonly occur, and the deficit of gas exchange in the bronchopulmonary vasculature in severe cases may indeed be enough to precipitate fatal hypoxia. Similarly, because of the same faulty exchange, CO_2 retention may cause PCO_2 rises, with pH changes, primary respiratory alkalosis or acidosis, and secondary metabolic upsets. In most cases, these are moderately to well compensated, but in severe cases compensation may fail.

149

LOCAL EFFECTS

The coagulative necrosis in a full-thickness burn in addition to involving the skin includes most of the skin appendages and often some of the subcutaneous fat. Whereas dermal collagen is homogeneous as early as 24 hours after burning, the elastic tissue fibers are unchanged and cannot be distinguished from those of normal elastic tissue [5].

When the depth of injury has become defined, inflammatory exudate appears at the junction of viable and nonviable tissue. In the burn without infection it often does not occur until the third week after burning. At that time there is an increase in vascular proliferation with clearly recognizable granulation tissue formation at the junction zone. Elastic tissue fibers, which would appear to be relatively resistant to burning, remain essentially normal at this late stage and can be seen to cross the junction between living and dead tissue [5]. The actual depth of injury seems to be defined by patent capillaries deep to the burn, and it is presumably these vessels that are the origin both of the neutrophilic infiltrate which forms the zone of subeschar liquefaction and of the granulation tissue that together allow the separation of the eschar [2].

REFERENCES

1. Artz, C. P., and Moncrief, J. A.   *The Treatment of Burns* (2nd ed.). Philadelphia: Saunders, 1969.
2. Foley, F. D.   Pathology of cutaneous burns. *Surg. Clin. North Am.* 50:6, 1970.
3. Jelenko, C., III.   Systemic response to burn injury: A survey of some current concepts. *J. Trauma* 10:10, 1970.
4. Stone, H. H., Martin, J. D., Jr., and Claydon, C. T.   Management of the pulmonary burn. *Am. Surg.* 33:616, 1967.
5. Vistnes, L. M., and Hogg, G. A. The burn eschar: A histopathological study. *Plast. Reconstr. Surg.* 48:56, 1971.

PATHOPHYSIOLOGY AND TREATMENT OF FLUID DERANGEMENT

JOHN K. MCKENZIE

THE BURN WOUND

The skin function of retaining fluid and heat is lost after burning, especially with full-thickness burns, and to this problem is added the formation of an enormous third space due to the large mass of injured tissue.

In any burn vascular permeability in the burned area rapidly increases and allows an outpouring of high-protein edema fluid (up to 5 percent protein) with an electrolyte composition similar to that of plasma. The protein is plasma protein and mainly albumin, as shown by experiments with radiolabeled serum albumin. This leakage is difficult to estimate but may be at least 50 percent of the extracellular fluid (ECF) volume in a patient with a 50 percent surface area burn. Some edema also occurs in unburned areas when the burn is large.

After about 48 hours, vascular permeability appears to return to normal, so that protein loss ceases and fluid begins to be reabsorbed. However, hypoproteinemia is usually still present because of catabolic factors and deficient protein manufacture.

Burned tissue cells, like cells in other wounds, tend to take up sodium and lose potassium. Hyperkalemia is common in the first few days, and urine potassium excretion is high if renal function is satisfactory.

The highly permeable blood vessels will be likely to lose plasma, producing red cell "sludging" and high viscosity [23]. Very poor perfusion of the burned area can be expected until the vessels return to normal. Direct red cell injury and continuing mechanical red cell hemolysis due to endothelial damage lead to anemia [9]. The tissue cell damage itself together with poor perfusion will result in anaerobic metabolism and metabolic acidosis. Shock states and renal function tend to be worse when metabolic acidosis is present [10].

Histamine output in the urine is greatly increased soon after burn injury [5] and is known to stimulate increased vascular permeability. However, this action lasts only a few hours, much less than the time of the vascular outpouring seen in burns [14]. Increased serotonin production also appears to have a short course. Bradykinin has a much longer period of release. Prostaglandins, which may be stimulated by kinins, also seem to be produced in experimental burns in dogs [13].

GENERAL RESPONSES TO THE BURN WOUND

The rapid fall in circulating plasma volume markedly decreases cardiac output. Further, release of a myocardial depressant factor or toxin has been postulated [3]. The best evidence for a burn "toxin" comes from Allgöwer et al., who found that in animals burned by high-temperature dry heat a lipoprotein can be isolated from the skin which is not present in normal skin [1]. Active or passive immunization against this material has notably lowered mortality from standard burns in experimental animals.

Peripheral resistance rises rapidly with the loss of volume while a high hematocrit value due to hemoconcentration is the rule.

Renal Effects

Hypovolemia quickly leads to reduced renal perfusion with a large fall in renal blood flow usually lasting several days [22], although glomerular filtration rate (GFR) is less affected. This drop in perfusion, together with increased sympathetic nervous activity, leads to activation of the renin-aldosterone system. Moreover, the low volume will stimulate thirst and antidiuretic hormone. Urine volume will therefore be low, the urine being concentrated, low in sodium, and high

in potassium. If hypovolemia is severe and prolonged, renal blood flow may be reduced to the point that acute renal failure occurs. If the burn wound is deep, with considerable red cell or muscle cell breakdown, large amounts of hemoglobin and myoglobin may be released which can deposit in the renal tubules [23]. It is debatable whether this mechanical tubular obstruction, the associated hypovolemia, or vasoactive products of hemoglobin and myoglobin breakdown lead to acute renal failure.

Other Endocrine Changes

Adrenal medullary hormone excretion is sharply increased in severe burns [4]. Cortisol and adrenocortical hormone excretions are usually elevated, and adrenal cortical insufficiency is rare.

TREATMENT OF THE INITIAL SHOCK PHASE

Colloid or Not?

There has been much argument as to what kind of fluid should be used to replace fluid losses in burns. Markley and co-workers [16] as well as Swedish workers [25] and others [21] have pointed to the cheapness, simplicity, and effectiveness of purely electrolyte solutions, whereas other groups, particularly in the United Kingdom, have used a large percentage of colloid, in the form of dextran, plasma, or albumin. Animal experiments [21] have not shown any necessity for colloid administration for survival in the early shock phase after burns. However, colloid is relatively effective in improving cardiac output and peripheral resistance in dogs [20], but only at much higher rates of administration than are normally used in human therapeutic protocols. In addition, GFR appears better maintained and recovers better in burned animals receiving albumin [11]. In one study [6], where enough plasma and albumin were used both in the early shock phase and later, to maintain a serum protein concentration of at least 5 gm per 100 ml, there was apparent improvement in survival especially with burns covering more than 30 percent of body surface area.

The type of colloid to be administered has also been debated. Dextran has been recommended as an inexpensive, easily available material without the danger of hepatitis associated with plasma [8]. However, dextran of higher molecular weight interferes with blood typing while the low-molecular-weight material tends to be less effective because it is rapidly excreted. Both types of dextran are associated with the formation of dense urinary casts, and there is some evidence they may cause obstruction in the renal tubules [11]. Use of high-molecular-weight dextran in dogs has been shown to be linked with consistently poor recovery of GFR after treatment of postburn shock [11]. Polyvinylpyrrolidone (PVP) has been used but may cause nephrotic syndrome and accumulate in reticuloendothelial tissues. Gelatin solutions, which can be relatively nontoxic and nonantigenic, have provided satisfactory osmotic activity for two to three days. In general, if colloids are to be given, some form of human plasma extract that is hepatitis free is desirable.

What Electrolytes?

The tonicity and alkalinity of the electrolyte solutions used in burn therapy are also a matter of argument. Markley and Smallman, in a series of animal experiments, showed that saline solution (0.85 gm per 100 ml) given by any route was superior to glucose, which only slightly improved mortality [17]. He next investigated the effects of a standard volume of hypotonic or hypertonic solution and found that moderately hypertonic saline (0.3M and 0.45M) was more effective than the same volume of isotonic (0.15M) saline or hypotonic (0.075M) saline [18].

If the volume of fluid administered was varied between 1 and 15 percent of body weight but the mass of NaCl was kept constant, higher volumes decreased mortality [18]. Hypertonic saline could be effective in much smaller volumes, but up to 30 percent

body weight of isotonic saline or NaCl-$NaHCO_3$ gave best survival at 48 hours following burning. Polk and Vanhinder have also reported that rats survived longer after some types of burns when hypertonic solutions were used [24]. Monafo and Pappalardo have had good results with a hypertonic lactated saline solution given both orally and intravenously [19]. Less volume of this solution is required for good urine output, and the tissues appear less swollen.

Monafo and Pappalardo suggested that an effective solution is

> Sodium 300 mEq per liter
> Chloride 100 mEq per liter
> Racemic lactate 200 mEq per liter.

With this solution the average total fluid administered in the first 48 hours in adults was 2.9 ml/liter body weight/1 percent of surface area burned. This compares with 4.6 ml per liter per 1 percent using isotonic Ringer's lactate and 7.4 ml per liter per 1 percent when colloid and other electrolytes were used. Under such a regimen, urine flow remained good (always greater than 30 ml per hour) and acidosis was not seen, blood pH being in the range of 7.45 to 7.50. Hypernatremia was frequent (Na 150 to 160 mEq per liter) but rarely greater than 160 to 170, at which level added water was given.

In the first day or two, antidiuretic hormone (ADH) secretion will be greatly increased, so that water administered as hypotonic solutions will not be lost in the urine. A considerable amount of water is lost through the burn wound by evaporation, especially if the exposure method is used. Nevertheless, in the first 48 hours the total amount of fluid involved in edema formation will usually much exceed evaporative loss. There appears to be merit, therefore, in the use of moderately hypertonic salt solutions for the first 48 hours.

Correction of Acidosis

Severe burns are associated with large volumes of poorly perfused tissue containing poorly functioning cells. Anaerobic metabolism resulting in metabolic acidosis therefore occurs. Normal saline (0.9% or 0.15M) contains 153 mEq per liter of sodium, but also 153 mEq per liter of chloride compared to normal serum levels of 100 to 110 mEq per liter. Use of large volumes of saline thus increases chloride ion concentration and tends to worsen the metabolic acidosis. Fox has compared the effect on burned and normal mice of the administration of equivalent quantities of isotonic electrolyte solutions and found that lactate or acetate solutions were far more effective than NaCl in promoting urine output as well as sodium, potassium, and urea excretion in burned animals [10]. Interestingly, NaCl was more effective than the other solutions in the animal without burns. Monafo and Pappalardo [19] and Thal [26] have stressed the improvement in cardiac output and perfusion that occurs in shock states when acidosis is corrected.

An Outline of Treatment of the Burn Shock Phase

Tables 9-1 and 9-2 show the classic Evans and Brooke Army Hospital formulas. Colloid is given at the rate of 0.5 ml per liter body weight per 1 percent burned surface area (determined as plasma colloid equivalents—see Table 9-3) for the first 24 hours and half the volume for the second 24 hours, since vascular permeability will be decreasing during the second 24 hours, and more colloid will be retained intravascularly. The hypoproteinemia that occurs later because of

TABLE 9-1. *Evans Burn Formula*

	First 24 hours
(a) 0.9% NaCl	1 ml/kg/1% burn
(b) Colloids	1 ml/kg/1% burn
(c) Free water (dextrose)	2000 ml

Second 24 hours
½ of (a) and (b) and all of (c)

Source: From Evans, E. I., et al., *Ann. Surg.* 135:804, 1952.

TABLE 9-2. *Brooke Army Hospital Burn Formula*

	First 24 hours
(a) Lactated Ringer's	1.5 ml/kg/1% burn
(b) Blood plasma or dextran	0.5 ml/kg/1% burn
(c) Free water (dextrose)	2000 ml

½ fluid in first 8 hours
¼ fluid in second 8 hours
¼ fluid in third 8 hours

Second 24 hours
½ of (a) and (b) and all of (c)

Source: From Reiss, E. J., et al., *J.A.M.A.* 152:1309, 1953.

catabolism can thus be counteracted to some extent. Administration of larger amounts of colloid in the first 24 hours may be unhelpful because over 90 percent is lost from the capillaries in the burned area. Electrolytes should be administered initially as isotonic solutions until vital signs are stable and urine output is 30 to 50 ml per hour. Hypertonic solutions containing liberal amounts of lactate or bicarbonate should probably be given thereafter during the first 48 hours.

TABLE 9-3. *Modified Burn Formula*

	First 24 hours
(a) Colloid	0.5 ml/kg/1% burned surface
(b) Lactated Ringer's	0.1 ml/kg/1%/hour until urine flow is greater than 30 ml/hour
(c) When urine flow is satisfactory, *hypertonic lactated saline* (Na 225, Cl 100, and racemic lactate 125 mEq/liter) at 0.05 ml/kg/1%/hour	

No free water (dextrose)

	Second 24 hours
(a) Colloid	0.5 ml/kg/1% burned surface
(b) Hypertonic lactated saline	1.0 ml/kg/1%

Reduce hypertonic lactated saline if urine output increases above 80 ml/hour. Give 5% dextrose if serum osmolality rises above 320 mOsm/kg, or serum Na$^+$ is greater than 155 mEq/liter.

Use of large amounts of isotonic or hypotonic solutions should be avoided, lessening edema and third space volume accumulation and still allowing an adequate urine output. However, as pointed out by Eklund, patients with poor renal function cannot excrete hyperosmolar urine [7]. Plasma hyperosmolality in this situation will not be corrected in the presence of a hypertonic load. It is thus crucial that early resuscitation be effective in ensuring good renal function if hypertonic solutions are to be used.

The hypernatremia of 150 to 170 mEq per liter frequently seen by Monafo would probably be avoided by the use of solutions containing, in addition to chloride (100 mEq per liter), between 200 and 250 mEq of sodium and 100 to 150 mEq of lactate or acetate [19].

POSTSHOCK PHASE

Hypercatabolism

In surviving the first 48 to 72 hours of shock the severely burned patient will have received large amounts of sodium, water, and probably colloid. With sufficient quantities of these, renal perfusion and urine output will be satisfactory. Depending on the type of fluid replacement, there will be a greater or lesser degree of edema.

With the return of vascular permeability toward normal and the maintenance of an adequate intravascular volume and oncotic pressure, interstitial fluid can be mobilized. As renin, aldosterone, and ADH levels fall to normal, the kidney can excrete salt and water and begin to retain potassium. However, depending on the severity of the burn and partly on what local burn care is used, other factors now begin to play a major role.

In all burns the large traumatized area becomes infected to a greater or lesser extent, and the resulting fever increases calorie requirement. Patients may have very large evaporational losses of water—up to 200 ml per hour per square meter of burned surface (i.e., between 3 and 10 liters of evaporated water per day [12]). This loss causes cooling, which requires 2500 to 6000 calories to counteract and maintain normal body temperature. The loss is greatest when treatment is by the open method and appears to be greater with use of some topical agents (such as Sulfamylon) than others (such as silver nitrate). The total heat loss can be reduced by increasing the environmental temperature and thus reducing heat loss from radiation. Use of an environmental temperature of 32°C has been shown to decrease markedly metabolic rate, weight loss, and mortality in burns [4].

Covering burned areas in rats with plastic sheeting or skin sharply reduces water and heat losses [15]. There is thus good reason for securing skin coverage as soon as possible, not only as a barrier to infection but to prevent water and heat losses and stop the resulting hypercatabolism.

Body Fluids During Hypercatabolism

The large water losses must be replaced or dangerous hypernatremia will result which, with the accompanying ECF deficit, may lead to reduced renal perfusion and poor renal function. Persistent hypernatremia in the first week of therapy appears to carry a poor prognosis [7]. Water requirements may be from 3 to 10 liters per day.

The metabolic cost of severe burn injury due to evaporation plus pyrexia due to infection is so great that caloric requirements may be difficult to maintain by oral means. Body energy stores of fat and protein will be utilized, therefore, and considerable muscle wasting occurs with gluconeogenesis causing urinary nitrogen losses in the order of 30 gm per day, equivalent to 187 gm of protein per day. The cell breakdown causes continued release and excretion of potassium and water while the ECF is relatively well maintained and so constitutes a larger percentage of total body fluid.

Once the catabolic state is established, potassium loss continues until skin coverage and control of infection are obtained, at which time anabolism commences [2]. In a similar way, phosphate and magnesium will also be lost and will not be regained until the anabolic phase starts. Sodium and chloride, on the other hand, after contributing to edema and being taken up by damaged cells, are not lost on a continuing basis after the initial edema has been reversed and the excess excreted.

It should be emphasized that the intracellular potassium, phosphate, and magnesium losses during catabolism represent "pseudo depletion" and cannot be replaced until anabolism and new cell formation occurs. However, protein and calorie intake should be encouraged and, with added vitamin supplements, should be provided in an imaginative form tailored to the patient's likes with frequent feedings [2]. There is some evidence that frequent oral feeding helps to prevent Curling's ulcer.

Intravenous hyperalimentation in burns offers another route of infection in patients whose defenses are already weakened. On the other hand, the development of satisfactory lipid and amino acid solutions allows safe administration, provides better intake, and can shorten the duration and severity of catabolism. Tube feedings are an uncomfortable substitute for eating and may cause extracellular hyperosmolality especially in a patient with reduced renal function.

In summary, the catabolic phase of burns may be lessened by the use of warm environmental temperatures, and the duration and severity improved by the use of high protein–high caloric alimentation.

REFERENCES

1. Allgöwer, M., Cueni, L. B., Stadtler, K., and Schoenenberger, G. A. Burn toxin in mouse skin. *J. Trauma* 13:95, 1973.
2. Artz, C. P., and Moncrief, J. A. *The Treatment of Burns* (2nd ed.). Philadelphia: Saunders, 1969.
3. Baxter, C. R., Cook, W. A., and Shires, G. T. Serum myocardial depressant factor of burn shock. *Surg. Forum* 17:1, 1966.
4. Birke, G., Carlson, L. A., Von Euler, U. S., Liljedahl, S. O., and Plantin, L. O. Studies on Burns: XIII. Lipid metabolism, catecholamine excretion, basal metabolic rate and water loss during treatment of burns with warm, dry air. *Arch. Chir. Scand.* 138:321, 1972.
5. Birke, G., Duner, H., Liljedahl, S. O., Pernow, B., Plantin, L. O., and Troell, L. Histamine, catecholamines and adrenocortical steroids in burns. *Acta Chir. Scand.* 114:8, 1957.
6. Dogo, G., and Visentini, P. Plasma in Anti-shock Therapy of Burned Patients: Clinical Findings and Considerations. In Bertelli, A., and Donati, L. (Eds.), *Pharmacological Treatment in Burns.* Amsterdam: Excerpta Medica, 1969.
7. Eklund, J. Studies on renal function in burns: III. Hyperosmolal states in burned patients related to renal osmolal regulation. *Acta Chir. Scand.* 136:741, 1970.
8. Evans, A. J. Baseline of Fluid Replacement During the First 48 Hours. In Matter, P., Barclay, T. L., and Konickova, Z. (Eds.), *Research in Burns.* Bern: Huber, 1971.
9. Evans, E. I., and Bigger, I. A. The rationale of whole blood therapy of severe burns. *Ann. Surg.* 135:804, 1952.
10. Fox, C. L., Jr. Evaluation of Various Salt Solutions. In Matter, P., Barclay, T. L., and Konickova, Z. (Eds.), *Research in Burns.* Bern: Huber, 1971.
11. Hoyle, C. L., McCall, D. A., Danford, R. O., Desuto-Nagy, G. I., and Hayes, M. A. Renal function in the early post-burn period. *Ann. Surg.* 169:404, 1969.
12. Jelenko, C. Studies in burns: 1. Water loss from the body surface. *Ann. Surg.* 165:83, 1967.
13. Jonsson, C. E., Arturson, G., and Anggard, E. Appearance of Prostaglandins in Lymph from Burned Tissue. In Matter, P., Barclay, T. L., and Konickova, Z. (Eds.), *Research in Burns.* Bern: Huber, 1971.
14. Koslowski, L. The Role of Histamine in Burns. In Bertelli, A., and Donati, L. (Eds.), *Pharmacological Treatment in*

Burns. Amsterdam: Excerpta Medica, 1969.

15. Lieberman, Z. H., and Lansche, J. M. Effects of thermal injury on metabolic rate and insensible water loss in the rat. *Surg. Forum* 7:82, 1956.

16. Markley, K., Bocanegra, M., Chiappori, M., Morales, G., and John, D. The influence of fluid therapy upon water and electrolyte equilibria and upon the circulation during the shock period in burned patients. *Surgery* 149:161, 1961.

17. Markley, K., and Smallman, E. Factors affecting shock mortality in mice burned by scalding. *Ann. Surg.* 160:146, 1964.

18. Markley, K., Smallman, E., and Millican, R. C. The efficacy and toxicity of iso-, hypo-, and hypertonic sodium solutions in the treatment of burn shock in mice. *Surgery* 57:698, 1965.

19. Monafo, W. W., and Pappalardo, C. *The Treatment of Burns: Principles and Practice.* St. Louis: Green, 1971.

20. Moncrief, J. A. Effect of various fluid regimes and pharmacological agents on the circulatory hemodynamics of the immediate post-burn period. *Ann. Surg.* 164:723, 1966.

21. Moylan, J. A., Mason, A. D., Rogers, P. W., and Walker, H. L. Post-burn shock: A critical evaluation of resuscitation. *J. Trauma* 13:354, 1973.

22. O'Neill, J. A., Jr., Pruitt, B. A., Jr., and Moncrief, J. A. Studies of Renal Function During the Early Post-burn Period. In Matter, P., Barclay, T. L., and Konickova, Z. (Eds.), *Research in Burns.* Bern: Huber, 1971.

23. Orloff, M. F., and Chandler, J. G. Fluid and Electrolyte Disorders in Burns. In Maxwell, M. H., and Kleeman, C. R. (Eds.), *Clinical Disorders of Fluid and Electrolyte Metabolism* (2nd ed.). New York: McGraw-Hill, 1972.

24. Polk, H. C., Jr., and Vanhinder, S. Saline Solutions for Burn Shock Resuscitation: An Experimental Dissection of Its Elements. In Matter, P., Barclay, T. L., and Konickova, Z. (Eds.), *Research in Burns.* Bern: Huber, 1971.

25. Sorensen, B., and Sejrsen, P. Saline solutions in the treatment of burn shock. *Acta Chir. Scand.* 129:239, 1965.

26. Thal, A. P. *Shock: A Physiologic Basis for Treatment.* Chicago: Year Book, 1971.

BURN WOUND INFECTION

CHARLES F. T. SNELLING AND ALLAN R. RONALD

Burn injury destroys the skin's natural effective barrier against bacterial invasion and alters the humoral and cellular defense mechanisms. Pathogens that normally are resident organisms or transiently contaminate the skin surface such as *Staphylococcus aureus* and group A streptococci, gain entry, and opportunists such as *Staphylococcus epidermidis, Pseudomonas aeruginosa,* and *Candida albicans* become aggressive invaders.

Certain definitions are necessary in order to consider this subject. *Contamination* refers to organisms on the burn surface without evidence of proliferation or invasion. *Colonization* indicates proliferation of organisms on the surface or within the eschar without invasion of unburned tissue. *Burn wound sepsis,* a concept first defined by Moncrief and Teplitz [15], is the presence of a significant number of organisms (more than 100,000 per gram of burn tissue) with invasion of adjacent and underlying unburned tissue. With gram-positive burn wound sepsis blood cultures are usually positive and yield high counts of organisms whereas with gram-negative colonization blood cultures may be negative or yield few organisms although the wound itself is heavily infected. The concept of burn wound sepsis focused attention on the mass of organisms in the burn wound itself and allowed the significance of gram-negative organisms in the eschar to be appreciated. Bacteremia, septicemia, and septic shock can complicate burn wound sepsis.

ORGANISMS OF BURN INFECTION

Initially group A streptococci and *Staphylococcus aureus* were regarded as the main burn wound pathogens. Wickman, in a careful study from the Karolinska Sjukhuset, Stockholm (a center where prophylactic antibacterial therapy was not used), reported a peak incidence of surface cultures yielding group A streptococci from 3 to 7 days following burn (20 percent of patients) and thereafter a steady increase in *Staphylococcus aureus* from 7 to 14 days following burn (60 percent of patients) [25]. *Pseudomonas aeruginosa* and *Proteus* considered together colonized in 20 percent of patients at 14 days and 40 percent of patients at 28 days following burning.

Other recent burn studies reporting the incidence of organisms colonizing in burn wounds are influenced by the use of prophylactic topical antibacterial agents. MacMillan has compared the organisms cultured from burns at the time of admission in different therapeutic eras [12]. In 1942–44 *Staphylococcus aureus* was recovered from 20 percent of patients' wounds while in 1958–64 it colonized in 45 percent of patients' wounds. In the early era group A streptococci were cultured from 14 percent of patients compared to 5 percent in the latter period. This difference resulted from the use of prophylactic systemic penicillin during the first postburn week. The incidence of *Pseudomonas aeruginosa* rose from 3 percent of patients (1942–44) to 24 percent of patients (1958–64).

Comparing organisms cultured during the first and third postburn weeks from the period 1942–44 und the period 1958–64 yielded the following patterns: In the recent era the percentage of patients colonized with *Staphylococcus aureus* and group A streptococci decreased from the first to third weeks, reflecting the availability of effec-tive antibiotics. In contrast, *Proteus* and *Pseudomonas aeruginosa* colonized in a greater percentage of patients' wounds by the third week, indicating the emergence and dominance of gram-negative organisms which were probably fostered by successful control of gram-positive infection.

Moncrief and Teplitz, reporting on Brooke Army Hospital experience from 1954 to 1962, found a fairly constant year-to-year incidence of deaths due to *Staphylococcus aureus* infection [15]. In the same period there was a dramatic rise in deaths due to *Pseudomonas aeruginosa* septicemia from less than 10 per year during the 1950s to 37 in 1962. This led to a close look at the burn wound itself plus blood and visceral organ cultures at the time of postmortem examination. In patients who died from *Pseudomonas aeruginosa* infection subcutaneous fat was massively invaded, leukocyte response was absent, and extensive invasion of lymphatics and later small vessels was noted. Less than 50 percent of the patients dying of *Pseudomonas aeruginosa* septicemia had visceral cultures positive for this organism. In contrast, at autopsy following death due to *Staphylococcus aureus* septicemia septic emboli were often found in the lung and kidney and organisms were cultured from vegetations of the heart valves. This study focused attention on the significance of *quantitative bacteriological examination* of the burn wound rather than relying on positive blood cultures in assessing the magnitude of burn wound infection.

Order et al. demonstrated that an experimental partial-thickness burn could be converted to full-thickness injury by immediate seeding with *Pseudomonas aeruginosa* [17]. Instead of gradual reestablishment of patency of vessels in the subpapillary plexus by one week following burning, as was seen in noninfected controls, a progressive arterial thrombosis and devitalization of tissue with conversion to full-thickness necrosis was noted by eight days. In contrast, a comparable inoculum of *Staphylococcus aureus* tended to remain and multiply within the burn eschar without invasion of or effect upon deeper viable tissues [24].

Fungal colonization has become common with the use of topical antibacterial agents, longer survival of large burns, and the use of intravenous hyperalimentation. *Candida* species are the most frequent, but the organisms causing mucormycosis, aspergillosis, and others are cultured. Law et al. reported that in 385 patients treated from 1964 to 1970, 55 percent had *Candida* wound colonization, 6 percent had positive blood cultures, and 15 patients died with evidence of disseminated candidiasis [11]. Amphotericin B therapy was often unsuccessful.

The burn wound is the major site of infection, but other significant portals exist. The urinary tract is vulnerable following indwelling catheterization. Septic thrombophlebitis is a complication of intravenous therapy. Central venous catheters and hyperalimentation act as ready portals of bacterial entry. Respiratory infection has been recognized as a frequent burn complication with serious consequences in mafenide-treated patients. Bacteremia and septicemia may lead to pyemia. Usually the organisms responsible for these infections mirror those colonizing the burn wound, and the body's response is limited by its ability to cope with the burn injury. Serum hepatitis can be a complication of blood and plasma transfusion.

ALTERATIONS IN NATURAL DEFENSE MECHANISMS IN BURNS

The keratin and basement membrane layers of the epidermis are effective mechanical barriers to invasion of organisms. If the keratin layer is intact, invasion is impossible. Normal intact skin surface protects itself by desiccation of organisms, desquamation of surface keratin, acidification of the surface by sweat, and bactericidal action of unsaturated fatty acids present in sebaceous secretion. The resident flora consist of *Staphylococcus epidermidis,* diphtheroids, and aerobic spor-

ing bacilli. These organisms compete for nutrients as well as producing antibiotic substances.

Burn injury destroys the epidermis and varying depths of the dermis, wiping out natural defense mechanisms. Burn injury alters the blood supply to the skin and prevents the delivery of host cellular and humoral factors. In experimental partial-thickness injuries, Order et al. demonstrated patency of part of the subpapillary arterial plexus with immediate delivery of inflammatory cells below the eschar and formation of granulation tissue at this level by the end of the first week [17]. In full-thickness injury there was a complete occlusion of the subpapillary plexus and absence of inflammatory response adjacent to the burn wound; granulation tissue was formed at a deeper, more remote level. A partial-thickness burn has better delivery of an effective inflammatory response. As the burn wound is essentially avascular for varying depths, organisms that colonize the eschar will be isolated from host defense mechanisms until such time as invasive burn wound sepsis ensues. Teplitz et al. demonstrated in a rat full-thickness burn wound model that *Pseudomonas aeruginosa* applied at the time of burn reached the interface with deeper viable tissue on the fourth day, after already achieving high concentration within the wound [24]. On the seventh day organisms had penetrated and caused necrosis of granulation tissue. In contrast *Staphylococcus aureus* did not show a tendency to invade.

Normal phagocytosis is altered in the following fashion: Complement levels are decreased in burn patients during the first postburn week, but not to levels sufficiently low to interfere with opsonization. All classes of immunoglobulins are depressed during the first postburn week. In adults Arturson et al. demonstrated a decrease of serum levels of IgG to 30 percent of normal and IgM to 49 percent of normal two to three days following burning [8]. IgM levels returned to normal by the seventh day while IgG levels returned to normal after 19 days and then continued to rise. The blister fluid levels of IgG were slightly lower than corresponding serum levels while IgM blister levels were much lower, this variation being due to the difference in molecular size of the two classes of immunoglobulins. The initial drop in immunoglobulin serum levels is due to both leakage from the intravascular into the interstitial space at the time of burn and decreased production. Subsequent increases result from increased production in response to specific bacterial antigens aided by a return to normal capillary impermeability. Therefore opsonization of bacteria will be decreased in the immediate postburn period. Ritzmann et al. demonstrated in infants and young children a slower return to normal levels for IgM and IgG [21]. Passive immunization with nonspecific gamma globulin has not been found to be effective in overcoming these deficits. The amounts that can be practically given are far below the amounts actually synthesized by the patient following the initial depression [22]. Specific human anti-*Pseudomonas* hyperimmune globulin therapy is currently undergoing clinical evaluation.

In the burned subject the primary response to antigen injections is variable; it appears to be principally related to the nature of the antigen and depends to a lesser extent on the size of the burn [7]. Heterologous alligator erythrocytes injected into burned patients failed to elicit a primary antibody response whereas this occurred in unburned controls [6]. In animals the same procedure produced a variable response depending upon the extent of burn [6, 7]. Primary immunization with *Pseudomonas aeruginosa* vaccine elicits a significant antibody response in both normal and burned humans and animals [4, 5, 7, 18]. A more rapid and vigorous anamnestic response to a booster dose of tetanus toxoid has been demonstrated in burned humans when compared to controls [6], and active tetanus prophylaxis is an established clinical practice in burns. In animals previously sensitized to

heterologous erythrocytes the anamnestic response was abolished after burning [7].

Primary immunization against *Pseudomonas aeruginosa* in humans has been clinically employed. Pierson and Feller used a monovalent vaccine effective for 76 percent of their *Pseudomonas aeruginosa* isolates [18] while Alexander et al. used a heptavalent vaccine effective for 87 percent of their isolates [4, 5]. Vaccination of large burns resulted in a reduction in mortality due to *Pseudomonas* sepsis of 86 percent when compared to a similar nonvaccinated group of large burns treated shortly before without vaccination [5]. A poor antibody titer response was observed in large burns when vaccination was begun after the sixth postburn day [5]. In children the best response was found if the vaccination was begun before postburn day 4 [16]. A measurable antibody response of the IgM and IgG fractions was demonstrated within four days of the first dose. Vaccinated patients continued to be colonized with *Pseudomonas aeruginosa* but showed an increased titer of antibody to the particular serotype colonizing their wounds when compared with unvaccinated controls [16]. The recommended dose for the commercially available heptavalent vaccine is 25 mg per kilogram of body weight as soon after receiving the burn as possible with repeat doses 5, 9, 16, and 23 days thereafter.

Rittenbury and Hanback studied the phagocytes and reticuloendothelial system in burned dogs [20]. They found a reduction in the phagocytic capability of the fixed reticuloendothelial cells of the liver, spleen, and lung in animals subjected to a lethal burn when compared to those subjected to a nonlethal burn. There was no difference between the two groups in regard to the phagocytic capability of the peripheral and subeschar leukocytes. McRipley and Garrison demonstrated reduced phagocytosis and capability for intracellular destruction of organisms by the fixed phagocytic cells of the spleen and liver in burned rats in the early postburn period [14]. Alexander demonstrated an early depression of phagocytic ability of the peritoneal phagocytes in the first 24 hours following the burn with a return to greater than normal ability 72 hours following burn [2]. He suggested that the stress reaction to thermal trauma produced increased levels of adrenocortical steroids which temporarily stabilized the lysosomal membranes preventing intracellular digestion of bacteria. Thus during the initial 24 hours postburn the patient increased susceptibility to infection.

Alexander studied the serum and leukocyte concentrations of the lysosomal enzymes β-glucuronidase, acid phosphatase, and lysozyme in patients with large burns [1]. Serum levels were variably elevated after burning while leukocyte concentrations of all were decreased, the maximum being at 6 to 10 days following the burn. Alexander et al. studied the ability of the neutrophil to kill phagocytosed bacteria and found that normal people have a periodic cycle of good and poor function as relates to intracellular killing ability which is variable and minor in extent [3]. This is probably related to lysosomal function. In eight patients with large burns neutrophil function fluctuated widely and irregularly. In several cases poor neutrophil function corresponded with a clinical episode of invasive burn wound sepsis.

The function of the thymus-dependent lymphocyte in cell-mediated immunity in burns has been studied. Lymphocytopenia has been observed in the early postburn period in burned animals [9] and patients. Prolonged allograft survival is a well-established observation and has been found to depend on the extent of the burn and the genetic similarity of host and donor [10]. Preliminary work in burned mice using B- and T-lymphocytes shows that B cells can respond slightly to *Pseudomonas* vaccine with subnormal concentration of T-lymphocytes but a maximal response requires the simultaneous presence of adequate concentration of T-lymphocytes [19]. The relationship of

these findings to burn wound sepsis remains to be determined.

MEASURES TO REDUCE THE INOCULUM OF BACTERIA

Reduction in the number of bacteria that can potentially contaminate a burn wound has been the object of a wide variety of recent endeavors. Special attention has been paid to the controlled environment (life island, isolator, and laminar airflow), protection of the patient from carriers (masks, caps, gowns, gloves, boot covers, and complete change of clothing), topical antibacterial agents which may attack surface organisms (silver nitrate) or actually penetrate burn eschar (mafenide, gentamicin, silver sulfadiazine), and subeschar injection of broad-spectrum antibiotics. Systemic penicillin started early is believed to sterilize the nasopharynx of group A streptococci carriers preventing autoinfection. Other efforts to kill the normal resident flora of the upper respiratory and gastrointestinal tracts have been generally unsuccessful primarily because of opportunistic infection with equally dangerous organisms. Careful monitoring of the hospital environment such as hydrotherapy equipment [23] and bedrails and sink drains [13] can detect reservoirs of pathogens. Monitoring of the sensitivity of organisms isolated from burn patients to antibiotics in current use will detect changes in bacterial population and may dictate changes in antibacterial use.

REFERENCES

1. Alexander, J. W. Serum and leukocyte lysosomal enzymes. Derangements following severe thermal injury. *Arch. Surg.* 95:482, 1967.
2. Alexander, J. W. Effect of thermal injury upon the early resistance to infection. *J. Surg. Res.* 8:128, 1968.
3. Alexander, J. W., Dionigi, R., and Meakins, J. L. Periodic variation in the antibacterial function of human neutrophils and its relationship to sepsis. *Ann. Surg.* 173:206, 1971.

4. Alexander, J. W., and Fisher, M. W. Immunological determinants of *Pseudomonas* infections of man accompanying severe burn injury. *J. Trauma* 10: 565, 1970.

5. Alexander, J. W., Fisher, M. W., and MacMillan, B. G. Immunological control of *Pseudomonas* infection of burn patients: A clinical evaluation. *Arch. Surg.* 102:31, 1971.

6. Alexander, J. W., and Moncrief, J. A. Alterations of the immune response following severe thermal injury. *Arch. Surg.* 93:75, 1966.

7. Alexander, J. W., and Moncrief, J. A. Immunological phenomena in burn injuries. *J.A.M.A.* 199:105, 1967.

8. Arturson, G., Hogman, C. F., Johansson, S. G. O., and Killander, J. Changes in immunoglobulin levels in severely burned patients. *Lancet* 1:546, 1969.

9. Casson, P. R., Gesner, B. M., Converse, J. M., and Rapaport, F. T. Immunosuppressive sequelae of thermal injury. *Surg. Forum* 19:509, 1968.

10. Chambler, K., and Batchelor, J. R. Influence of defined incompatibilities and area of burn on skin—Homograft survival in burned subjects. *Lancet* 1:16, 1969.

11. Law, E. J., Kim, O. J., Stieritz, D. D., and MacMillan, B. G. Experience with systemic candidiasis in the burned patient. *J. Trauma* 12:543, 1972.

12. MacMillan, B. G. Local care and infection of burns. *J. Trauma* 5:292, 1965.

13. MacMillan, B. G., Edmonds, P., Hummel, R. P., and Maley, M. P. Epidemiology of *Pseudomonas* in a burn intensive care unit. *J. Trauma* 13:627, 1973.

14. McRipley, R. J., and Garrison, D. W. Effect of burns in rats on defense mechanisms against *Pseudomonas aeruginosa. J. Infect. Dis.* 115:159, 1965.

15. Moncrief, J. A., and Teplitz, C. Changing concepts in burn sepsis. *J. Trauma* 4:233, 1964.

16. O'Neill, J. A., Nance, F. C., and Fisher, M. W. Heptavalent *Pseudomonas* vaccination in seriously burned children. *J. Pediatr. Surg.* 6:547, 1971.

17. Order, S. E., Mason, A. D., Walker, H. L., Lindberg, R. B., Switzer, W. E., and Moncrief, J. A. The pathogenesis of second and third degree burns and conversion to full thickness injury. *Surg. Gynecol. Obstet.* 120:983, 1965.

18. Pierson, C., and Feller, I. A reduction of *Pseudomonas* septicemias in burned patients by the immune process. *Surg. Clin. North Am.* 50:1377, 1970.

19. Pierson, C. L., Johnson, A. G., and Feller, I. Lymphoid cell transfer of resistance to experimental *Pseudomonas* infection in mice. *Abstracts*, Sixth Annual Meeting, American Burn Association, No. 16, 1974.

20. Rittenbury, M. S., and Hanback, L. D. Phagocytic depression in thermal injuries. *J. Trauma* 7:523, 1967.

21. Ritzmann, S. E., Larson, D. L., McClung, C., Abston, S., Falls, D., and Goldman, A. S. Immunoglobulin levels in burned patients. *Lancet* 1:1152, 1969.

22. Stone, H. H., Graber, C. D., Martin, J. D., and Kolb, L. Evaluation of gamma globulin for prophylaxis against burn sepsis. *Surgery* 58:810, 1965.

23. Stone, H. H., and Kolb, L. D. The evolution and spread of gentamicin-resistant pseudomonads. *J. Trauma* 11:586, 1971.

24. Teplitz, C., Davis, D., Mason, A. D., and Moncrief, J. A. *Pseudomonas* burn wound sepsis: I. Pathogenesis of experimental *Pseudomonas* burn wound sepsis. *J. Surg. Res.* 4:200, 1964.

25. Wickman, K. Studies on burns: XIV. Bacteriology 11. *Acta Chir. Scand.* 408 (Suppl.):1, 1970.

10

Shock

Clifford M. Herman

Shock is a common clinical problem, and so the diagnosis is often used with a familiarity that implies a generally accepted understanding of what is meant. However, difficulties become apparent as soon as one tries to define shock in precise etiological and physiological terms. Unlike many diseases in which a clear picture of cause-and-effect mechanisms is brought to mind simply by statement of the name, shock cannot be so easily understood. Therefore, a discussion of shock must begin with some useful definition.

Shock can be considered to be a condition in which there is a generalized breakdown in cell function. This may be caused by one or

more of these factors: (1) inadequate tissue perfusion, (2) inadequate oxygen supply, or (3) inability to utilize oxygen. An expansion of this definition is illustrated in Figure 10-1. This outline will serve as the framework for our discussion and should be kept in mind as the individual elements are considered in more detail.

The surgeon deals mainly with shock resulting from acute hypovolemia (whether from whole blood loss as in hemorrhage or from plasma loss as in burns or pancreatitis) and from the septic and other complications that may follow the original insult. In order to be most useful and less confusing, this chapter will *not* deal with primary cardiogenic shock, anaphylactic shock, or the shock referred to when a television actor witnesses a horrible scene or hears bad news. Rather, we will be concerned with shock from acute short-term hypovolemia, prolonged hypovolemia, and systemic sepsis.

The emphasis will be on prolonged hypovolemia and systemic sepsis, because a brief episode of acute hypovolemia is quite easily reversible if there is no associated disease of the cardiovascular or other vital organ

Supported by the Bureau of Medicine and Surgery Work Unit No. M4318.01.008BGG0. The opinions or assertions contained herein are the private ones of the author and are not to be construed as official or reflecting the views of the Navy Department or the Naval Service at large.

The experiments reported herein were conducted according to the principles outlined in the Animal Welfare Act (PL 89-544 as amended) and followed the guidelines prescribed in DHEW Publication No. (NIH) 72-73, formerly PHS Publication No. 1024, "Guide for Laboratory Animal Facilities and Care."

1. Inadequate Tissue Perfusion
    Decreased Blood Volume
    Decreased Cardiac Output
    Maldistribution of Cardiac Output
    Microcirculatory Dysfunction

2. Inadequate Oxygen Supply
    Pulmonary Dysfunction . . .   RBC Loading
    Red Cell Dysfunction . . . . RBC Release

3. Inability to Utilize Oxygen
    Sepsis

FIGURE 10-1. *The mechanisms of shock. A combination of derangements is usually responsible for the generalized breakdown in cell function.*

systems, as in the case of the previously healthy young person. The major problems lie with the older person with arteriosclerotic cardiac and peripheral vascular disease who is brought to the hospital only after several hours of hypotension from an injury or a spontaneous gastrointestinal hemorrhage. Blood loss often continues during preparation for surgery, and the anesthesia and surgical trauma are then added to an already stressed situation. If this patient survives the initial treatment, the development of sepsis, cardiac failure, pulmonary failure, and renal shutdown will then create a complex problem involving virtually every body system.

It will be helpful to begin with a review of the normal physiological responses to trauma and blood loss. The compounding of problems when hypovolemia is prolonged will then be examined. The chapter will end with a discussion of the physiological, biochemical, and immunological responses to posttraumatic sepsis. New information concerning acute changes in the way the red blood cell delivers oxygen to the tissues indicates that these phenomena apply to nearly any shock situation; hence the topic will be considered separately. For a different reason, mainly the absence of enough firm information which can define the causes for the pulmonary problem following shock, this topic too will be discussed separately.

One should keep in mind that blood loss from any cause produces essentially the same effects. Furthermore, the differences between systemic responses to an elective osteotomy and an accidental fracture are differences largely in degree of injury. Similarly, bacteremia will set in motion the same chain of events whether the source is an infected traumatic limb amputation or an infected cancer resection site. Since the body has a limited number of ways of reacting to an infinite variety of stresses, this commonality of response must be considered in a discussion of hemorrhagic and septic shock.

ACUTE HYPOVOLEMIC SHOCK

The acute loss of blood in a previously healthy person activates a series of events that are primarily circulatory in nature. Because the role of the cardiovascular system is simply to supply oxygen and nutrients to tissue cells and to remove products of metabolism and materials needed for control of other tissues and organs, the effects of these circulatory events occur at the cellular level. The composite events of acute hypovolemia shown in Figure 10-2 will be described in the following sections. The overall effects of this complex scheme are to enhance cardiac function, to ensure perfusion of vital organs, and to restore blood volume.

Neuroendocrine Responses

A fall in arterial blood pressure due to blood loss activates stretch receptors in the carotid sinus, aortic arch, and left atrium, causing them to send impulses via the ninth and tenth cranial nerves to the vasomotor center in the medulla. The result is an increase of sympathetic nervous system activity directed mainly to the heart, arterioles, and small veins. An increased release of norepinephrine from the adrenal medulla augments these cardiovascular effects [8].

The activation of the stretch receptors also causes the release of antidiuretic hormone (ADH) from the pituitary, resulting in increased renal tubular reabsorption of water. The juxtaglomerular apparatus in the kidney [1], stimulated mainly by the narrowing of

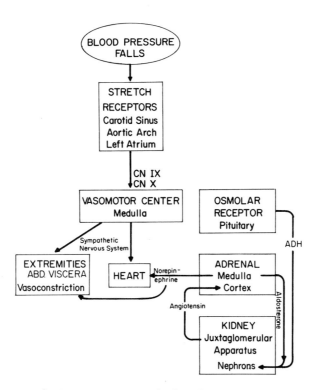

FIGURE 10-2.   *Neuroendocrine responses in shock. The sequence of events follows the arrows beginning with a fall in blood pressure. Osmolar receptors in the pituitary are activated separately by changes in serum osmolality resulting from the renal responses.*

pulse pressure which occurs in hypovolemia, releases renin, a proteolytic enzyme that forms angiotensin I from plasma protein precursors. Angiotensin I is converted to angiotensin II in the pulmonary circulation, leading to increased production of aldosterone from the adrenal cortex. The aldosterone acts in concert with ADH to enhance renal sodium and water retention.

Cardiovascular Responses

Cardiac

The effects of the neuroendocrine activity on the heart are both inotropic and chronotropic, augmenting the rate and force of cardiac contraction. Whether an actual increase in cardiac output follows depends on the effectiveness with which the decreased blood volume has been diverted from the periphery to the central circulation and on the ability of

the heart to respond to this demand for increased work.

Arterioles and Veins

The sympathetic responses cause constriction of arterioles and veins in the skin, extremities, and abdominal viscera. The accompanying increase in venomotor tone enhances the effective blood volume by squeezing blood from large venous reservoirs (such as the splanchnic bed) into the central circulation. Because the coronary and central nervous system circulations will constrict very little under intense sympathetic stimulation, the effect is to divert the flow of diminished blood volume to these vital areas.

Capillary Beds

The capillaries are the only site of communication between the cardiovascular system and the tissues, so it is important to review the forces that govern the transfer of fluid, gases, and all other materials out of and into the vascular space [15]. At the arterial end of the capillary the normal hydrostatic pressure of 40 to 50 torr (mm Hg) exceeds the pressures acting to keep water in the capillary (plasma colloid osmotic pressure of 25 to 30 torr plus tissue turgor of -2 to -5 torr), causing movement of water from the capillary to the interstitial space. The hydrostatic pressure drops along the capillary until, at the venous end, it becomes low enough ($+10$ to -15 torr) to allow an inflow of water back into the vascular space.

These mechanisms represent a primary defense against acute, short-term hypovolemic shock. The sympathetic arteriolar and venous constriction causes a fall in capillary pressure. The plasma oncotic pressure and tissue turgor then exceed the hypostatic pressure throughout the length of the capillary, causing a net movement of extracellular fluid into the capillary and thus restoring plasma volume. This process of transcapillary refilling occurs after even moderate blood loss (approximately 1500 ml in the adult), and can contribute 50 to 120 ml per hour to the circulating plasma volume. The extent and duration of the process are, of course, limited, and the capillary fluid transfer events in prolonged, severe hypovolemia will be reviewed later.

Tissue Metabolism

Since the most critically needed material for cellular metabolism is oxygen, the initial tissue effects of decreased perfusion are compensatory responses to an oxygen lack [3]. These events cannot yet be examined directly in the cells; they are best understood, therefore, by observing the changes in the blood that reflect the cellular activity.

In the face of decreased cardiac output and peripheral vasoconstriction in acute hypovolemic shock, tissue oxygenation is at first maintained by an increase in oxygen extraction which shows as an increase in

arterial-venous oxygen difference. With normal pulmonary function and saturation of arterial blood, the increased extraction is due entirely to a fall from the normal mixed venous PO_2 of about 40 torr to levels of 20 or even lower. It should be recognized here that changes in oxygen extraction vary markedly from organ to organ because of the selective vasoconstriction in some tissue beds more than in others. Therefore, the PO_2 of mixed venous blood (from the right atrium or pulmonary artery) shows the net overall response of the body as a whole and represents a disproportionate contribution by the skeletal muscle mass and abdominal viscera. This will be dealt with subsequently in more detail in the discussion of mechanisms of tissue oxygenation.

Inadequate tissue perfusion that progresses to the point of failing to meet the oxygen needs results in partial arrest of cell glycolysis at the anaerobic phase [4]. Lactate cannot be fully metabolized to carbon dioxide and water and therefore begins to appear in elevated levels (over 15 mg per 100 ml) in arterial blood. Accompanying this rise is an increase in cell hydrogen ion production which is buffered primarily by the blood bicarbonate system. When hypoperfusion is moderate and not prolonged, the HCO_3^- : H_2CO_3 ratio of 20:1 may be maintained by hyperventilation to eliminate carbon dioxide, leaving the blood pH at the normal level of 7.4.

The supply of glucose for tissue metabolism will be maintained initially through the mobilization of liver glycogen by catecholamine stimulation. With adequate pancreatic perfusion and release of insulin, the glucose will be utilized effectively in the moderately hypovolemic patient who is resuscitated within a reasonable period of time.

The Clinical Picture

The early picture after acute blood loss shows the expected signs of circulatory compensation. The patient is pale, with cold extremities on account of vasoconstriction of the skin vessels, and the heart rate is usually over 100. Urine output is low (less than 20 ml per hour), and cardiac output measured before treatment is less than the normal 2.5 liters per minute per square meter of body surface area.

Blood pressure is usually low, with systolic less than 100 torr. However, the exact level will depend on the patient's normal pressure, the degree of compensation to the hemorrhage, and the health and ability of his heart to respond to the stress. This is one reason why blood pressure is not a reliable factor in the definition of early hypovolemic shock. When compensation seems effective in maintaining a relatively normal blood pressure by intense vasoconstriction, it will often be seen to drop, along with a further increase in heart rate, if the patient sits up.

Analysis of blood gases usually shows a normal Pa_{O_2} with a low venous blood oxygen tension. While pHa is initially maintained relatively normal, this is often the result of lowering of both HCO_3^- and CO_2, often with visible hyperventilation [2].

The extent to which the individual patient compensates for blood loss also depends on the duration of the hypovolemic period [12]. When treatment is not instituted until an hour or more for a moderate hemorrhage and even less for a more massive one, the compensatory mechanisms break down and tissue damage occurs. These developments, which should be viewed as a continuum with the earlier responses described above, are discussed in the following sections.

PROLONGED HYPOVOLEMIC SHOCK

Circulatory Responses

The prompt administration of fluid and blood given rapidly and in adequate amounts will usually reverse the responses to hemorrhage, even in elderly patients. When treatment is delayed, or when the volumes of replacement fluid are inadequate, the situation becomes more complex and much more difficult to correct. While volume replacement is the only primary treatment for acute hypovolemia, it should also be emphasized that the early use of vasoactive drugs is not only ineffective but can also compound the problems. These drugs are mentioned, therefore, mainly to be condemned. Vasopressors given in an attempt to elevate the blood pressure in a patient who remains hypovolemic because of inadequate volume replacement will only prolong and reinforce the peripheral vasoconstriction and will worsen tissue damage. At the same time, the heart is being driven even harder by the drugs to increase its work in order to circulate more rapidly the insufficient blood volume available for it to pump. The result is a vicious cycle of progressive tissue death with heart failure now superimposed on what might have been a readily reversible condition if adequate volume replacement had been carried out. Because they can mask the needs for more fluids, and because in themselves they can worsen the situation, drugs should never be considered as part of the initial, primary treatment of hypovolemic shock.

When hypovolemia is allowed to persist, the vasoconstriction which lowered capillary pressure and thereby promoted transcapillary refilling from the extravascular space to augment plasma volume begins to fail. Furthermore, postcapillary venous pressure rises to the point where the net influx of fluid into the capillaries ceases. The elevated levels of norepinephrine and angiotensin also increase capillary venous pressure and so interfere with capillary refilling [1].

In addition, bradykinin and possibly other vasoactive peptides that are activated in the blood in ischemic states compound the problem by causing an increase in capillary permeability to fluid and protein. The net effect of all these events is an actual loss of plasma from the capillaries. The resulting interstitial edema further inhibits tissue perfusion and aggravates the cellular hypoxia.

Cardiac function under such circumstances becomes difficult to maintain and must be monitored closely. While cardiac output, as measured by a variety of indicator dilution techniques, is vital information for patient management, it is also essential to be able to determine continuously the ability of the heart to pump the fluid volumes needed for treatment of the hypovolemia. The best approach would be to measure left atrial filling pressure as an indicator of left ventricular function, but direct measurement of left atrial or left ventricular pressure is not possible at this time. Balloon-tipped catheters designed to be quite readily floated into the pulmonary artery through a peripheral vein have, however, provided a substantial advantage [5]. The pressure at the catheter tip with the balloon inflated (pulmonary artery "wedge pressure") has been found to approximate very closely the left atrial pressure. By watching this pressure carefully to avoid increases above safe levels, one can rapidly infuse large fluid volumes with good assurance that left ventricular failure and pulmonary edema will be avoided.

Tissue and Organ Effects

When the treatment of hypovolemia is delayed until the circulatory compensations can no longer be sustained, tissue damage becomes increasingly evident. The effects of inadequate perfusion occur first in the organs from which blood flow has been selectively diverted to maintain the central circulation. The ability of skeletal muscle to metabolize anaerobically is exceeded, and the lactate and other acid products accumulate in the stagnant tissue vascular beds. Actual cell breakdown results in the release of intracellular potassium, creatine, and eventually myoglobin.

This tissue death in the periphery is further compounded by events in the splanchnic organs. Hypoperfusion of the pancreas, along with catecholamine suppression of insulin release, at first causes hyperglycemia. However, liver hypoperfusion becomes coupled with exhaustion of hepatic glycogen stores,

resulting eventually in hypoglycemia, thereby depriving the peripheral tissues of a vital energy substrate. The loss of bowel wall integrity has been said to allow entry of endotoxin into the circulation, adding endotoxemia as an ultimate cause of further circulatory collapse, but this concept has not been fully substantiated in man.

Hypoperfusion of the kidneys initially results in a cessation of urine formation. Prolongation of this condition leads to renal damage ending in acute tubular necrosis which may or may not be reversible when blood volume is eventually restored. This possibility must be kept in mind when resuscitation fails to restore urine output in the face of what appears to be adequate volume replacement, in order to avoid the real danger of fluid overload in a patient with no renal function.

While coronary and central nervous system perfusion are at first selectively maintained, the heart will show signs of ischemic damage and failure when low blood flow becomes prolonged. The ability of the myocardium to withstand the stress depends mainly on the presence and degree of preexisting arteriosclerotic occlusive disease. Cerebral function is most sensitive to ischemia in the central nervous system, and early obtunding of the senses progresses to coma and eventual loss of muscle reflexes and more primitive brain stem functions.

SEPTIC SHOCK

Circulatory dysfunction and collapse seen in septic patients is in many ways more complex than shock from uncomplicated blood loss. The difficulties are aggravated by the profusion of studies of many different laboratory animal models, some of which use live bacteria and others of which employ endotoxin to simulate the clinical syndrome.

For the purposes of this discussion, it will be most helpful to concentrate mainly on the studies of septic patients, citing laboratory data where they help to clarify specific mechanisms. The major clinical problems with systemic sepsis today are caused principally by gram-negative organisms, although there is increasing awareness of the importance of the enteric anaerobes [6].

Cardiac Responses

Heart failure has been described by many authors in patients with septic shock. Others have found cardiac outputs elevated well above normal in septic patients with no signs of failure. The animal studies have been similarly confusing [7]. While there is much still to be learned, it is possible to form a coherent picture of the cardiac effects of sepsis based on current knowledge.

The response of the heart to systemic gram-negative sepsis must be viewed as a dynamic changing phenomenon within the context of time. Just as the general condition of the septic patient can fluctuate over short periods of time, his cardiac function is subject to the same instability. It makes little sense to take one measurement of cardiac output at some arbitrary point in the course of the illness and call it characteristic of the disease. For example, a low cardiac output late in septic shock means nothing more than that, when a patient is approaching death, all of his vital systems are likely to be failing.

The bulk of the existing evidence indicates that the early cardiac response to systemic gram-negative sepsis is an elevation in cardiac output. The primary event seems to be a decrease in peripheral vascular resistance, with pooling of blood in the capillary and venous circulations. Blood pressure falls, and when this condition is treated by volume expansion, cardiac output often rises to levels as high as twice normal. Coronary artery disease will, of course, limit the extent, but the basic response is an elevation in cardiac output. Thus early in septic shock the previously healthy patient exhibits elevated cardiac output, decreased total peripheral vascular resistance, and a requirement for large amounts of fluids and blood to support the circulation.

This situation has been described as the *hyperdynamic phase* of septic shock.

If the source of the sepsis is not removed or brought under control, the cardiac response cannot be sustained, and signs of decreasing cardiac performance then develop. The volumes of fluid required to maintain blood pressure and urine output become less well tolerated, producing elevations in pulmonary artery pressure that will threaten to induce congestive heart failure and pulmonary edema. Digitalis and other adrenergic drugs become needed to drive the heart and support the peripheral circulation.

Experimental studies to elucidate the effect of sepsis on the heart have yielded interesting but conflicting data. One series of experiments in dogs has shown the heart to be extremely resistant, functioning well long after the peripheral circulation has failed in septic shock. Others have described early heart failure. Extensive work has been directed at defining a material said to form in the splanchnic bed during low flow states which has a primary depressant effect on myocardial function, but the evidence for this in man is unconvincing.

The important point is that cardiac function in the patient in septic shock is a dynamic, rapidly changing process. Close monitoring by frequent measurements of blood pressure, pulmonary artery pressure, cardiac output, and urine output is necessary, and the treatment must be directed at the problem as it is seen by the bedside at any particular time.

Major Vessels

The peripheral circulation in sepsis shows a picture of decreased resistance on the arterial side. When blood volume is adequately supported, the patient often exhibits a widened pulse pressure, due mainly to decreased diastolic pressure. On the venous side, pooling is found in the major capacitance beds in the splanchnic and peripheral circulation. While direct observations of these phenomena cannot yet be made, measurements using isotope tracers on plasma albumin and on red cells suggest that in large segments of the vascular space circulation is slow and functionally sequestered.

Capillary Beds

The capillaries are subjected to a combination of hydrostatic, biochemical, and inflammatory factors in septic shock [14]. The net effect is to cause a generalized loss of integrity with leaking of fluid and plasma protein into the interstitial space.

Tissue Metabolic Effects

The effect on the cells is less specific. As described above under Prolonged Hypovolemic Shock, cellular changes are the result of hypoperfusion [16]. The lack of oxygen and the inadequate removal of metabolic products result in metabolic acidosis which becomes reflected in the circulating blood, as in hemorrhagic shock, with elevated lactate and hydrogen ion concentrations.

There is often a narrowing of the normal (5 volumes per 100 ml) arterial-venous oxygen difference, the result of an elevated venous oxygen tension. The cause for this decreased extraction of oxygen by the tissues is not clear. Some workers have postulated the opening of precapillary shunts that divert blood flow from the cells. Others have described an uncoupling of mitochondrial oxidation and phosphorylation in septic shock. It is not known definitely whether endotoxin exerts any direct effect on cellular metabolism, or whether the depressed metabolism is simply the indirect result of inadequate perfusion. However, the end result in the patient is a breakdown in cellular oxidative energy metabolism.

Immunological Events

The recent intense research in immunology, spurred by transplantation and cancer research activity, has generated a wealth of new information and concepts. It is becoming apparent that immunological mechanisms are involved in the body's responses to virtually all threats by foreign agents. This realization has stimulated a renewed interest in the immunological responses to microorganisms, which gave birth originally to the field of immunology a hundred years ago. A concept is emerging that views the responses to gram-negative bacteria and to endotoxin as primarily an activation of immunological systems. Rather than attacking cells directly, the damaging effects of sepsis may well be the result of activation of these systems, which then causes the widespread phenomena of septic shock. This concept of sepsis will be developed in the following sections.

The Humoral Mediators of Inflammation

The materials that affect vascular tone, capillary permeability, blood coagulation, and the activities of white blood cells and platelets comprise a large group of extremely potent peptides [9]. Figure 10-3 shows the variety and ubiquity of these agents. Without going into unnecessary detail, we note that the amines are mainly the catecholamines (epinephrine and norepinephrine), histamine, and serotonin. The principal kinin is bradykinin, a potent vasodilator which also increases capillary permeability; it is the end product of the sequential activation of prekallikrein and kallikreins. Hageman factor (HF, factor XII) has been found to be involved not only in the initiation of blood clotting but also in the activation and functioning of essentially all of the other agents in the list. Plasmin is the activated form of plasminogen, which

AMINES
KININS
KININOGENASES (Kallikreins)
HAGEMAN FACTOR (XII)
PLASMIN (Fibrinolysin)
COMPLEMENT
COLLAGEN & FIBRINOGEN FACTORS
LYMPHOKINES
PMN LYSOSOMAL ENZYMES
PROSTAGLANDINS

FIGURE 10-3. *Agents of inflammation. The order of listing does not imply any sequence of activation.*

breaks down fibrin formed in the blood and tissues.

Serum complement was originally described as a participant in the defense against microorganisms and was best known in the various serological tests for syphilis. It has now been discovered to be an exceedingly complex family of enzymes and agents with extremely diverse actions. Nine separate components have been described and labeled C1 to C9; each is composed of several subcomponents which are active both separately and together. The complement system plays a key role in the body's responses to gram-negative sepsis and endotoxemia, as will be seen in the context below.

Collagen, fragments of fibrinogen and fibrin, and materials now being found to be released from lymphocytes (macrophage inhibition factor, leukocyte chemotactic factor, capillary permeability factor) all participate in the response to sepsis. Polymorphonuclear leukocytes which are attracted to sites of inflammation release lysosomal enzymes. These not only have the local effects of assisting in breakdown and removal of bacteria but also enter the general circulation,where they exert widespread and indiscriminate tissue damage.

Prostaglandins are another newly described family of potent agents, the functions of which are confusing in their variety and apparent contradictions. They constrict or dilate blood vessels, aggregate or disaggregate platelets, and exhibit many other complex actions. It is too early to be certain of the exact mechanism, much less to think in terms of attacking them therapeutically, but there is no question that they are importantly involved in septic shock.

The events that stimulate the release and activation of these mediators of inflammation are listed in Figure 10-4. Without going into further detail, we should point out that these inflammatory responses are quite nonspecific and are remarkably sensitive to an enormous variety of stresses and threats to the body's integrity.

BLOOD LOSS
CATECHOLAMINE RELEASE
BLOOD EXTRAVASATION
BLOOD ACTIVATION
FLUID VOLUME EXPANSION
TRANSFUSION
ANESTHETICS & DRUGS
FAT EMBOLISM
SEPSIS

FIGURE 10-4. *Stimuli in trauma. All of these events, alone or in combination, can initiate activation of all the humoral mediator systems.*

Figure 10-5 attempts to integrate the interrelationships among these mediators into a coherent picture. The central role of Hageman factor is apparent, and its activation by any of the factors listed in Figure 10-3 triggers the entire spectrum of inflammation. Beginning in the upper right corner of the diagram in Figure 10-5, the familiar role of HF in triggering the coagulation process is shown. Clockwise, the active subunits of HF are seen to activate the kinin-forming system. At the left side of the diagram, the HF converts plasminogen to plasmin in a counter-reaction to the blood clotting process. The plasmin, along with kininogen and probably also HF itself, in turn initiates the serum complement sequence, which generates a myriad of functional components as it proceeds to formation of the C9 complex that ultimately causes cell lysis.

Many of the agents formed during activation of this network also cause platelets to aggregate and adhere to capillary endothelium. In such a state the platelets release serotonin, histamine, and vasoactive nucleotides, the most potent of which is adenosine diphosphate (ADP). These peptides are vasodilators, and their release causes a redirection of blood flow through the surrounding capillary beds.

Polymorphonuclear leukocytes are also affected by these activated blood materials. They stick to vascular endothelium in most of the same locations as do the platelets, mainly in the pulmonary circulation, where they cause increased capillary permeability and contribute to the local inflammatory response.

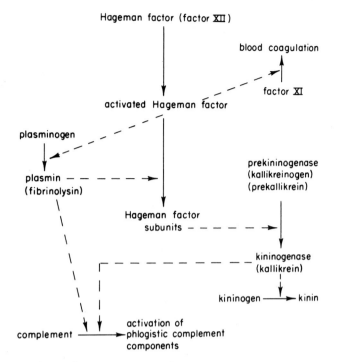

FIGURE 10-5.   *Interrelationships among the mediator systems. While HF activation is portrayed as the central event, the pathways can all be initiated by activation of any component anywhere in the network.*

Endotoxin Actions

Most of the damage in gram-negative sepsis is caused by the endotoxin released from the bacterial cell wall when the organisms disintegrate. According to a growing body of evidence, endotoxin does not damage cells directly and independently. Rather, it activates the mediator systems described in the previous section. The activated mediators then produce the injuries. It is obvious from the diversity of the mediators that the effects of their activation will be very widespread and will affect many body systems. This is indeed the case.

Endotoxin seems to require the presence of complement in order to initiate its actions. The requirement for preformed antibody is not established; in fact there is evidence that it is not essential. At any rate, the initial action of endotoxin is to activate C3 complement by an alternate pathway bypassing the earlier complement components. All of the other

HF-related systems are activated in turn through the network shown in Figure 10-5, resulting in kinin liberation, platelet aggregation, fibrin formation, fibrinolysis, and further generation of anaphylatoxin and other materials from the complement system. The network is interlaced with positive feedbacks, activation of one system reinforcing the activation of others in a series of vicious cycles.

The result is a diffuse disturbance of capillary blood flow that disrupts perfusion in all tissues. While the reticuloendothelial system works continuously to phagocytize and clear endotoxin, the widespread complex nature of the derangements makes it very difficult to overcome. Circulatory support and antibiotics are only partly effective, and usually only the drainage or excision of abscessed tissue tips the balance definitively in favor of the body's defenses. In view of the intricacy of the problem, it is not surprising that septic shock is so confusing in its appearance and so hard to treat.

Disseminated Intravascular Coagulation

Disseminated intravascular coagulation (DIC), seen in a variety of surgical situations, is probably most common in the patient with systemic sepsis. Because it is one of the few manifestations of the diffuse mediator activation that is amenable to some kind of treatment, we shall examine the mechanisms involved in a little detail.

Figure 10-6 presents an array of the many events that can activate the blood clotting process. In essentially all cases there is a concomitant activation of the fibrinolytic system. The balance between thrombin action, which converts fibrinogen to fibrin on the one hand, and plasmin action, which breaks down fibrin on the other hand, is shown at the bottom of the diagram.

The degree of imbalance between the two mechanisms varies from patient to patient. In those whose fibrinolytic response to intravascular coagulation is adequate, the fibrin is broken down as rapidly as it forms, and the appearance of fibrin degradation products in

the blood may be the only evidence of what is going on. When fibrin formation is too active and overwhelms the fibrinolytic process, actual clotting occurs in small vessels. This Shwartzman-type reaction commonly takes place in the kidneys but is seen in many vascular beds.

Whether or not fibrinolysis keeps pace with the rate of clotting, there is always an accelerated usage of the clotting factors. When the consumption of clotting factors becomes severe, spontaneous bleeding or exaggerated bleeding from wounds occurs. This paradox of bleeding caused by a basic hypercoagulability is a most ominous complication of sepsis. Heparinization is a courageous but necessary measure—the only feasible treatment known. The earlier institution of heparin therapy at the first signs of DIC is now being explored as a possible means of preventing the full development of consumption coagulopathy and bleeding.

RED CELL OXYGEN TRANSPORT

The availability of oxygen to the cells is a central factor in all degrees and types of shock. The amount of oxygen which is pre-

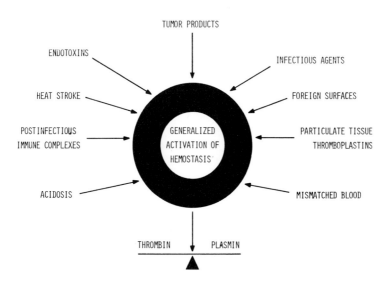

FIGURE 10-6. *Activation of blood clotting. The balance between the clotting process and the reactive fibrinolysis that usually develops concurrently is represented at the bottom of the figure.*

sented to a given tissue per unit time is a function of (1) blood flow, (2) blood oxygen content (physically dissolved or hemoglobin bound), and (3) red blood cell release. In shock, all these factors are called into play to increase tissue oxygenation, with varying effectiveness and varying potential benefit limited by the physiology of the system involved.

To consider the first mechanism, an increase in oxygen delivery to tissues can be produced by an increase in blood flow. For an additional flow to the whole body, there must naturally be greater cardiac output. For an increase to certain organs, a redistribution of cardiac output can take place. As described earlier, both of these mechanisms occur in shock, the results being limited by the blood volume, by the ability of the heart to perform extra work, and by the adequacy of vascular constriction in the less essential tissues.

More oxygen can also be made available to the tissues by an increase in the oxygen content of the blood perfusing them. However, this is a strictly limited potential mechanism for the following reasons: Oxygen dissolves very poorly in blood, with only 0.0031 ml going into solution for each millimeter of mercury of PO_2. Therefore, at an arterial blood PO_2 of 650, which is as high as occurs even in a person breathing 100% oxygen, the blood will contain only 2 ml of oxygen per milliliter in solution. The futility of expecting to raise significantly the content of physically dissolved oxygen in blood by elevating the PO_2 is apparent.

The major amount of oxygen is, of course, carried bound to hemoglobin, with each gram of hemoglobin binding 1.38 ml of oxygen. This mechanism is also limited as a means for increasing the availability of oxygen to the tissues. In a patient with a reduced red cell mass from acute hemorrhage, transfusion is vital for restoration of normal hemoglobin-oxygen-carrying capacity. However, there is considerable evidence that a hematocrit value much above 40 will increase the viscosity of the blood, thereby impeding its flow through the microcirculation and probably

offsetting the potential benefits of the added oxygen capacity. Therefore, while restoration of red cell mass is necessary in the treatment of shock, the advantage cannot be pursued beyond that limit.

It has recently become recognized that changes in the way hemoglobin releases oxygen in the capillaries represent another mechanism for increasing the availability of oxygen to the tissue cells [13]. A review of the dynamics and the controlling influences of the oxyhemoglobin dissociation curve will help to elucidate these phenomena.

The significance of the sigmoid shape of the curve can be seen by consideration of Figure 10-7. A drop of 10 torr (from 100 to 90) at the upper part of the curve, where oxygenation occurs in the lungs, is associated with only a very small decrease in the saturation of hemoglobin. The same 10 torr decrease (from 40 to 30) at the lower part of the curve, which represents the situation in the tissue capillary beds, causes a much greater drop in saturation. This results in the release of 5 ml of oxygen per 100 ml of blood, an amount that is adequate for most tissues in a normal resting state. Thus, there is a kind of pulmonary reserve ensuring that the hemoglobin will be well saturated even in the face of some pulmonary dysfunction with lowered alveolar oxygen tension.

The point on the curve labeled P50 is the oxygen tension at which the hemoglobin is 50% saturated. This point is a convenient way of describing the location of the curve in a horizontal axis, as it identifies the steepest part of the curve, which shows the greatest change when the curve shifts in either direction. The P50 of normal human blood under normal conditions is 27 torr, and shifts from this location will now be considered.

The position of the oxyhemoglobin dissociation curve is not static but rather is quite mobile in a horizontal direction. While the shape remains unchanged, the curve shifts readily to the left or to the right in a variety of conditions shown in Figure 10-8.

The influence of pH and PCO_2 on the curve

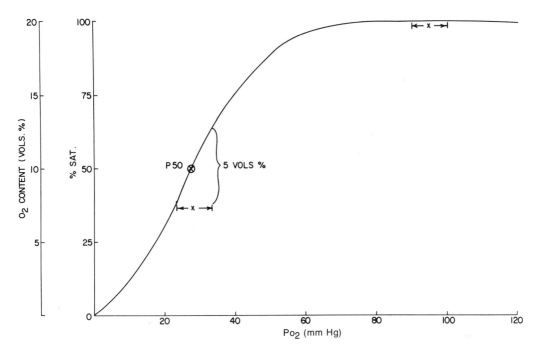

FIGURE 10-7. *The oxyhemoglobin dissociation curve. P50 is the Po₂ at which hemoglobin is 50% saturated. The x's represent a decrease of 10 torr in Po₂ and indicate the consequent change in saturation, as measured on the vertical axis of the graph.*

location is the familiar Bohr effect. The role of red cell 2,3-diphosphoglycerate (2,3-DPG) in shifting the curve has been more recently described. This material is found in highest concentration as a glycolytic cycle intermediate in the red cell, where it competes with oxygen for binding sites on the molecule. The effect of an elevation of 2,3-DPG in the red cell is to decrease the affinity of hemoglobin for oxygen, causing it to release oxygen more readily at any given Po₂. This condition is represented in Figure 10-9 as a right-shifted curve. A lowered 2,3-DPG in concentration results in the opposite effect of a left-shifted curve, which gives off oxygen less readily to the tissues.

The physiological consequences of these shifts in the curve observed in the listed conditions can be appreciated more fully by an analysis of Figure 10-9. The solid curve is the normal location at a P50 of 27, and the dashed-line curves represent 4 mm shifts to either side. In the upper area, the numbers refer to the amount of oxygen that can be extracted on passage of blood through tissues where the Po₂ is 40 torr (the normal value in skeletal muscle, for example). Blood with the right-shifted curve will give up 6.4 volumes per 100 ml of oxygen, while the left-shifted curve gives up only 3.2 volumes per 100 ml, all at the same rate of blood flow. It is thus apparent that the patient with a right-shifted curve will enjoy delivery of twice as much oxygen into his tissues as the patient with the left-shifted curve, with *no increase* in blood flow.

This advantage is of the greatest potential importance for the heart. While such tissues as skeletal muscle normally function at a Po₂ of about 40 torr and extract about 5 volumes per 100 ml of oxygen from the blood, the heart is quite different. In the presence of a left-shifted dissociation curve, or when blood flow is diminished, skeletal muscle can adjust

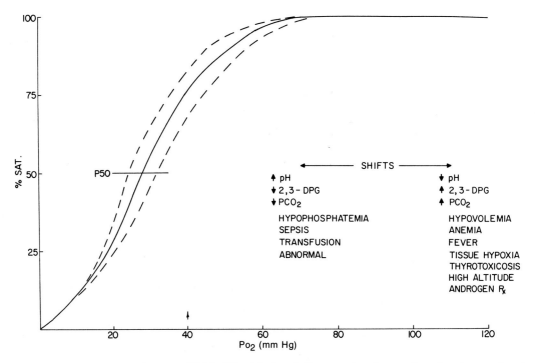

FIGURE 10-8.   *Determinants of P50. The left-hand list contains factors found to be associated with left shifts of the curve, while the conditions in the right-hand list are associated with a shift to the right.*

its operating PO_2 downward and simply extract more oxygen in that way by sliding down the curve. The PO_2 of femoral vein blood has been found to go as low as 10 torr in very low flow states, reflecting this adaptation of muscles. The heart, on the other hand, normally operates at a much lower PO_2 (20 to 22 torr) and correspondingly extracts over 11 volumes per 100 ml of oxygen from the coronary blood flow. Therefore, the reserve available to the myocardium is much less, being already closer to the point on the lower end of the dissociation curve where oxygen cannot be removed at a physiological PO_2. Any increase in oxygen delivery to the myocardium must be accomplished by an increase in coronary blood flow.

As one would deduce on teleological grounds, a right shift in the dissociation curve would seem to be beneficial to the heart when an increased demand for oxygen cannot be met by an increase in coronary blood flow. This conclusion has some support in a study of patients with coronary arteriosclerosis and exertional angina. When treadmill stress caused the onset of angina, the blood coming into the coronary sinus from the coronary veins was found to develop a right shift in the dissociation curve.

Attempts to take some therapeutic advantage of such shifts are currently under way. Freshly donated blood has a much higher P50 and 2,3-DPG (right shift) than stored bank blood, and studies are exploring for any benefit in transfusion of fresh as opposed to aging blood for massive hemorrhage. Also, it is now possible to shift the curve to the right pharmacologically by in vitro treatment of blood with phosphate and other substrates. Blood treated in this way to elevate P50 and 2,3-DPG well above normal (truly "super cells") has been found to be of significant benefit to

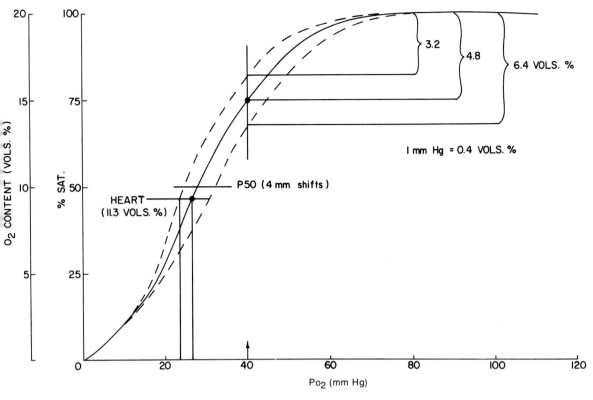

FIGURE 10-9. *Oxygen content and P50. The consequences of 4 torr shifts in either direction are shown to allow release of more oxygen with a right shift and less with a left shift.*

patients undergoing open heart surgery.

Work is proceeding to define the methods and indications for therapeutic manipulations of the location of the oxyhemoglobin dissociation curve. In the meanwhile, the observation of right shifts of the curve in hemorrhagic shock, fever, anemia, and at high altitude seems to substantiate this concept as an important adaptive mechanism for enhancing tissue oxygenation.

THE LUNG IN SHOCK

Over the past decade, and especially with the impact of the Vietnam War, a great deal of interest has been generated in the phenomenon of pulmonary failure following nonthoracic trauma [11]. In the late 1960s a voluminous literature described this syndrome as "shock lung," and it was variously attrib-

uted to each or all of the factors listed in Figure 10-10. Further clinical and laboratory investigation has clarified some of the uncertainties about the etiology.

No single factor has been established as the sole cause of pulmonary failure after trauma. It is rarely possible to study patients who have had only one of the stresses listed in Figure 10-10, but studies using animal models for each of them separately have been largely unsuccessful or have suffered from questionable clinical relevance. Perhaps the most important observation is that, when care is taken to minimize or prevent as many of the proposed causative events as possible, the incidence of pulmonary failure seems to be substantially reduced. With increased awareness of the potential dangers, and especially by avoidance of fluid overload, it is now becom-

MICROEMBOLI
TISSUE
TRANSFUSED BLOOD
FAT
DIC
OXYGEN TOXICITY
RESPIRATORS
FLUID OVERLOAD
SEPSIS
SEDATION & ANESTHESIA

FIGURE 10-10. *Pulmonary failure following trauma. Each of these factors has been described as causing post-traumatic pulmonary failure, although they are rarely found singly in any patient.*

ing apparent that the greatest risk of post-traumatic pulmonary failure is in the septic patient. The pulmonary consequences of the inflammatory mediator activations described earlier are still not understood well enough to offer much basis for more definitive prevention or treatment.

The clinical picture is better defined. The patient typically may have a moderately low arterial PO_2 (70 to 90) in the first few hours following surgical or accidental trauma. This improves with mobilization, lessening sedation, and institution of pulmonary physiotherapy. On the second to fifth day there is a decrease again in arterial oxygenation, particularly when gram-negative wound infection develops.

The oxygenation difficulty is usually found to be due to an imbalance between ventilation and perfusion, with blood going through the lungs without participating in gas exchange. This pulmonary shunting initially responds to use of a ventilator, but eventually it becomes impossible to maintain adequate Pa_{O_2} even on 100% inspired oxygen. The lungs become stiff, requiring increasing ventilator force to overcome the noncompliance.

Pulmonary failure following nonthoracic trauma remains a difficult complication to

overcome, with a high mortality for the fully developed syndrome. Improved treatment, and eventually an effective method of prevention, will depend on further understanding of the vascular derangements of shock.

REFERENCES

1. Abel, F. L., and Wolf, M. B. Increased capillary permeability to 125I-labelled albumin during experimental hemorrhagic shock. *Trans. N.Y. Acad. Sci.* 35:243, 1973.
2. Bear, R. A., and Gribik, M. Assessing acid-base imbalance through laboratory parameters. *Hosp. Practice* 9:157, 1974.
3. Cohen, P. J. The metabolic function of oxygen and biochemical lesions of hypoxia. *Anesthesiology* 37:148, 1972.
4. Cunningham, J. N., Shires, G. T., and Wagner, Y. Cellular transport defects in hemorrhagic shock. *Surgery* 70:215, 1971.
5. Ellertson, D. G., McGough, E. C., Rasmussen, B., Sutton, R. B., and Hughes, R. K. Pulmonary artery monitoring in critically ill surgical patients. *Am. J. Surg.* 128:791, 1974.
6. Gorbach, S. L., and Bartlett, J. G. Anaerobic infections. *N. Engl. J. Med.* 290:1177, 1974.
7. Hinshaw, L. B. Role of the heart in the pathogenesis of endotoxin shock. *J. Surg. Res.* 17:134, 1974.
8. Jakschik, B. A., Marshall, G. R., Kourik, J. L., and Needleman, P. Profile of circulating vasoactive substances in hemorrhagic shock and their pharmacologic manipulation. *J. Clin. Invest.* 54:842, 1974.
9. Kaplan, A. P. The Hageman factor dependent pathways of human plasma. *Microvasc. Res.* 8:97, 1974.
10. Selkurt, E. E. Current stages of renal circulation and related nephron function in hemorrhage and experimental shock. *Circ. Shock* 1:3, 1974.
11. Neville, J. F. Respiratory Gas Exchange—Normal and Abnormal. *Surg. Clin. North Am.* 54(5):943, 1974.
12. Watkins, G. M., Rabelo, A., Bevilacqua,

R. G., Brennan, M. F., Dmochowski, J. R., Ball, M. R., and Moore, F. D. Bodily changes in repeated hemorrhage. *Surg. Gynecol. Obstet.* 139:161, 1974.

13. Watkins, G. M., Rabelo, A., Plzak, L. F., and Sheldon, G. F. The left shifted oxyhemoglobin curve in sepsis. *Ann. Surg.* 180:213, 1974.

14. Wilhelm, D. L. Mechanisms responsible for increased vascular permeability in acute inflammation. *Agents Actions* 3:297, 1973.

15. Wraight, E. P. Capillary permeability to protein as a factor in the control of plasma volume. *J. Physiol.* (Lond.) 237:39, 1974.

16. Wright, C. J., Duff, J. H., McLean, A. P. H., and MacLean, L. D. Regional capillary blood flow and oxygen uptake in sepsis. *Surg. Gynecol. Obstet.* 132:637, 1971.

IV

*Alternative Factors Producing
Tissue Abnormality*

INTRODUCTION

It is not only the hostile external environment that produces tissue breakdown. Many other factors are also responsible for the production of tissue changes. Some of them are known, some can be guessed at, and others remain an enigma.

Part IV brings together some of these factors and, more important to the reconstructive surgeon, the changes they cause in tissue.

Because the skin is such a large area of our surgical endeavor, it seemed logical to examine it in some detail before going on to another important aspect of the raison d'être *of reconstructive surgeons: skin tumors. As we progress to hamartomas we get into the soft tissue below the skin as well as the skin itself, until with the changes of growth and the results of aging our examination must include the entire body and its constituent tissues. The reason cosmetic surgery is so popular in today's society is easy to understand when one reads the last chapter in this section.*

11

The Skin

B. Herold Griffith

The skin is the largest and most versatile organ in the body. In the average adult man, the skin weighs about 4 kg (14 to 17 percent of lean body weight), has a volume of 3.6 liters, and has a surface area of over 1.8 square meters. It is larger than either the brain or the liver. Dubois and Dubois's [6] standard formula for calculating the surface area in man is:

(1) stratum corneum, (2) barrier area, (3) granular area, and (4) the cellular epidermis, composed of the stratum malpighii and the stratum germinativum. The underlying dermis is made up of connective tissue, blood vessels, nerves and specialized epithelial derivatives, and the epidermal appendages (sweat glands, sebaceous glands, and hair follicles).

$$\text{Surface area (in sq cm)} = (\text{body weight in kg} \times 0.425) \times (\text{height in cm} \times 0.725) \times 71.84$$

The essential functions of the skin are (1) protection—a barrier against the loss of body fluids and the ingress of foreign substances, (2) sensation, (3) regulation of body temperature and fluid metabolism, (4) regulation of blood pressure, (5) sexual attraction, and (6) identification. The skin is also a signpost for the recognition of local and systemic diseases. It has a remarkable ability to regenerate itself and thereby heal its wounds [5].

ANATOMY

The skin is composed of *epidermis*, derived from the ectoderm, and *dermis*, a mesodermal derivative. The epidermis has several layers:

The full thickness of the skin—epidermis plus dermis—varies from 0.5 mm on the eyelids to 3 to 6 mm on the palms and soles. The epidermis is 0.12 mm thick except on the palms and soles, where it may be 0.8 mm thick. The dermis is 5 to 10 times as thick as the epidermis [6].

PROTECTIVE FUNCTION

The principal function of the skin is protection and depends on special features of the epidermis. First, a film of emulsified material is spread rather evenly over the surface. It assists with antisepsis, lubrication, absorption of toxic agents, control of hydration, and buffering of acids and alkalies. The film contains (1) lactic acid, urea, amino acids, uric acid, and ammonia from the sweat glands, (2) triglycerides, fatty acids, and wax alcohols from the sebaceous glands, and (3) sterols, pentoses, amino acids, phospholipids, and complex polypeptides which come from the process of cornification. The composition of the film varies from area to area of the body. The sole of the foot, for example, like the palm of the hand, has no sebaceous glands and therefore lacks some strongly fungistatic fatty acids. This lack may account for the fact that fungus infections are most common on the sole. In winter, when sweat and sebaceous gland activity are diminished, the skin is dry, scaly, and easily fissured. The application of petrolatum or wool fat corrects these deficiencies [12].

The activity of the sebaceous glands reaches its peak in adolescence and diminishes as the glands gradually involute with age. Dietary, hormonal, and emotional factors all play roles in the activity of the sebaceous glands.

The stratum corneum is 40 to 60 μ thick over most of the body but thickens as the result of trauma and is even thicker prenatally in areas that will be subjected to the most trauma. It reaches 600 μ in thickness on the palms and soles. This horny layer continually desquamates and is replaced by cells that migrate up from the lower layers of the epidermis. As the cells pass through the granular layer, they lose their nuclei and become very compact. They are held together by "spot welds" called *desmosomes*. Within the epidermal cells are cytoplasmic filaments called *tonofibrils*, believed to be forerunners of keratin. A lipid monolayer surrounds the keratin fibers in the stratum corneum [10].

The stratum corneum is remarkably impervious to water, water vapor, and diatomic gases such as nitrogen and oxygen. Only 5 to 10 ml of water pass through 1 square meter of lipified keratin per hour under a vapor pressure of 26 to 35 mm Hg. Removal of the lipid from the stratum corneum permits a 30- to 60-fold increase in the rate of flow of water through it, making it as porous as a nylon stocking. Dehydrated but lipified human skin offers so little resistance to the passage of diatomic gases that, under a pressure of 1 atmosphere, 1 mole of air passes through 1 square meter of dehydrated skin in three minutes. When the skin is rehydrated, it becomes so resistant that it takes 1 mole of air 150 days to pass through it at 1 atmosphere of pressure. The skin's resistance to the passage of water is therefore lipid dependent, while its resistance to the passage of gases is hydration dependent. It is this water-retaining capacity of the skin that makes it possible for man to live in air [10].

The density of the keratin mesh in the cells and the tight packing together of the cells themselves prevent most bacteria and large chemical molecules from entering the skin. With desquamation of the keratin, these noxious substances are cast off. Smaller molecules that get through the stratum corneum are blocked by the next layer, the *barrier area*, which has a negative charge. It repels anions and attracts and holds cations, thereby preventing their further penetration. A break in the continuity of the stratum corneum, such as occurs with a scratch or laceration, destroys the barrier's effectiveness and may permit harmful substances to enter the body [12]. It has been estimated that the average person sustains one scratch per week. These injuries are prevented from causing serious harm by virtue of the great healing capacity of the skin.

Although the epidermis is an effective barrier, certain substances do penetrate easily: metallic nickel, mustard gas, and the oleoresin of poison ivy, for example. Breaks in the integrity of the barrier layer in some dermatoses permit the entry of locally applied steroids such as hydrocortisone and triamcinolone. The steroid inhibits inflammation and allows the barrier to be repaired quickly. Most other drugs and hormones do not enter normal intact skin.

The *granular layer* participates actively in

keratinization, but the details of its function are not known. The *cellular epidermis* also contributes to the protective function of the skin. Its desmosomes are essential for holding the skin together. The dissolution of the strong intercellular bonds between the layers of the epidermis and at the dermal-epidermal junction, which occurs in second-degree burns and about 30 skin diseases, leads to blistering. The exact nature and source of the enzymatic factors responsible for this are not yet known. The peeling off of only a few of the many layers of the stratum corneum results in a strong stimulation of mitoses in the stratum germinativum [13]. Scattered among the epithelial cells of the stratum germinativum are the *pigment cells*, which afford important protection against ultraviolet radiation [15].

The *dermal-epidermal junction* appears, on electron microscope study, to be essentially a basement membrane that cements the epidermis to the dermis. This bond can be broken by heating the skin to 50°C and by the action of certain chemicals [12].

Protection against harmful bacteria is provided by the anatomical barrier of the epidermis, local tissue antibodies, and the rich vascular supply of the dermis, which furnishes the skin with antibodies, phagocytes, and the mechanism for inflammation [5]. Protection against physical trauma is afforded by the tough but pliable stratum corneum on the outside, the strong intercellular bonds which resist shearing within the epidermis, and the resiliency of the dermis and the underlying subcutaneous fibroadipose tissue [11].

PIGMENTATION

The color of the skin is largely due to the hemoglobin in the vessels of the dermis and the melanin in the epidermis. *Melanin* is a term used for a group of pigments that are formed by the oxidation of phenols. They are found uncombined as well as conjugated with proteins. In other animals, many phenolic substances act as precursors; in man tyrosine is the precursor. Melanin ranges in color from yellow in the reduced state, through orange and brown shades, to black in the oxidized state. It is chiefly responsible for the differences in the color of skin, eyes, and black hair of man. In brown, red, and blond hair the pigment is pheomelanin.

The only known function of melanin in man is to filter out ultraviolet radiation and prevent its harmful effects on the dermis. This function can be complemented by a thick stratum corneum. The protective action of melanin is believed to be due to its properties as a stable free radical that acts as a repository of photoactively produced electrons. Melanins in general are inert, insoluble, nonhydrolyzable, and chemically intractable. In man, tyrosine melanin is bound to protein through sulfhydryl groups. It is a strong reducing agent capable of reducing gold and silver salts.

In man all melanin is produced by melanocytes. These unicellular secretory glands can hydroxylate tyrosine to melanin. The melanocytes of the skin arise as melanoblasts from the neural crest; those in the retina, from the outer layer of the optic cup. Melanoblasts are first found in human skin in the tenth week of fetal life. They migrate to various places, but only those in the epidermis persist. They can be seen only when they are forming pigment. The number of melanocytes is believed to be the same in all races. It is only the amount of pigment within them that makes differences in the color of the skin [15].

SENSATION

The skin supplies the body surface with countless receptors for feeling pain, touch, heat, and cold. When the receptors are stimulated, the sensation is the product of temporal and spatial summation peripherally and in the spinal cord, and the interaction of central factors such as experience and emotion [18].

The dermal nerve networks and their related nerve endings make up most of the nervous tissue in the skin. The nerve networks are in all levels of the dermis. At any point, a nerve network is made up of nerves that come in from several directions. Deep in the dermis the nerves are large and heavily myelinated. Higher in the dermis there are many non-myelinated and lightly myelinated fibers. In the subepidermal area most of the network consists of nonmyelinated fibers. The function of the networks is to gather stimuli from many fibers in a given area and to transmit the information to the cord and brain. They are the receptors for touch, temperature, pain, and itch [18].

There are also *intraepithelial nerves*, which lie between the epithelial cells as high as the granular layer. Their function appears to be to increase acuity, and they are seen mainly in thick skin. *Nonspecific nerve endings* in the dermal papillae seem to function in the same way as the general dermal networks. As yet no definite relation has been established between the nerve endings and the melanocytes, in spite of their common embryological origin.

Around the hair follicles are abundant nerve networks, probably carry-overs from the fur of lower animals—that is, the first structure to be stimulated. Sensory hairs or "whiskers" of lower animals serve as tactile antennae [5].

Mucocutaneous end-organs are located in the subpapillary area of the dermis of the eyelid, lip, tongue, gum, oral cavity, prepuce, penis, clitoris, labia, and perianal area, but not in the nipple, areola, or vagina. They appear to be only touch receptors, though they may also receive the sensation of cold.

Meissner's corpuscles are located in the distal extremities, particularly on the pads of fingertips. They are highly sensitive touch receptors. The *hederiform endings of Merkel-Ranvier* exist in humans only in the distal glabrous skin and are also tactile receptors. The *Vater-Pacini corpuscles* are the largest sensory receptors in the skin and are located in the subcutaneous tissue of the fingers, palms, toes, soles, nipples, external genitalia and perianal area, and in numerous deeper positions. They are pressure receptors but may be used for vascular control as well, through connections with the glomus bodies.

There is great variation in the type and number of nerve endings in different areas of the skin. Transplanted skin never has more nerve endings after it has become established in its new site than it had in its original location.

The autonomic nervous system is represented in the skin by the sympathetic nerves. Parasympathetic fibers may be present, but they have not been conclusively demonstrated. The sympathetic fibers come mainly from the thoracic cord and reach the skin via the blood vessels and cutaneous nerves that supply the dermal networks. They innervate the vessels, myoepithelial muscles, sweat glands, and arrectores pilorum muscles [18]. The sebaceous glands do not appear to have any innervation.

TEMPERATURE REGULATION

The normal oral body temperature is 98.6°F (37°C). The rectal temperature is 0.6°F higher, and the axillary temperature is at least 1°F lower. The skin is normally cooler, and the internal organs are warmer. The skin, covered with clothes, averages 85° to 93°F (29.5° to 33.9°C). Body temperature varies 2° to 3°F during the day with the peak in the afternoon. Warm-blooded animals such as man are said to be *homoiothermic* and can maintain a narrow range of temperature despite wide environmental differences. Cold-blooded animals are *poikilothermic*; their body temperatures change with changes in their environment.

The body continually produces heat by metabolic activity, the rate being minimal in sleep and maximal with strenuous muscular activity. The rate of heat loss must equal the rate of heat production in order to maintain a constant temperature. Environmental temperature affects the rate of heat loss and production. In a hot environment and during strenuous exercise the evaporation of sweat is essential to dispose of excess heat. Sweating is an "emergency measure," as is shivering at the other extreme of temperature. In the average moderate range of temperatures the rate of heat loss is adequately controlled by variation of the rate of blood flow through the skin. Most of the heat production occurs deep in the body, with insulation by the overlying skin and fat. The excess heat is transported by the blood to the skin, where it can be dissipated. Heat is lost from the body by (1) radiation (50%), (2) conduction (less than 1%), (3) convection (15%), (4) evaporation of sweat (30%), (5) warming of inspired air (3%), and (6) urine and feces (2%). The average man doing light work produces 3000 Cal per day. Basal metabolic rate normally produces 1 Cal per kilogram of body weight per hour [5].

Heat loss depends largely on adjustments in the blood-vascular system and is under the control of the autonomic nervous system. By redistribution of blood, the skin temperature may be adjusted to any temperature from about 59°F (15°C) to 100°F (37.8°C) at a room temperature of 93°F (34°C). The amount of blood flowing through the skin may amount to 12 percent of the total cardiac output; with exertion, 30 to 35 percent. Blood flow through the fingers increases from 1 ml per minute per 100 gm of tissue in a cold room to 80 to 90 ml per minute per 100 gm of tissue in a hot room. These changes may be initiated in one or all of four ways: (1) a change in the temperature of the blood flowing through the cerebral centers, principally the hypothalamus, (2) reflex through centers in the brain and cord in response to changes in skin temperature which are picked up by temperature receptors in the skin, (3) local axon reflexes, and (4) direct stimulation of the vessels by changes in the environmental temperature.

Changes in blood volume also affect heat loss. An increase in blood volume, with the blood being diluted by fluid drawn into the circulation from the tissues (mainly the skin, muscles, and liver) lowers heat. Blood is expelled from the spleen. The total circulating blood volume can be increased by 10 percent in two to four hours on exposure to enough heat to cause diffuse cutaneous vasodilata-tion. Also, increased cardiac output provides a rapid flow of blood through the dilated vessels of the skin.

The human skin, regardless of color, is an almost perfect *black body radiator*; that is, it radiates almost all infrared rays (98 percent). When the vessels are constricted, the skin and subcutaneous fat are as efficient an insulating mechanism as a thin layer of cork. The greater thickness of the subcutaneous layer in women accounts for their greater ability to withstand cold than men have. The radiating surface of the body is only about 85 percent of the total surface area since the axillae, inner arms and thighs, and other opposed surfaces do not lose heat by radiation. Clothing also retards the radiation of heat, as does the layer of air between the body and the clothing. But convection currents can be set up when there is a significant difference between the body and its environment, and the temperature of the skin can be altered thereby. The main factor influencing heat loss by convection, however, is the movement of air, the loss increasing with the square of the wind velocity.

The nearer the environmental temperature approaches the body temperature, the smaller is the loss of heat by convection and radiation, reading 0° at 98.6°F. When the environmental temperature exceeds the body temperature, heat loss must take place by evaporation of sweat and exhalation of heated air. The evaporation of 1 ml of water uses up 0.58 Cal. At room temperature heat loss from the skin and lungs is 17 Cal per hour, about two-thirds of which is from insensible perspiration. At a room temperature of 35°C or above, almost all heat is lost by evaporation. Insensible perspiration is independent of the sweat glands and consists of water which is extravasated from the cutaneous capillaries and seeps through the epidermis. Water moves out of the skin into air of less than 90 percent relative humidity or into a salt solution of greater than 10 percent concentration. As much as 18 gm of water per square meter per hour can be lost in this way. Nevertheless, persons who are born without sweat glands or whose sweat glands do not function properly because of spinal cord injuries may be essentially poikilothermic in a hot environment. An increased respiratory rate, which is produced by a rise in the temperature of the air, causes an increase in the loss of heat via inspired air, which is 95 percent saturated with water. The loss of heat by insensible perspiration and by sweating is impaired by high environmental humidity. Heavy occlusive drapes which are placed over a patient on the operating table can interfere with the normal loss of body heat and result in serious overheating.

Sweat glands are of two types, eccrine and apocrine. The *eccrine glands* are present in all areas of the skin except the lips, glans penis, clitoris, and inner surface of the prepuce. They are small tortuous glands that lie deep in the dermis and open onto the surface of the skin via small independent pores. There are 100 to 340 eccrine glands per square centimeter of skin or a total of about 2,000,000 in the adult. Their secretion, sweat, is a weak aqueous solution of sodium chloride (0.2% to 0.5%), together with urea and small quantities of lactic acid and potassium. The pH varies from 4.2 to 7.5. Muscle activity increases the salt concentration, and heavy exertion in a high temperature can deplete the body's chloride unless salt is ingested to restore the balance. As much as 2 gm of salt can be lost per hour by profuse sweating.

The sweat glands are cholinergic, but under the control of the sympathetic nervous system. Their responses are anomalous in that they are stimulated by pilocarpine, acetylcholine, and muscarine and are inhibited by atropine. Acetylcholine appears to act through direct stimulation of the gland (muscarine-like action) by initiation of axon reflexes (nicotine-like action). The glands are not excited by epinephrine or paralyzed by ergotoxine. The usual stimulus to the excretion of eccrine sweat is a rise in blood temperature, which acts *directly* on the nervous centers (mainly the hypothalamus) and reflexly by stimulation of heat receptors in the skin.

Cutting of the nerves going to the area abolishes the sweating response to a rise in body temperature [1]. Sweating is not dependent on the circulation. Although it is usually associated with vasodilatation, it may occur with constricted vessels—"cold sweat" in response to fear, fatigue, nervousness, or mental work. In situations like these sweating occurs mainly on the forehead, palms, and soles.

The secretion pressure of sweat is 250 mm Hg. Sweat is therefore a true secretion, not a simple filtrate. The rate of secretion may be very great, up to 2 liters or more per hour with heavy work. At ordinary room temperature sweat evaporates as it forms and thus goes undetected.

The *apocrine sweat glands* are large tortuous glands whose ducts empty into hair follicles in the axillae, groin, umbilical area, periareolar areas, perineum, and perianal area. Unlike the eccrine glands, they are undeveloped in childhood and become active only with puberty. Their exact hormonal control is unknown, but in women they enlarge premenstrually, regress during menstruation, and atrophy after the menopause. Their yellow, translucent secretion contains proteins and carbohydrates. It is produced continuously but empties onto the skin only after adrenergic sympathetic stimulation, especially from emotional stress, which causes a contraction of the myoepithelium about the glands. The secretion is sterile initially, but its decomposition by bacteria gives rise to its unpleasant, characteristic odor. The apocrine glands do not appear to have any useful function, but the cerumen glands of the ear canal and the mammary glands, which are modified apocrine glands, have obvious uses. The main significance of the apocrine glands is that they are often the site of chronic smoldering infections (hidradenitis suppurativa) which may require radical surgical excision.

CIRCULATORY FUNCTIONS

The blood flow through the vessels of the skin is regulated by an interaction of the sympathetic nervous system, local tissue mediators, and factors that influence the intrinsic properties of the vessels themselves. The vessels of the skin do not arborize as do those in other tissues. The small arteries, upon entering the skin, give rise to a series of long arterioles, which interconnect to form an extensive interarteriolar network. Adjacent arterioles give off cross-branches that interconnect by a series of fine capillaries. Most of the precapillaries and capillaries that actually nourish the skin are branches of these arcades. A comparable interconnecting meshwork of large and small venules is associated with the arterioles. The venous plexus lies in the subcutaneous tissue and is more extensive than the arteriolar network. The numerous direct connections between the venular and arteriolar plexuses allow blood to be shunted back to the venous system without having to pass through the capillaries [12].

The capillaries immediately below the epidermis are direct offshoots of the arteriolar arcades. Each branch is surrounded by several coiled muscular elements before it divides into two or three capillary loops. These are essentially capillary sphincters. Some capillary branches come off the deeper arterial plexus and enter the dermis proper. It is these vessels that continue to supply blood to the skin when the arteriovenous shunts are open (see also Chapter 15).

The small vessels of the skin have marked vasomotor activity, in contrast to those in other tissues. The arteriolar arcades are particularly sensitive to constrictor and dilator agents, which allow minimal stimuli to trap blood in the capillary networks. The venules are highly responsive to changes in temperature. A fall of 1° to 2°C results in a 10- to 20-fold increase in reactivity to epinephrine—a greater response than occurs in any other tissue [5].

The small vessels of the skin are under the control of both the central and sympathetic nervous systems. In fact, the vessels of the skin are the most responsive units to neurogenic constrictor and dilator influences. In hemorrhagic shock the interarcading arterioles go into almost total constriction within minutes of the start of blood loss and remain constricted until the blood pressure is restored by transfusion. In these situations the precapillary sphincters close and the circulation in the dermis is negligible, making the skin pale and cool. Its moist "clammy" feel is due to sympathetic stimulation of the sweat glands. A slow flow continues in the deeper venous plexuses because of the deeper arteriolar-venular shunts. With continued hypotension there is a backflow in the venous plexuses, with resultant stagnation of blood in the venules, and the skin becomes cyanotic. The vasoconstriction within the skin during stress is mediated mainly by neurogenic factors.

Necrosis of the skin can follow prolonged vasoconstriction due to prolonged hypovolemic shock or bacterial endotoxins. Lesions in the skin produced by endotoxin, epinephrine and endotoxin, or epinephrine and 5-hydroxytryptamine can be prevented by autonomic blocking agents, especially Phenergan, Dibenzyline, and chlorpromazine [12].

Necrosis of the skin and subcutaneous tissues may result from prolonged mechanical compression of an area which is sufficient to keep the vessels collapsed and the tissues deprived of blood. It is commonly seen in patients with paraplegia, who have no warning sign of discomfort to alert them to the need for changing position. It is also seen in old or debilitated patients who remain in one position in bed for too long a time. When the necrotic tissue sloughs in one of these patients, an ulcer results—properly called a *pressure ulcer* or *pressure sore* [4].

Prolongation and survival of cells that have been deprived of their blood supply can be favored by local hypothermia, which lowers the temperature and metabolic rate and thus the oxygen requirement. Increasing the oxygen tension in the blood also helps.

Tissues vary in their oxygen needs. Skin does not have as high a need as brain, skeletal muscle, etc. The range of the skin's needs is not great and depends mainly on temperature. Even so, the blood flow through the skin is at least 100 fold—from 0.5 to 1.0 ml per minute per 100 cc of tissue in full vasoconstriction, to over 100 cc of tissue in full vasodilatation. This wide range, of course, is not needed just for the skin but serves the whole body. The main purpose is the regulation of temperature, but the regulation of blood pressure is another function. Unique arteriovenous shunts in the skin of the digits permit the blood to bypass the resistance of the capillary beds. The myoepithelial cells of the glomus bodies of these shunts are heavily supplied with cholinergic nerve endings. The shunts are of prime importance in temperature regulation, even though they function like similar shunts in the mesentery and stomach, which play no role in temperature control. They open and close apparently automatically, resembling the safety valves on a boiler. A sudden rise in blood pressure, which may be caused by marked vasoconstriction elsewhere, raises the pressure in the shunts and automatically opens them, thereby preventing an excessive rise of pressure in the entire system.

IDENTIFICATION

There is considerable variation in the skin's texture, color, topography, and thickness from area to area and from person to person. Some of the differences have obvious advantages, such as the rough surfaces of the feet and hands that facilitate grip. Most of the patterns are genetically determined. Since they are unique for each individual, they are a means of personal identification. Physical features, racial coloring, lines of expression, tattoos, and scars from infections, injuries, and operations are special possessions of each individual. *Dermatoglyphics*—the pattern of whorls, loops, ridges, lines, and arches of the palms of the hands—is of particular interest to law enforcement agencies. No two people, not even identical twins, have the same dermatoglyphics. The chance that two people will have the same fingerprints is estimated to be 1 in 24 billion—long odds in today's world. The patterns are noted in the fetus at three to four months of gestation. The dermatoglyphics of a person's right and left hands are different as well, suggesting that handedness may be established in the first trimester of fetal life. Women's fingerprints differ from men's, having more arches and fewer whorls.

SKIN BIOMECHANICS

The intrinsic lines of tension within the skin seem to be due, at least partially, to the orientation and polarity of the dermal collagen. The extensive work of Gibson and his coworkers is helping to clarify these forces and may have important implications in the planning of surgical procedures [2, 3, 7] (see also Chapter 16, Tissue Dynamics and Surgical Geometry). They have noted that at certain sites skin extends farther in one direction than in others, on application of uniaxial loads. If the orientation of maximum extensibility is known in the locality of a defect, then the excision can be planned to optimize the possibility of direct wound closure. If the defect is small enough to permit direct closure in any direction after excision, appropriate orientation of the excision will be helpful in minimizing the tension across the healing wound. Their experimental studies have shown that the mechanical properties of skin are largely dependent upon the spatial arrangement of collagen and elastic fibers in the dermis. When placed under tension in any given direction, the fibers eventually become aligned in tht direction, over a spectrum of strain typified by the "limit strain." For 60 percent of the sites tested there was found to be a definite preferred orientation of the architectural pattern indicated by the significant difference between axes of limit strain. At sites where there was a significant difference between axes of limit strain, the direction of minimum limit strain correlated closely with Langer's lines. This finding supports the belief that Langer's lines are *not* lines of tension, but probably lines of preferred orientation of the dermal fibers [3].

Gibson and Kenedi, in studying skin tensions in man, and with the tensometer and extensometer in their laboratory, have determined that a small incision across a band of blanching in the base of a rotated flap relieves the blanching and improves the blood supply in general. Only a minor part of this effect appears to be due to the opening of the incision. Most of it is due to changes in the mechanism of force transmission within the dermis, because of changes in orientation of the collagen and elastic fibers. Their work lends scientific support to the long-held clinical view that local flaps should be made as large as possible to increase their chance of survival [2].

SIGNPOSTS OF DISEASE

Often the first clue to a systemic disease is a change in the skin. A few of the diseases that have early dermatological manifestations are (1) the exanthems (e.g., varicella, variola, rubella, rubeola), (2) allergies (e.g., urticaria, eczema, drug reactions), (3) diabetes (xanthelasma, necrobiosis lipoidica diabeticorum, etc.), (4) the lymphomas, leukemias, and mycosis fungoides, (5) amyloidosis, (6) porphyria, (7) syphilis, (8) tropical diseases (e.g., leprosy, leishmaniasis, yaws), and (9) congenital deformities (e.g., mongolism).

THE PHYSIOLOGY OF
SKIN GRAFTS

Skin can be transplanted either as a pedicle flap or as a free graft. A *flap* is a piece of tissue that is transferred from one area to an adjacent or distant site with its blood supply maintained intact (see Chapter 15). A *free graft* is one that is cut completely loose from its original ("donor") site and transplanted as a free piece of tissue to another location on the body.

Free grafts of skin are of three types: autografts, homografts (allografts), and heterografts. An *autograft* is transplanted from one site to another in the same person. A *homograft* is transplanted from one individual to another of the same species. A *heterograft* is

taken from an individual of one species and placed on an individual of another species. A *zoograft* is a piece of tissue transplanted from an animal to a human.

An autograft can be expected to "take" in its new location and survive permanently, provided there is no physical, technical, or bacteriological complication. A homograft will often "take" in its new site as well as an autograft, only to be rejected later as a foreign substance. Acquired immunity is the main factor responsible for this loss. The permanent "take" of a homograft will occur in the case of identical twins (*isograft*) where the tissues of the two individuals are genetically the same. It may also occur when the recipient has congenital agammaglobulinemia and is incapable of producing antibodies against the homograft. Homografts are useful at times for temporary coverage of extensive burns. They last long enough for the patient's general condition to improve sufficiently for him to withstand autografting later, after the homografts have been rejected.

A heterograft, like a homograft, is a foreign substance and will not survive permanently. But it, too, may be useful for temporary coverage of a wound. Skin from young pigs is now being used in many situations where homografts might have been used a few years ago.

In repairing a defect in the skin, one should, whenever possible, use adjacent tissue to assure a good match of texture and color. If this is not a possible solution, a distant donor site must be used. In most instances a free skin graft is the material of choice, but where it cannot be used a pedicle flap is required [5].

Skin grafts are of two general types, full-thickness and split-thickness. The *full-thickness (whole-thickness) graft* (Wolfe-Krause graft) consists of the entire epidermis and dermis. It withstands trauma better than the thinner split graft because of the stability afforded by the dermis. It also, for the same reason, contracts less than does a split graft. However, since it is thicker, the full-thickness graft "takes" less readily than the split graft, and conditions must be optimal before it dare be used. The recipient bed must be free of infection and well vascularized. Another disadvantage of the full-thickness graft is the fact that its donor wound extends into the subcutaneous tissue and must be sutured or covered with a split graft [8].

A *split-thickness skin graft* is composed of the full thickness of the epidermis and a variable thickness of the dermis. The thickness used depends on the situation. As a general rule, the thinner the graft the more readily it "takes." Thin split grafts (Ollier-Thiersch), which consist of all the epidermis and superficial dermis, and thick split grafts (Blair), which contain all of the epidermis and about half of the underlying dermis, are particularly useful for covering granulating wounds containing bacteria. The thicker Blair-Brown grafts, made up of the epidermis and about two-thirds of the dermis, have great value in most large wounds where local conditions are ideal.

The rates of contracture of skin grafts vary directly with the skin laxity in the particular region, being minimum (11 to 27 percent) in the scalp, arms, and legs; medium (41 to 48 percent) in the abdomen, chest, and back; and high (52 to 80 percent) in the neck, eyelids, and dorsum of the hand. Rapid contracture occurs in the first two to three weeks, and the contracture is generally complete in one to one and a half months. Contracture of skin is least along lines of cleavage compared to lines perpendicular and diagonal to them, and the difference is highly significant [14].

The *take* of a graft warrants some discussion. A free graft which is cut loose from its original blood supply will survive for a limited time in the free state. Inside a sterile container in saline-moistened gauze a free graft can be kept viable for up to three weeks in a refrigerator at 4°C. At normal skin temperature it must get nourishment from the blood promptly. The process of vascularization of the graft and attachment to the recipient bed is called the "take" of the graft. Anastomoses develop between the vessels of the graft and those of the bed, by growth of endothelial buds from the cut ends of the vessels in each. This process starts shortly after grafting and is well advanced by the third day. In thin- and intermediate-thickness grafts there are good vascular connections by the fifth day; in full-thickness grafts, by the sixth or eighth day.

The rapidity with which the vascular connections occur depends upon several factors: (1) the vascularity and regenerative capacity of the recipient site, (2) the metabolic activity of the transplanted skin, and (3) the distance the capillary sprouts from the wound bed must traverse to reach the vessels of the graft [16]. Prior to the establishment of vascular connections, the graft is nourished by the diffusion of gases and nutrient fluids across the graft-bed interface, a process that has been called *plasmatic circulation*, or more properly *plasmatic imbibition* [16]. The richer vascularity of the superficial dermis probably accounts for the more rapid vascularization of thinner grafts than of thicker ones. The ingrowth of new vessels into the graft from the bed is probably negligible, the main blood supply of the graft coming from the anastomosis of existing vessels. Hence the persistence of the *original* color of grafts in Caucasians after transplantation [17]. This phenomenon must be kept in mind in the selection of donor sites for grafts that are to be placed on the face, since the face normally has a pinker color than the extremities or the trunk. Grafts from the postauricular area and the neck are best suited for the face. In the full-thickness graft that is accurately sutured into its recipient site, there is evidence that anastomoses develop between the vessels at the edges of the defect as well as between the vessels of the undersurface of the graft and those of the underlying bed.

While the graft is becoming vascularized, the fibrin clot between the graft and the recipient bed becomes organized, and the graft becomes secured to the bed by fibrous connections. During this period of anchorage, the graft must be protected from movement which could tear loose the new vascular and fibrous connections. Also, it must be firmly held against the bed so the blood or serum cannot accumulate under it and prevent the connections from being established.

A bed that cannot produce granulation tissue, such as bare cortical bone, cartilage, or tendon, or a bed that is avascular as a result of scarring or radiation injury, is an unsuitable site for a free graft. Further, because fat is poorly vascularized, the undersurface of a graft must be deprived of fat before it is applied to the recipient site, to assure that good vascular connections can develop.

The healing of the donor site of a split-thickness graft is important to consider. From this wound the epidermis and part of the dermis have been removed, leaving a large "raw" surface devoid of the normal source of surface epithelium, the stratum germinativum. If the graft has not been cut too thick, the remaining dermis of the donor site contains many epidermal elements—the hair follicles and the sebaceous and sweat glands with their ducts. These structures are lined with cuboid and columnar epithelial cells, which under the new conditions grow up and across the healing dermis, undergoing *squamous metaplasia* in the process; thus the wound becomes covered with stratified squamous epithelium. This epithelium thickens over the succeeding two or three months, forming a stable cover. Donor sites frequently remain red for some months following grafting, but fading to normal or paler than normal color occurs in time. In Negroes and other dark-skinned patients hyperpigmentation of donor sites often replaces the initial hypopigmentation within three to six months, and at times the hyperpigmentation persists indefinitely. Hydroquinone cream, rubbed into the hyperpigmented skin, is at times effective in reducing the pigmentation, since this drug interferes with the production of melanin by the melanocytes.

If the donor site is protected and does not become infected, it heals within 8 to 14 days, depending upon its location and the thickness of the graft. If the graft has been cut so thick that an insufficient number of appendages remain in the donor site to provide for reepithelialization, the donor wound cannot heal spontaneously except by slow migration of cells (about 1 mm per day) from the edges toward the center, a most unsatisfactory process. In this situation the donor site must be covered with another thin split graft, unless it is small enough to be sutured, lest a hypertrophic scar result.

REFERENCES

1. Best, C. H., and Taylor, N. B. *The Physiological Basis of Medical Practice* (8th ed.). Baltimore: Williams & Wilkins, 1966.
2. Gibson, T., and Kenedi, R. M. The Significance and Measurement of Skin Tensions in Man. In *Transactions of the Third International Congress of Plastic Surgeons.* New York: Excerpta Medica, 1964. P. 387.
3. Gibson, T., Stark, H., and Evans, J. H. Directional variation in extensibility of human skin in vivo. *J. Biomech.* 2:201, 1969.
4. Griffith, B. H. Advances in the treatment of decubitus ulcers. *Surg. Clin. North Am.* 43:245, 1963.
5. Griffith, B. H. The Skin. In Preston, F. W., and Beal, J. M. (Eds.), *Basic Surgical Physiology.* Chicago: Year Book, 1969. Pp. 423–432.
6. Leider, M., and Buncke, C. M. Physical dimensions of the skin. *Arch. Dermatol.* 69:563, 1954.
7. Lister, G. D., and Gibson, T. Closure of rhomboid skin defects: The flaps of Limberg and Dufourmentel. *Br. J. Plast. Surg.* 25:300, 1972.
8. McGregor, I. A. *Fundamental Techniques of Plastic Surgery* (3rd ed.). Baltimore: Williams & Wilkins, 1965.

9. Montagna, W. *The Structure and Function of Skin.* New York: Academic, 1962.

10. Moyer, C. A., and Allen, J. G. *Surgery: Principles and Practice* (3rd ed.). Philadelphia: Lippincott, 1965. Pp. 342–343.

11. Rothman, S. *Physiology and Biochemistry of the Skin.* Chicago: University of Chicago Press, 1954.

12. Rothman, S. (Ed.). *The Human Integument: Normal and Abnormal.* Washington: American Association for the Advancement of Science, 1959.

13. Rushmer, R. F., Buettner, K. J. K., Short, J. M., and Odland, G. F. The skin. *Science* 154:343, 1966.

14. Sawhney, C. P. Contracture of skin grafts and its relation to cleavage lines of skin. *Br. J. Plast. Surg.* 24:233, 1971.

15. Scanlon, E. F. Melanin. In Preston, F. W., and Beal, J. M. (Eds.), *Basic Surgical Physiology.* Chicago: Year Book, 1969. Pp. 433–442.

16. Smahel, J. Biology of the stage of plasmatic imbibition. *Br. J. Plast. Surg.* 24:140, 1971.

17. Smahel, J., and Ganzoni, H. Contribution to the origin of the vasculature in free skin autografts. *Br. J. Plast. Surg.* 23:322, 1970.

18. Winkelman, R. K. *Nerve Endings in Normal and Pathologic Skin.* Springfield, Ill.: Thomas, 1960.

12

Neoplasms of the Skin

Richard L. Kempson

The skin gives rise to a greater number of neoplasms than does any other organ—partly because it is the largest organ, but also because the skin is in contact with carcinogens in the environment. Not only does the skin develop many neoplasms, but they are of widely varying types. This diversity has caused diagnostic and classification problems for the pathologist and the clinician. The purpose here will be to present some of the recent concepts in carcinogenesis of the skin, a working classification of the more common skin neoplasms, a brief résumé of the clinical behavior of certain skin tumors, and the role of the pathologist in the diagnosis and management of the patient with a mass involving the skin.

INDUCTION OF NEOPLASMS

Although the mechanisms of neoplastic induction are poorly understood, it is known that both benign and malignant neoplasms may be produced in the skin of animals and man by ionizing radiation including ultraviolet radiation, oncogenic viruses, and chemical carcinogens [13, 18]. Other factors, as yet undefined, such as aging may also cause neoplastic transformation. For man, ultraviolet radiation is probably the most important and frequent carcinogenic agent to affect the skin, resulting in a variety of epithelial and melanocytic neoplasms [13]. Other types of ionizing radiation are also carcinogenic but cause fewer tumors than ultraviolet light. Chemical carcinogens undoubtedly account for some of the skin neoplasms found in man. In fact, much of our fragmented and incomplete knowledge of the sequence of events in carcinogenesis comes from studies of chemical carcinogenesis in the skin of experimental animals. Only a few human neoplasms, mainly warts and molluscum contagiosum, are known to be virus induced, but perhaps others will be discovered in the future. For many skin neoplasms, however, the carcinogen is totally unknown.

While ultraviolet light is apparently the principal factor in the production of human skin neoplasms, chemicals are a major cause of human cancer and are increasingly important in our industrial society [18]. A large number of chemicals come into contact with the skin of most individuals, and the carcinogenic potential of the majority of them is unknown. Over the past 75 years much knowledge concerning the carcinogenic potential of some chemicals, particularly the hydrocarbons, to cause tumors in the skin of animals has been accumulated. Progress is being made, but the basic mechanisms of chemical carcinogenesis are still largely undiscovered. Pertinent questions are whether carcinogenic chemicals transform normal cells to cancer cells, select for preexisting cancer cells, or activate latent oncogenic viruses. It is known that at least some of the chemical carcinogens are not themselves capable of inducing tumors but must be metabolically converted to chemically active compounds. This activation is carried out by microsomal enzymes in the presence of NADPH and oxygen and allows the activated compound to be covalently bound to macromolecules, probably DNA, RNA, or protein [18]. For example, the amine oxides are the chemically active forms of certain of the polycyclic hydrocarbons, and they are bound to DNA and RNA. Recent tissue culture experiments also suggest that chemical carcinogens directly transform benign cells to malignant ones rather than selecting for preexisting malignant cells [18]. It appears too that the active forms of at least some chemical carcinogens are mutagenic; that is, they alter the structural sequence of DNA. Tumor promoters enhance the neoplastic potential of carcinogens by unknown mechanisms, and it has been recently postulated that the promoter is essential for the phenotypic expression of neoplastic transformation [31]. Chemically induced neoplasms in experimental animals characteristically progress from cellular atypia to papillomatous lesions to metastasizing carcinoma.

One of the more exciting advances in the area of skin neoplasia is the discovery of the relationship between ultraviolet light, DNA repair, and skin carcinogenesis in man. Abundant evidence has been presented that sunlight is carcinogenic and will produce basal cell carcinomas, squamous cell carcinomas, and malignant melanoma [13]. In animals ultraviolet light is both carcinogenic and cocarcinogenic. The mechanism of ultraviolet carcinogenesis is not yet known, but the important demonstration has been made of the formation of pyridine dimers in the nucleic acid of cells exposed to ultraviolet light. When such dimers are formed in normal cells, they are excised and normal DNA is replicated [33]. In 1968 Cleaver demonstrated a deficiency of this repair system in dermal fibroblasts from a patient with xeroderma pigmentosum, a congenital disease of the skin in which the patients have a high incidence of skin neoplasms [8]. It has been postulated that, in patients with xeroderma pigmentosum, cancers may result from increased mutation rate due to failure to remove the pyridine dimers from damaged DNA. This defect is apparently not present in all patients with xeroderma pigmentosum [33]. Since all normal individuals can repair DNA normally, this is not the mechanism of skin cancer production in non-xeroderma pigmentosum individuals. Possibly, however, repeated ultraviolet injury in normal persons may lead to faulty DNA repair in individual cells and subsequent errors in DNA replication. Occasionally such faulty cells may proceed to replicate and produce neoplasms [13].

In summary, the mechanisms of skin carcinogenesis and the causative agents for many human skin tumors remain largely unknown. Epidemiological, clinical, and experimental studies indicate that ultraviolet light is an important carcinogen. One of the ways it may induce neoplastic transformation is through the medium of faulty DNA repair of pyrimidine dimers in individual cells. Chemicals are also undoubtedly important in human tumor induction. Metabolic activation, covalent binding of active components to DNA and RNA, and protein, and subsequent mutogenic transformation of DNA may be important steps in the neoplastic process. Most carcinogenic chemicals must be placed in contact with the skin for long periods of time before tumor develops. Promoters enhance the neoplastic potential of the carcinogen, and tumor development commonly proceeds through cellular atypia to papilloma to carcinoma. Only a small number of human skin tumors are known to be caused by a virus.

CLASSIFICATION OF SKIN NEOPLASMS

Before attempting to understand the clinical behavior of skin neoplasms, one must have some concept of how they are classified. Given below is a working classification of the more common ones, followed by a discussion of many of them. It is hoped that this will serve as a framework for understanding the various types of skin neoplasms. Detailed histological descriptions of the tumors appear in standard dermatopathology textbooks.

I. Epidermal tumors
1. Fibroepithelial papillomas (skin tags)
2. Verrucae
3. Seborrheic keratosis
4. Actinic keratosis
5. Bowen's disease
6. Basal cell carcinoma
7. Squamous cell carcinoma
II. Adnexal tumors
A. Hair follicle
1. Trichoepithelioma
2. Keratoacanthoma
3. Keratinous cysts
4. Pilomatrixoma
B. Eccrine sweat glands
1. Poroma
2. Eccrine acrospiroma
3. Eccrine spiradenoma
4. Dermal eccrine cylindroma
5. Chondroid syringoma
6. Syringoma
7. Syringoadenoma papilliferum
8. Adenocarcinoma
C. Apocrine sweat glands
1. Hidradenoma papilliferum
2. Cystadenoma
D. Sebaceous glands
1. Sebaceous hyperplasia
2. Nevus sebaceous of Jadassohn

III. Melanocytic tumors of the skin
A. Nevi
1. Intradermal, junctional, and compound nevi
2. Spindle and epithelioid nevi
3. Blue and cellular blue nevi
4. Halo and balloon cell nevi
5. Congenital nevi
B. Premalignant lesions
1. Lentigo maligna (Hutchinson's freckle)
C. Malignant melanoma
1. Superficial spreading melanoma
2. Nodular melanoma
3. Lentigo maligna melanoma
IV. Dermal tumors
A. Scars and fibromatosis
1. Hypertrophic scars and keloid
B. Fibrous histiocytomas
1. Subepidermal nodular fibrosis
2. Dermatofibrosarcoma protuberans
3. Atypical fibroxanthoma
4. Juvenile xanthogranuloma
C. Lymphoreticular lesions
1. Cutaneous lymphoplasia
2. Malignant lymphoma
3. Mycosis fungoides
D. Tumors of the supporting structures
1. Vascular neoplasms: angiomatous, pericytial, and glomus tumors, and angiosarcoma
2. Smooth muscle neoplasms
3. Schwann's cell neoplasms and neuromas
4. Fibrous neoplasms and fibromatosis
E. Neoplasms of unknown histogenesis
1. Kaposi's sarcoma

EPIDERMAL TUMORS

Seborrheic keratoses, the most common epidermal neoplasms encountered, are greasy, often pigmented, lesions that protrude above the surface of the skin. They display numerous histological patterns, but the combination of horn cysts and basaloid cells and the superficial location of the lesion usually allow easy diagnosis. We consider inverted follicular keratosis a form of seborrheic keratosis [28]. Many different types of epidermal lesions characterized by verrucous epidermal hyperplasia are found in the skin, the best known being verruca vulgaris and verruca plantaris. Verrucous hyperplasia is also found in many forms of chronic dermatitis. Several of the congenital epidermal nevi are verrucous. Actinic keratosis represents one form of damage to the skin from sunlight. Histologically the lesions are characterized by hyperkeratosis and parakeratosis, varying degrees of atypia, disarray of the epidermal cells, and chronic inflammation and basophilic degeneration in the dermis. The epidermis may be atrophic, hypertrophic, or of normal thickness, and in some instances acantholysis is found. Actinic keratosis is a specific clinicopathological entity, and strict criteria should be used for its diagnosis. It is generally considered to be a premalignant lesion. Bowen's disease is a form of squamous cell carcinoma in situ characterized clinically by scaly erythematous lesions occurring more frequently on non-sun-exposed surfaces [17]. Histologically, there is extensive disarray of the squamous epithelium with immature cells high in the epidermis, nuclear atypia, and frequent mitoses, some of which are atypical. Large cells with irregular hyperchromatic nuclei known as *Bowenoid cells* are common, as are shrunken eosinophilic cells, which are called *dyskeratotic cells.* Bowen's disease cannot be diagnosed by histological changes alone; it is a clinicopathological entity, and the lesion must clinically be that of Bowen's disease before a histological diagnosis is made. Basal cell carcinoma of the skin is the most prevalent neoplasm found in man and may present in several clinical and histological patterns. Although metastases are very rare, recurrence does occur; however, the recurrence rate is low. Even when the tumor extends to the surgical margins, only about one-third of the lesions will recur [16].

Squamous cell carcinoma must be distinguished from other squamous proliferative lesions, particularly keratoacanthoma, inverted follicular keratoma, and pseudo-epitheliomatous hyperplasia. The differentiation can be difficult, and the pathologist must be supplied with detailed clinical information as to the length of time the lesion has been present and its clinical appearance. Shave biopsies of squamous proliferative lesions may be impossible to interpret accurately because the base of the lesion is usually not present [14]. There has been a tendency to overdiagnose squamous carcinoma in the past, and a conservative approach is warranted since the metastatic rate of squamous cell carcinoma of the skin is low (e.g., in Lund's series only 7 of 780 squamous carcinomas metastasized [23]). Factors favoring a diagnosis of squamous cell carcinoma in a squamous proliferative lesion of the skin are (1) duration over three months, (2) atypia and actinic changes in surrounding epithelium, (3) ulceration without a central keratin plug, (4) wide and haphazard invasion of the dermis with infiltration under the surrounding epidermis, (5) poor differentiation, and (6) location on ears, forehead, or face near the ears. In Lund's series the only squamous cell carcinomas in actinically exposed areas that metastasized arose from the ear, the skin near the ear, or the forehead [23]. However, the incidence of metastases of squamous cell carcinomas arising in non–actinically damaged skin was greater than in actinically damaged areas. In some instances pathologists cannot be certain of the diagnosis of a squamous proliferative process. In this circumstance it is better to label the lesion as a squamous proliferative lesion rather than underdiagnose or overdiagnose squamous cell carcinoma. Such lesions can be treated by complete excision.

ADNEXAL TUMORS

Trichoepithelioma is a benign tumor of hair follicle origin. It should be separated from basal cell carcinoma, with which it shares some histological features. Hair follicle differentiation allows the distinction to be made without difficulty. Keratoacanthoma is a benign self-limited squamous proliferative lesion frequently confused with squamous cell carcinoma [35]. Keratoacanthoma most often arises from normal skin, has a rapid period of growth to a dome-shaped keratin-filled lesion, and then regresses. Sections of the entire lesion are usually diagnostic, but, when only a biopsy is done, it may be impossible to separate keratoacanthoma from squamous cell carcinoma. Perineural and muscular invasions are of no diagnostic significance since they may be found in both keratoacanthoma and squamous cell carcinoma [23]. Some keratoacanthomas pursue an aggressive course and the term *malignant keratoacanthoma* has been suggested for such lesions.

Keratinous cysts may be divided into two types: epidermal and pilar [24, 25]. These cysts are frequently erroneously labeled *sebaceous cysts*, a term which should not be used since they are not cysts of the sebaceous glands. Keratinous cysts of the epidermal type are the most common and occur wherever there is hair-bearing skin. They are lined by cornified squamous epithelium with a granular layer and are filled with keratin. Keratinous cysts of the pilar type represent 10 percent of the keratinous cysts and usually occur on the scalp or forehead. They are lined by noncornifying squamous epithelium which may shed cells into the center of the cyst. Keratinous cysts of the scalp may become very large and form massive layers of squamous epithelium. These are known as *proliferating keratinous cysts* or *giant hair matrix tumors* and should not be confused with squamous cell carcinomas [9]. *Pilomatrixoma* is the better term for the benign tumor derived from the hair root frequently classified as "calcifying epithelioma of Malherbe" [15].

Tumors differentiating as eccrine sweat gland structures present numerous, diverse, and often confusing histological patterns. All the eccrine sweat gland tumors are benign, except for the sweat gland adenocarcinoma, which may be hard to recognize unless there is invasion of the perineural space, metastasis, or abnormal mitosis. Fortunately, sweat gland carcinomas are extremely rare. The benign eccrine sweat gland tumors are numerous, and the nomenclature is characterized by a multitude of names for the same tumor. We have adopted the nomenclature of Helwig, which we think is reproducible and covers most of the main types [19]. Eccrine poroma occurs chiefly, and almost exclusively, on the palms and soles. It is composed of proliferating sheets of basaloid keratinocytes in the epidermis and superficial dermis. It must be separated from seborrheic keratosis and basal cell carcinoma, both of which are exceedingly rare on the palms and soles. Eccrine acrospiroma is a distinctive tumor that has also been designated as clear cell hidradenoma, dermal duct tumor, or porosyringoma. Eccrine acrospiromas present as painless masses and histologically are composed of cells with eosinophilic to clear cytoplasm. Basaloid cells and squamous differentiation are common. The tumor cells grow in sheets, and duct formation is rather often seen. Eccrine spiradenoma usually presents as a painful mass in any part of the skin but is rare in apocrine areas. This tumor has a diagnostic two-cell pattern allowing ready histological identification. Ninety percent of dermal cylindromas occur on the head and neck, and most of them are small single lesions although the literature emphasizes the multiplicity and large size which can be attained. Striking eosinophilic basement membranes surround the basal cells in this tumor. Syringoma is a flat papule-like lesion that occurs chiefly on the face and neck. Chondroid syringoma, also known as mixed tumor of the skin, appears predominately in the head and neck area and has a histological pattern identical to that of mixed tumor of the salivary glands. Syringoadenoma papilliferum occurs chiefly as a verrucous lesion. It often presents as a "birthmark" which develops verrucous areas and may bleed. Approximately 20 percent of the patients will have a contiguous nevus sebaceus, and 10 percent will have an associated basal cell carcinoma. Histologically there are numerous clefts and papillae lined by a double row of cells. The stroma characteristically contains many inflammatory cells.

Adenocarcinoma of the sweat glands may be difficult to distinguish from the benign tumors unless obvious invasion or metastasis has taken place. In some instances recurrence or metastases will have to develop before an eccrine tumor can be accurately diagnosed as adenocarcinoma. Metastatic adenocarcinoma from the internal organs must also always be considered in the differential diagnosis of both benign and malignant sweat gland tumors.

Apocrine tumors are less prevalent than the eccrine variety; only two tumors occur with any frequency in the skin. Hidradenoma papilliferum appears only on the vulva and perineal areas of women and is histologically and clinically different from syringocystadenoma papilliferum. Apocrine cystadenoma is found almost exclusively on the face and is also known as *hidrocystoma* [27].

True neoplasms of the sebaceous glands, adenoma or carcinoma, are very rare except for carcinoma of the glands of Moll in the eyelid. The so-called adenoma sebaceum, occurring in tuberous sclerosis, is an angiofibroma. The sebaceous glands are normal or atrophic. The chief cause for a mass involving the sebaceous glands is hyperplasia. This occurs mainly on the nose and cheeks of older individuals and has been described as "senile sebaceous hyperplasia." It is a relatively common lesion and results in unsightly yellow nodules on the nose and face. Nevus sebaceus is a hamartomatous malformation composed of numerous enlarged sebaceous glands associated with apocrine glands and defective hair follicles. It occurs on the scalp and face and presents as a papillomatous mass due to the sebaceous gland enlargement. Basal cell carcinoma is found in approximately 20 percent of cases of nevus sebaceus.

MELANOCYTIC TUMORS

Melanocytic tumors are composed of cells with the inherent capacity to synthesize melanin. Melanogenesis takes place in organelles known as *melanosomes*, and their identification ultrastructurally identifies a cell as a melanocyte. The cells of the melanocytic series are derived from the neural crest, which gives rise to pigment-producing epidermal melanocytes as well as the dermal neval cells. The origin of the melanocytic nevus cell is uncertain, but most opinion supports the dual origin of Masson, who postulated that neval cells result both from the drop-off of epidermal melanocytes into the dermis and from differentiation of dermal Schwann cells into neval cells [26a]. The superficial neval cells are generally considered to originate from the epidermal melanocytes, which lose their melanocytic capacity and dendritic processes as they migrate into the dermis. Deeper neval structures may assume neuroid features, and Masson has theorized that they are derived from Schwann cells. Malignant melanomas are the malignant neoplasms of melanocytic origin, and the vast majority are derived from the epidermal melanocytes rather than the neval melanocytes [5].

Nevi are present in all persons, but their number is variable. Nevi are best classified on the basis of the location of the neval cells. Junctional nevi are characterized by neval cells at the dermoepidermal junction, and dermal nevi by neval cells in the dermis; compound nevi are composed of neval cells in both locations. Spindle cell and epithelioid nevi are compound nevi found mainly in children, but also in adults, in which the cells are spindled or epithelioid; thus they bear some resemblance to malignant melanoma [10]. Spitz first recognized these as benign lesions and suggested the designation "juvenile melanoma," a term which should not be used since spindle cell nevi occur in adults and neither lesion is a melanoma [36]. We have not seen a pure epithelioid cell nevus in an adult, but mixed forms occur in both children and adults.

Spindle cell nevi are composed of spindled elongate cigar-shaped cells present in a "falling rain" pattern at the dermoepidermal junction and extending into the dermis. The epithelioid cell nevus is composed of larger cells with polygonal eosinophilic cytoplasm. Giant cells may be found in either type but are more common in the epithelioid cell nevus.

Blue nevi are intradermal nevi composed of proliferating, often heavily pigmented, spindle-shaped dermal melanocytes. The margins of the lesion are indistinct. Cellular blue nevus is a larger, more cellular lesion. Some of the neval cells in cellular blue nevus have large rounded vesicular nuclei. Junctional activity is absent in both types of blue nevi, and mitoses are infrequent or absent. Although on rare occasions lymph node metastases have developed from a cellular blue nevus, distant metastases apparently are very rare. Therefore, both blue nevus and cellular blue nevus should generally be considered benign lesions, with the latter capable of metastasizing to regional lymph nodes [34].

Halo nevus is a clinical descriptive term for a melanocytic nevus surrounded by an area of depigmentation. A heavy infiltrate of chronic inflammatory cells in the lesion is characteristic. When over 50 percent of a nevus is composed of cells with foamy cytoplasm and pyknotic nuclei, it is designated a balloon cell nevus. It should be carefully distinguished from malignant melanoma containing balloon cells.

Congenital nevi tend to be large, and the neval cells are often present around appendages, nerves, and vessels as well as in the subcutaneous tissue—features that can cause diagnostic difficulties to the neophyte pathologist. Neuroid structures are also common in such nevi. The giant pigmented nevus is of special importance to the plastic surgeon because it is, by definition, a large, often disfiguring, lesion. In addition, malignant melanoma will develop in about 10 to 30 percent of giant congenital nevi.

Whether ordinary nevi carry a greater risk of developing malignant melanoma than normal skin is controversial. While some authors have concluded that most, if not all, malignant melanomas arise in junctional nevi,

recent studies indicate that melanomas do not universally stem from nevi; in fact, in one series only 8 to 10 percent of malignant melanomas arose in preexisting nevi [5]. Thus there is little support for the widespread theory that junctional nevi are premalignant. Even on the palms and soles, where the incidence of malignant melanoma is supposed to be especially high, a study of 10,000 healthy men showed the incidence of melanoma to be too low to advocate routine removal of plantar and palmar nevi [40]. Nevi that are enlarging, changing appearance, ulcerated, bleeding, or in a position to be irritated should be removed because it may be difficult to separate nevus from malignant melanoma. Routine removal of nevi to prevent melanoma, except large congenital nevi which are resectable, is not warranted and is certainly impractical. When a pigmented lesion of the skin is removed, it should be removed with a margin of grossly uninvolved skin whenever possible, and a cold knife should be used for the excision. Lesions that are too large to be excised without extensive surgery may be subjected to biopsy. There is no evidence that biopsy changes the prognosis of malignant melanoma. The separation of nevi from malignant melanoma is often difficult histologically, and distortion by the cautery may render the tissue unsuitable for diagnosis. Although malignant melanoma does occur in children it is very rare. Great caution should be utilized before making a diagnosis of malignant melanoma in a prepubertal individual.

Lentigo maligna (Hutchinson's freckle) is a flat brown-black freckle-like lesion ordinarily found on the sun-exposed skin, particularly the face, of the elderly; however, the lesion may appear on the trunk and in younger patients [6]. Histologically lentigo maligna is characterized by a proliferation of atypical melanocytes of irregular size and shape at the dermal-epidermal junction. Retraction of the cytoplasm and pleomorphic nuclei are common. Lentigo maligna must be considered a premalignant melanocytic lesion since malignant melanoma often develops in the lesion.

Of 85 cases of lentigo maligna reported by Wayte and Helwig, malignant melanoma was present in 45 at the time of excision [39]. It is likely that all lentigo maligna will develop malignant melanoma if left untreated long enough. However, evolution to melanoma is apparently slow and requires many years in most patients. Because of the frequent location of lentigo maligna on the head and neck, and the large size of the lesions before patients seek medical treatment, therapy is often difficult and has consisted in excision with or without skin grafts, dermabrasion, fulguration, biopsy and observation, and topical chemotherapy. If only a biopsy is done, the lesion must be observed carefully and repeat biopsies should be utilized to sample areas which are changing color or in which masses develop.

Concepts of the histopathology of melanoma and the significance of the depth of invasion have changed in the last decade primarily owing to the classic studies of Clark et al. in the United States and McGovern in Australia [5, 26]. It is now generally accepted that there are, in addition to melanoma arising in congenital nevi, three types of malignant melanoma, each with a different clinical and histological appearance and with different clinical behavior. These three are superficial spreading melanoma, nodular melanoma, and lentigo maligna melanoma [29]. The prognosis differs depending upon the histological type of melanoma.

Superficial spreading melanoma is the major type, may occur in any part of the skin, and is slightly more common in the female. Clinically, it has a variegated color but is essentially a brown to gray to black lesion with areas of red, white, and blue coloration. The lesions are almost always elevated, and many have an arciform shape with one part of the lesion forming the arc of a circle while the other part is flat and irregular. Tumor nodules and ulceration of the surface may be present. Histologically superficial spreading malignant melanoma is characterized by intraepidermal spread of melanoma cells at least three rete pegs beyond the area of invasion [5]. In contrast to lentigo maligna, the cells in superficial spreading malignant melanoma are uniform, have foamy to granular cytoplasm, and tend to form theques at the dermal-epidermal junction. Nodular melanoma is almost universally blue-black and may present as a nodule, a flat plaque, or an exophytic mass. Histologically the melanoma cells do not extend three rete pegs on either side of the area of invasion. Lentigo maligna melanoma arises in lentigo maligna and is characterized by a nodule or an area of ulceration or a more darkly pigmented area within a part of a lentigo maligna [6]. Histologically lentigo maligna melanoma is recognized by the presence of atypical melanocytes invading the dermis in an otherwise typical lentigo maligna. The invading melanocytes are often spindle shaped, and less atypia and fewer pleomorphic tumor cells are found than in the other two types of melanoma.

The other significant contribution by Clark and co-workers is confirmation of the observation, noted by others in the past, that the depth of invasion of malignant melanoma is of great importance in determining the prognosis and possibly the therapy [5]. They distinguish five levels of invasion which have become generally accepted. Level I invasion is melanoma confined to the epidermis and is rarely, if ever, seen. Level II invasion is extension of the tumor into the papillary dermis; level III invasion is extension to the junction between the papillary and reticular dermis; level IV is invasion into the reticular dermis; and level V is tumor extending into the subcutaneous tissue. Breslow and others have shown that the measurement of tumor thickness by using an optical micrometer is more accurate than estimating the level of invasion. Care must be taken to ensure that sections are from the thickest part of the tumor and that the measurements are taken from the granular layer rather than the dermo-epidermal junction [3, 4, 4a].

By combining the type of melanoma, the depth of invasion, and the size of the tumor, one can arrive at a reasonably good estimate of the prognosis and the effectiveness of therapy. With each of the histological types, and regardless of the level of invasion, approximately 30 percent of patients with superficial spreading melanoma will die as the result of their tumor whereas the figure is 56 percent for nodular melanoma and less than 10 percent for lentigo maligna melanoma [5]. However, the most important prognostic factor is the microlevel of invasion, and when this is determined it is noted that the deeper the tumor the worse the prognosis. In most series survival is between 90 and 100 percent for level II tumors and 60 to 80 percent for level III invasion [38]. It is unusual for a melanoma under 1 mm in diameter to metastasize, and Breslow has reported that level III melanomas less than 0.76 mm in thickness have an excellent prognosis while those greater than that have an almost 50 percent metastasis or recurrence rate [4]. These are known as *thin* and *thick level III melanomas.* A recent report by Breslow and Macht has shown that 62 patients with melanomas less than 0.76 mm thick remained free of disease even though resection margins were less than 0.5 cm in 22 percent. Thus "wide" excision does not seem indicated for patients whose tumors are less than 0.76 mm thick. For tumors 0.76–1.50 mm thick a 2-cm margin appears sufficient; data are insufficient to reach conclusions for tumors with invasion greater than 1.50 mm [4a].

Every pathology report of a malignant melanoma should contain the following information: the type of melanoma, the level of invasion in mm, the diameter of the tumor, the number of mitoses per 10 high-power fields, and, if it is an excision specimen, whether the margins are free of tumor. Clinicopathological studies based on such data reveal that elective lymph node dissection adds nothing to survival of patients with level II and thin level III lesions and should not be performed unless the nodes are clinically positive or the primary tumor is immediately adjacent to the regional lymph node group [38]. On the other hand, there seems to be increased survival in patients with more extensive melanomas who have been treated with elective lymph node dissection as compared to those treated by excision alone, but the series are small, differences are often not statistically significant, and the value of elective lymph node dissection remains controversial. The treatment of the primary melanoma, with invasion greater than 0.76 mm, whether superficial spreading or nodular, is "wide" excision. Whether this means a 2-cm margin of normal skin or a 4-cm margin is not well defined, but the extent of the excision should be based on the depth of invasion, the size of the melanoma, and the location of the primary tumor. The survival in melanoma appears to be better if the fascia under the lesion is left intact. If the regional lymph nodes are clinically involved, node dissection is indicated, but the prognosis will be poor if the nodes are shown histologically to contain melanoma. Lentigo maligna melanoma is indolent, rarely metastasizes, and should be treated by the most conservative measures that will allow removal of all the tumor. Elective lymph node dissection is not indicated for lentigo maligna melanoma.

DERMAL TUMORS

Differentiation of scars, hypertrophic scars, and keloids is often useful because of the high incidence of recurrence of keloids. Although there is some overlap, histological differences are usually great enough to allow accurate diagnosis.

The fibrous histiocytomas are a diverse group of lesions that present as masses in many different tissues including the skin [20]. Some are undoubtedly reactive while others are neoplasms, both benign and malignant. The cells forming the fibrous histiocytomas differentiate as both fibroblasts and histiocytes, and foam cells are common. Fibrous histiocytomas occurring in the skin include subepidermal nodular fibrosis, atypical fibroxanthoma, dermatofibrosarcoma protuberans, and juvenile xanthogranuloma. The giant cell tumor of the tendon sheath is also a fibrous histiocytoma. Many of the other fibrous histiocytomas are soft tissue tumors.

Subepidermal nodular fibrosis is the term used for the common dermal fibrous histiocytoma in which there are varying numbers of fibroblasts, histiocytes, and blood vessels. When the lesion is predominately fibrous, it is commonly designated as a *dermatofibroma.* When the tumor is composed almost entirely of histiocytes, it may be labeled as a *histiocytoma;* when the blood vessels are prominent, as *sclerosing hemangioma.* We prefer the term *subepidermal nodular fibrosis* regardless of the ratio of tumor cell types [2]. Clinically, subepidermal nodular fibrosis presents as a firm, often pigmented dermal mass. On cross section it is seen to be white to yellow and to blend into the surrounding dermis. Atypical fibroxanthoma is a fibrous histiocytoma which contains anaplastic malignant-appearing cells in a fibrous stroma [21]. It occurs most frequently on the sun-damaged skin of the elderly and may be confused clinically and pathologically with malignant neoplasms. Although atypical fibroxanthoma may recur and has, on rare occasions, metastasized to regional nodes, it is almost always a benign lesion cured by adequate excision.

Dermatofibrosarcoma protuberans, which we prefer to call *storiform fibrous histiocytoma*, occurs in both skin and soft tissues. It is a fibrous histiocytoma with a high recurrence rate but rarely metastasizes [37]. Clinically it presents as an elevated, often large, mass and histologically is composed of swirling masses of thin fibroblasts arranged in a cartwheel or "storiform" pattern.

Cutaneous lymphoid infiltrates may be divided into four different clinical and histological entities [7]. Only one of the four regularly presents clinically as a tumor nodule, namely, cutaneous lymphoplasia. This lesion is ordinarily found on the face as a red nodule. Histologically it is composed of lymphocytes, follicular centers, plasma cells, and scattered histiocytes. Although most examples of cutaneous lymphoplasia are easily recognized as benign, occasional examples present cellular atypia of a significant degree to cause difficulty in separating them from malignant lymphoma. Such lesions are often designated as *lymphomatoid papulosis* and are known to be clinically benign, even though they are anaplastic histologically. Since differentiation of cutaneous lymphoplasia and malignant lymphoma can be a problem, the diagnosis of malignant lymphoma should rarely be made on the basis of a skin biopsy alone [7].

Malignant lymphoma may involve the skin but, except for mycosis fungoides, usually does so secondary to systemic lymphoma. Except for mycosis fungoides, histiocytic lymphoma is the most common lymphoma to present as a primary skin tumor. Primary cutaneous lymphocytic lymphoma and Hodgkin's disease are distinctively rare, and great care should be used before making such a diagnosis especially in view of the difficulty in telling lymphomatoid papulosis from malignant lymphoma. Malignant lymphomas usually present as large firm nodules or masses, and there is no significant difference in the clinical presentation of the various nonmycosis lymphomas.

Mycosis fungoides is a form of malignant lymphoma which originates in the skin [12]. Clinically patients may present with one of three patterns: erythematous scaly lesions, plaques, or tumors. The course of the disease is often long, and the diagnosis may be difficult to establish when the patient is in the erythematous stage. Biopsy is usually diagnostic in the plaque stage and almost always diagnostic in tumors. Histologically there is a dermal infiltrate containing lymphocytes, plasma cells, and atypical lymphocytes derived from T cells with convoluted nuclei known as *mycosis cells.* Mycosis cells are also often present in the epidermis. Although mycosis fungoides is limited to the skin for long periods of time, spread to regional lymph nodes, spleen, and other organs is common in the terminal stages of the disease [32].

TUMORS OF THE SUPPORTING STRUCTURES

Vascular neoplasms of the skin may be divided into hemangiomas, angiosarcoma, glomus tumors, and hemangiopericytoma. The hemangiomas are discussed elsewhere. The glomus tumor occurs most frequently in the subungual area but may be found in other areas of the skin and soft tissues. It is classically painful, particularly in the subungual area, and is benign, although rare examples have recurred. The tumor cells are derived from the neuromyoarterial apparatus and ultrastructurally have many resemblances to smooth muscle [22]. Hemangiopericytoma, a tumor of the vascular pericytes, is rare in the skin and subcutis. Histologically the tumor cells are elongate and arranged in a characteristic "woven" pattern. Approximately 10 percent of the hemangiopericytomas will metastasize, and aggressive neoplasms can usually be recognized because of increased cellularity, prominent mitoses, and areas of hemorrhage and necrosis [11a]. Metastases often develop many years after the initial excision. Angiosarcoma of the skin is bluish violaceous plaque-like lesion which occurs mainly on the scalp and face of the elderly. The neoplasms are relentlessly aggressive and local spread and recurrences are the rule. Metastases occur in approximately one-third of patients. Histologically they are characterized by numerous vascular channels lined by atypical cells [35a]. Postmastectomy lymphangiosarcoma has identical histologic features and is separated from cutaneous angiosarcoma by history.

Smooth muscle tumors, both leiomyomas and leiomyosarcomas, occur in the skin. Leiomyomas are characteristically painful. Fibromatosis and fibrosarcoma are both rare in the skin but may be found in the superficial soft tissues and in the soft tissues of the head and neck. *Fibromatosis* is the term given to a group of fibrous proliferative lesions characterized by an infiltrative pattern of growth, lack of atypical cells, few mitoses, and frequent local recurrences. Several different clinicopathological entities are included in the category of fibromatosis. These include palmar (Dupuytren's) and plantar (Lederhose's) fibromatosis, congenital torticollis, musculoaponeurotic fibromatosis (desmoid), generalized fibromatosis, and localized fibromatosis not otherwise classified. The term *aggressive fibromatosis* is best not used as a specific diagnostic term since many of the forms of fibromatosis may be aggressive [1]. Musculoaponeurotic fibromatosis occurs in many sites but most commonly in the abdominal wall, the shoulder girdle, the head and neck area, and the thigh [11]. Histologically it is similar to other forms of fibromatosis except that the fibrocytes infiltrate skeletal muscle. This is perhaps the most aggressive of any of the types of fibromatosis and is best treated by wide radical excision, but usually without sacrifice of major blood vessels, nerves, or an extremity. Although about 50 percent of musculoaponeurotic fibromatosis will recur, loss of life due to this tumor is rare. Palmar and plantar fibromatosis may be sufficiently cellular and contain enough mitoses to be confused histologically with fibrosarcoma. The history should be sufficient to make a correct diagnosis. Cicatricial and postirradiation fibromatoses indicate a specific etiology; and Gardner's syndrome is the association of soft tissue fibromatosis with multiple colonic polyps.

Fibrosarcoma is a tumor of fibroblasts capable of metastasizing. It occurs in many sites and generally in adults. Microscopically fibrosarcomas are composed of closely appositioned fibroblasts with elongate nuclei. The fascicles of cells are arranged in bundles that intersect at acute angles, and mitoses are usually greater in number than five or six per 10 high-power fields. The dividing line between the cellular forms of fibromatosis and fibrosarcoma is not well defined, and care should be taken to include in the fibrosarcoma category only those tumors thought to be capable of metastasizing.

Kaposi's sarcoma is a malignant neoplasm of uncertain histogenesis. Although it characteristically is a tumor of the skin presenting as a bluish nodule, it can be primary in other tissues. The course of Kaposi's sarcoma is usually prolonged, and radiation and chemotherapy are of therapeutic value. The histological features of Kaposi's sarcoma are specific but are frequently confused with those of other neoplasms, particularly fibrosarcoma, melanoma, hemangioma, and angiosarcoma.

CLINICOPATHOLOGICAL CORRELATION

Accurate histological diagnosis requires the highest degree of cooperation and coordination between clinician and pathologist. The pathologist must be given full clinical information and a summarization of the operative findings. Sending specimens to the surgical pathology laboratory unaccompanied by an adequate summarization of clinical findings is to be condemned and is a practice that will lead to errors in diagnosis. For example, it is not possible to correctly distinguish keratoacanthoma from squamous carcinoma without an accurate history, and the surgical pathologist should not attempt to do so. Verbal communication with the surgical pathologist is desirable in many cases, particularly those in which the clinical presentation is unusual, or in which unusual sections are needed. Unfortunately it is the custom in many hospitals to send specimens to the laboratory with only the patient identification and the origin of the specimen noted or with an inadequate history. In this event the pathologist should immediately communicate with the surgeon to obtain the necessary history and operative findings. Special features to be noted in the specimen and special sections to be taken should be indicated on the request slip or on a drawing. Whenever the pathologist discovers unusual features in the specimen which do not correlate with the clinical findings, he should immediately notify the surgeon.

When the specimen is received in the laboratory, the gross changes are described, it is fixed, and blocks are selected for microtome sectioning. In addition to establishing a diagnosis, one should section the margins of the specimens containing neoplasms to determine the adequacy of excision. For skin excision specimens, we sample the margins in four areas as seen in Figure 12-1. For certain highly malignant neoplasms, such as melanoma, it is advisable to sample all of the margins. Not only should the surgical pathologist determine whether a lesion is benign or malignant, but in most instances he will be able to classify the disease process, determine the adequacy of excision, and give a reasonable estimate of the prognosis and future biological behavior. Most surgical

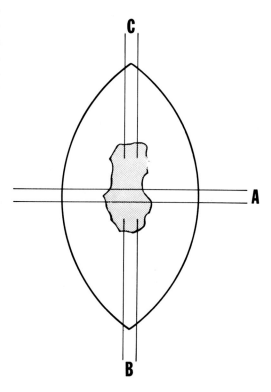

FIGURE 12-1. *Double lines at A, B, and C are sections taken routinely from skin excisions to sample the tumor and its margins. More extensive margin sampling is indicated for highly malignant neoplasms, such as melanoma. Surgical margins nearest to the lesion should always be sampled.*

pathologists are fully cognizant of the results of therapy and the best methods of treating a specific entity. It must be realized, however, that not all lesions are diagnosable, and in rare instances a lesion will not be classifiable.

Accurate histological diagnosis of tissue specimens requires adequate sampling of the lesion and prompt, proper fixation of the specimen. A pathologist cannot make a diagnosis from a tissue specimen that does not contain the lesion. If a lesion is ulcerated, removal of tissue from the center often results in a necrotic specimen that is not interpretable. The cautery will burn tissue, and specimens obtained with it may not be adequate. If cells are burned, traumatized, degenerated, or necrotic, they cannot be interpreted, and the specimen is worthless for establishing a diagnosis. A cold knife biopsy of as large a fragment of a lesion as is possible with normal surrounding tissue will give the best specimen [1]. In general, shave biopsies of skin lesions, particularly squamous lesions, result in an inadequate specimen. In our opinion, biopsy by complete excision should be done on pigmented lesions of the skin when the lesion is small. Following their removal, tissues must be rapidly and satisfactorily fixed to stop autolysis and drying. It is the responsibility of the surgeon to see that the specimen he has carefully and meticulously removed is placed into the proper fixative if a pathologist is not in the operating room.

Frozen section is a method of rapid sectioning of tissue to obtain microscopical sections for diagnosis. The only reason for obtaining a frozen section is to make a therapeutic decision in the operating room [1]. Frozen sections should not be used to satisfy the surgeon's curiosity, or because one is too impatient to wait until the following day when permanent sections are available. Frozen sections are accurate, but they have disadvantages, and they are not meant to be used to replace well-prepared permanent paraffin sections. In general, tissues, such as the skin, which are readily available for biopsy using local anesthesia should not be frozen to establish a diagnosis but should be submitted for permanent sections. We do not think pigmented lesions of the skin should be diagnosed by frozen section. The most common use of frozen sections is to establish a diagnosis at the time of operation or to determine whether margins are adequate. We do not think routine frozen section diagnosis to determine the margins of basal cell carcinoma is indicated because of the low rate of recurrence even in insufficiently excised basal cell carcinomas. Frozen sections are useful when a basal cell carcinoma is in a cosmetically difficult area, or when a skin graft is contemplated.

Today many surgical pathologists utilize electron microscopy, immunofluorescence, histochemistry, and tissue cultures as aids in diagnosis in addition to light microscopy. These procedures require special handling and fixation of the specimen, and consultation with the pathologist whenever an unusual lesion is encountered will be helpful. When a difficult lesion is encountered, the surgeon may be requested to obtain another specimen so that these procedures can be performed to establish a diagnosis.

REFERENCES

1. Ackerman, L. V., and Rosai, J. *Surgical Pathology* (5th ed.). St. Louis: Mosby, 1974.
2. Black, W. C., McGavran, M. H., and Graham, P. Nodular subepidermal fibrosis. *Arch. Surg.* 98:296, 1969.
3. Breslow, A. Thickness, cross sectional areas, and depth of invasion in the prognosis of cutaneous melanoma. *Ann. Surg.* 172:902, 1970.
4. Breslow, A. Tumor thickness in evaluating prognosis of level III melanomas. *Lab. Invest.* 32:418, 1975. (Abstract.)
4a. Breslow, A., and Macht, S. D. Tumor thickness and optimal size of resection margins in cutaneous melanoma. *Lab. Invest.* 36:331, 1977.
5. Clark, W. H., Jr., From, L., Bernardino, E. A., and Mihm, M. C. The his-

togenesis and biologic behavior of primary human malignant melanomas of the skin. *Cancer Res.* 29:705, 1969.

6. Clark, W. H., Jr., and Mihm, M. C. Lentigo maligna and lentigomaligna melanoma. *Am. J. Pathol.* 55:39, 1969.

7. Clark, W. H., Jr., Mihm, M. C., Reed, R. J., and Ainsworth, A. M. The lymphocytic infiltrates of the skin. *Hum. Pathol.* 5:25, 1974.

8. Cleaver, J. E. Defective repair replication of DNA in xeroderma pigmentosum. *Nature* (Lond.) 218:652, 1968.

9. Dabska, M. Giant hair matrix tumor. *Cancer* 28:701, 1971.

10. Echevarria, R., and Ackerman, L. V. Spindle and epithelioid cell nevi in the adult. *Cancer* 20:175, 1967.

11. Enzinger, F. M., and Shiraki, M. Musculoaponeurotic fibromatosis of the shoulder girdle (extra abdominal desmoid); analysis of 30 cases followed up for ten or more years. *Cancer* 20:1131, 1967.

11a. Enzinger, F. M., and Smith, O. B. H. Hemangiopericytoma: An analysis of 106 cases. *Hum. Pathol.* 7:61, 1976.

12. Epstein, E. H., Levin, D. L., Croft, J. D., and Lutzner, M. A. Mycosis fungoides. *Medicine* (Baltimore) 15:61, 1972.

13. Epstein, W. L., Fukuyama, K., and Epstein, J. H. Ultraviolet light, DNA repair and skin carcinogens in man. *Fed. Proc.* 30:1766, 1971.

14. Fisher, E. R., McCoy, M. M., and Wechsler, H. L. Analysis of histopathologic and electron microscopic determinants of keratoacanthoma and squamous cell carcinoma. *Cancer* 29:1387, 1972.

15. Forbis, R. J., and Helwig, E. B. Pilomatrixoma. *Arch. Dermatol.* 83:606, 1961.

16. Gooding, C. A., White, G., and Yatsuhashi, M. Significance of marginal extension in excised basal cell carcinoma. *N. Engl. J. Med.* 273:923, 1965.

17. Graham, J. H., and Helwig, E. B. Bowen's disease and its relationship to systemic cancer. *Arch. Dermatol.* 80:133, 1959.

18. Heidelberger, C. Current trends in chemical carcinogenesis. *Fed. Proc.* 32:2154, 1973.

19. Helwig, E. B. Benign Tumors of the Sweat Glands. In Helwig, E. B., and Mostofi, F. K. (Eds.), *The Skin*. Baltimore: Williams & Wilkins, 1971. Pp. 455–475.

20. Kempson, R. L., and Kyriakos, M. Fibroxanthosarcoma of the soft tissues. *Cancer* 29:961, 1972.

21. Kempson, R. L., and McGavran, M. H. Atypical fibroxanthomas of the skin. *Cancer* 17:1463, 1964.

22. Kuhn, C., and Rosai, J. Tumors arising from pericytes; ultrastructure and organ culture of a case. *Arch. Pathol.* 88:653, 1969.

23. Lund, H. Z. Epidermal Tumors: Some Special Considerations. In Helwig, E. B., and Mostofi, F. K. (Eds.), *The Skin*. Baltimore: Williams & Wilkins, 1971. Pp. 476–489.

24. McGavran, M. H. The pathologic anatomy of the human pilosebaceous unit. *Cancer* 17:65, 1964.

25. McGavran, M. H., and Bennington, B. Keratinous cysts of the skin. *Arch. Dermatol.* 94:499, 1966.

26. McGovern, V. J. The classification of melanoma and its relationship with prognosis. *Pathology* 2:85, 1970.

26a. Masson, P. My conception of cellular nevi. *Cancer* 4:9, 1951.

27. Mehregan, A. H. Apocrine cystadenoma. *Arch. Dermatol.* 90:274, 1964.

28. Mehregan, A. H. Inverted follicular keratosis. *Arch. Dermatol.* 89:229, 1964.

29. Mihm, M. C., Clark, W. H., Jr., and From, L. The clinical diagnosis, classification, and histogenetic concepts of the early stages of cutaneous malignant melanoma. *N. Engl. J. Med.* 284:1078, 1971.

30. Mundth, E. D., Guralnick, E. A., and Raker, J. W. Malignant melanoma: A clinical study of 427 cases. *Ann. Surg.* 162:15, 1965.

31. Raick, A. N. Cell differentiation and tumor promoting action in skin carcinogenesis. *Cancer Res.* 34:2915, 1974.

32. Rappaport, H., and Thomas, L. B.

Mycosis fungoides: The pathology of extracutaneous involvement. *Cancer* 34:1198, 1974.

33. Robbins, J. H., Kraemer, K. H., Lutzner, B. W., Festoff, B. W., and Coon, H. G. Xeroderma pigmentosum. *Ann. Intern. Med.* 80:221, 1974.

34. Rodriguez, H., and Ackerman, L. V. Cellular blue nevus. *Cancer* 21:393, 1968.

35. Rook, A., and Champion, R. H. Keratoacanthoma. *Natl. Cancer Inst. Monogr.* 10:257, 1963.

35a.Rosai, J., Sumner, H. W., Kostianovsky, M., et al. Angiosarcoma of the skin: A clinicopathologic and fine structural study. *Hum. Pathol.* 7:83, 1976.

36. Spitz, S. Melanomas of childhood. *Am. J. Pathol.* 24:591, 1948.

37. Taylor, H. G., and Helwig, E. B. Dermatofibrosarcoma protuberans. *Cancer* 15:717, 1962.

38. Wanebo, H. J., Woodruff, J., and Fortner, J. G. Malignant melanoma of the extremities: A clinicopathologic study using levels of invasion (microstage). *Cancer* 35:666, 1975.

39. Wayte, D. M., and Helwig, E. B. Melanotic freckle of Hutchinson. *Cancer* 21:893, 1968.

40. Wilson, F. C., Jr., and Andersonk, P. C. A dissenting view on the prophylactic removal of plantar and palmar nevi. *Cancer* 14:102, 1961.

13

Hamartomas

Ernest N. Kaplan

From early medical history it has been recognized that disorders of growth which manifest as local tumors, regional distortions of form, or variations of color and texture are caused by a variety of pathological conditions. Congenital malformations, hyperplasias, and neoplasms are general biological conditions into which specific diagnostic entities can be categorized. However, the distinction between them is not absolute. Rather, they are subject to individual interpretation and definition. Willis discussed the interconnection between these disorders of growth in *The Borderland of Embryology and Pathology* [43].

Beginning with the initial replication of the human zygote, there follows an amazingly complex yet well-ordered sequence of cell division and differentiation that produces human form and function. The genetic information determining the normal role of the cell can be altered or the expression of the genetic information modified by the internal or external environment. The variant genetic products—a malformation (hamartoma), neoplasm, or hyperplasia—are determined by the etiological agent, timing within the life cycle, and severity of the cellular modification. This chapter defines the characteristics of each category of growth disorder, classifies the specific diagnostic entities, examines the theories of teratogenesis and oncogenesis, and describes the clinical behavior of common congenital hamartomas seen by plastic surgeons.

DEFINITIONS

Hamartomas are congenital malformations comprised of normal tissues but of faulty composition. Their cell types are those normally found at that site but are either excessive in numbers or abnormal in their relationship to other tissues. The individual cell can retain fairly normal (mature or embryonic) histology and function. The hamartoma follows a pattern of growth and maturation that is proportional to surrounding tissues; any enlargement is frequently due to distention by its vascular, ductal, or cystic components as a result of faulty relationships and not to an abnormal neoplastic cellular proliferation, although true neoplasia can develop within a hamartoma. Occasionally a hamartoma such as hemangioma does manifest a true disproportionate cellular growth during postnatal maturation.

A *neoplasm* is an uncontrolled new growth of tissue. Its cells are permanently altered and have the capability of multiplication and function independent of the usual directives and restraints of the genetic information of the normal cell type. Neoplasms enlarge faster than the surrounding tissue and replace normal tissue by expansion, direct extension, or metastasis. The cells of the neoplasm resemble those of the parent tissue from which they have been derived and can retain the specialized cellular function. The distinction between benign and malignant neoplasms is based upon the individual cellular morphology and clinical and histological patterns of growth and dissemination.

Hyperplasias and *hypertrophies* are similar categories of growth disturbances. A *hyperplasia* is a localized increase in the number of normal cells in a normal arrangement of tissue. The growth disturbance may affect a specific cell type rather than every cell type within an organ or part. Tissue hyperplasias are caused by a physiological response to an environmental stimulus or internal pathophysiological process. There is no DNA alteration. Hyperplasia is controlled by the genetic information within the cell and can resolve after the original environmental stimulus has been removed. The stimulus may be physical, chemical, infectious, or hormonal. Thyroid goiter secondary to iodide deficiency is an example of reversible hyperplasia. Epithelial hyperplasia in response to recurrent trauma is another example.

Hypertrophy is the enlargement or overgrowth of an entire organ or part due to an increase in size or number of all its constituent cells or increase in volume of the extracellular matrix. Thus, the uterine enlargement during pregnancy and hemihypertrophy related to arteriovenous fistulas are examples of hypertrophies. (See Table 13–1.)

TABLE 13-1.   *Classification of Hamartomas*

Embryological Origin	Histological Diagnosis
Ectodermal	Epidermal (linear) nevus
	Sebaceous nevus
	Hair follicle nevus
	Sweat gland nevus
	Basal cell nevus
Neuroectodermal	Neurofibromatosis
	Melanocytic nevus
Mesodermal	Lymphangioma (cystic hygroma)
	Hemangioma (port wine, capillary, cavernous, etc.)
	Fibrous dysplasia
	Angiolipoma (tuberous sclerosis)
	Lipoma
Combinations	
Ectodermal and meso	"Vascular hamartoma"
Ectodermal and endo-meso	Teratomas
Ecto or endo and meso	Dermoid, branchial cleft
Endodermal-meso	Thyroglossal duct

BIOLOGY OF HAMARTOMAS

We have defined hamartoma as a congenital tissue conglomerate made up of normal cell types that are normally found at that site but are either excessive in numbers or abnormal in their relationship to other tissues. Many of the systemic hamartomas show a considerable tendency to autosomal dominant inheritance. Warkany, in his book *Congenital Malformations* [38], has chosen to limit the term *hamartoses* to dominantly inherited disorders characterized by having hamartomas as a part of the disease. Examples of the hereditary hamartoses are von Recklinghausen's neurofibromatosis, tuberous sclerosis, and Hippel-Lindau disease. Other syndromes are associated with hamartomas but are not considered hamartoses because of lack of evidence of dominant hereditary traits. They include the Sturge-Weber syndrome (port wine hemangioma of trigeminal nerve distribution with associated intracranial hemangioma and calcification), Maffucci's syndrome (cavernous hemangioma and dyschondroplasia), isolated hemangiomas or lymphangiomas, giant nevi, dermoids, and teratomas.

Although the teratologists, surgeons, pediatricians, and pathologists of the past century had extensive knowledge of the morphology and pathology of congenital malformations, their ideas concerning etiology were rather limited and based on superstitions and speculation rather than scientific theories. Hippocrates had attributed "crippling of the fetus" to a fall or injury of the mother, and common superstition attributes malformations to maternal misbehavior, frights, or mental impressions. For example, the birth of a child with a giant nevus gave rise to the opinion that it is dangerous for a woman to look at monkeys during pregnancy. Ballantyne was among the first to attribute malformations to maternal illness and trauma and identified amniotic changes as the common root of all congenital malformations [1]. As new theories were introduced, it seemed more likely that amniotic abnormalities were the result rather than the cause of malformations. Nutritional deficiency as a cause of congenital malformations has been widely expounded. Considerable animal experimentation supports this theory [39, 40, 41], but there is little or no proof that nutritional deficiency is a significant factor in human teratogenesis.

Chemical compounds, particularly drugs, had been widely used in experimental teratology to cause congenital malformations. The last vestige of doubt of the teratogenic capabilities of drugs was dispelled by the recognition of thalidomide [25], steroids [2], antimetabolites [27], and vitamins [6, 45] as undeniable causes for malformations. Radiation [19] and other agents have likewise been implicated.

Infectious biological agents are another clearly defined cause for malformations. The classic example is that of the anomalies related to the rubella virus. Probably many other viruses can produce malformations; however, the direct cause-effect relationships have not been adequately identified. In fact, viruses have been postulated as the common link that is required to induce alterations in embryological or neoplastic disorders of growth. Little is known about the normal and abnormal mechanisms that are interposed between conception and birth or about exactly how teratogens result in congenital malformations. These theories have emphasized the role of postconceptional modification as the chief source of deformities.

Early in the nineteenth century, Meckel pointed out that hereditarily transmitted anomalies could not be explained by mechanical causes [38, p. 23]. Chromosomes as carriers of hereditary information were recognized in the 1880s, and the basic laws of mendelian inheritance were proposed and published in 1866. In 1909 the independent role of the "genes" located on the chromosome was described by Johannsen. Only recently has the mode of transmission of this genetic information been more clearly understood. It is believed that deoxyribonucleic acid (DNA) in the cell nucleus is the source of the genetic information. The role of ribonucleic acid (RNA) as a link in the transmission of the genetic information has also received considerable attention. Messenger RNA is thought to carry information from the nuclear DNA to the cytoplasmic ribosomes. Transfer RNA aids in transport of amino acids to the ribosomes, where the amino acids are aligned and proteins synthesized.

The unitary theory of congenital malformations proposes that any modification of the ultimate expression of the DNA-RNA system can result in malformation. This may occur by the transmission of abnormal genetic information in the nuclear DNA from parents to offspring, by postconceptional alteration of the DNA and/or RNA, or by any one of the aforementioned chemical, physical, or biological factors.

ECTODERMAL HAMARTOMAS [13, 34]

Hamartomas of epidermis or epidermal appendages are generally referred to as *nevi* of that skin structure which they most closely resemble. The most common ectodermal nevi are the epidermal nevus, sebaceous nevus, and basal cell nevus. Somewhat less common are the hair follicle nevus, sweat gland nevus, and collagen nevus.

Epidermal Nevus

The epidermal nevus (linear nevus, nevus unius lateris, verrucous nevus) is a hamartoma of the malpighian epidermal layer. Histologically it is characterized by hyperkeratosis and acanthosis. The nevus has a yellow-brown, verrucous, elevated appearance reminiscent of a seborrheic keratosis or a wart with a distribution that tends to be arranged in linear bands or streaks. Malformations of the central nervous system are a common association, and basal cell tumors have been reported. Because it is a superficial lesion, either dermabrasion or excision can be effective treatment.

Sebaceous Nevus

This hamartoma of the sebaceous glands (nevus of Jadassohn) has a yellow-tan, seborrheic appearance. A reported 20 percent incidence of basal cell carcinoma is associated with it. The sebaceous nevus should be distinguished from the adenoma sebaceum, which is the cutaneous angiofibroma associated with tuberous sclerosis. Excision and closure with flaps or grafts is the required treatment. Dermabrasion is ineffective because of the depth of the sebaceous hamartoma.

Basal Cell Nevus

This is an autosomal dominant trait characterized by diffuse cutaneous hamartomas that resemble basal cell carcinomas and, furthermore, have a strong tendency to form true basal cell carcinoma. The clinical appearance of the hamartoma is of multiple irregular cutaneous nodules. Associated anomalies include pits of the palmar and sole skin, jaw and vertebral cysts lined with squamous epithelium, and a facies characterized by a broad, flat nose.

NEUROECTODERMAL HAMARTOMAS

Neurofibromatosis

Also known as von Recklinghausen's disease [7, 16], this dominantly inherited syndrome is typified by the presence of multiple hamartomas or benign neoplasms of the skin and other organs. Primarily involved are the neural ectodermal tissues.

Café au Lait Spots

Usually the earliest, but least significant, cutaneous lesion is the café au lait spot. This is a light tan, ovoid, flat lesion caused by an increase in the number of melanocytes and an excessive production of melanin. Furthermore, biopsies and electron microscope histological examinations have revealed that there are giant pigment granules in the melanocytes of a café au lait spot and possibly within all the melanocytes of the skin of an individual with neurofibromatosis. Such examinations should distinguish the café au lait of neurofibromatosis from the café au lait spot that occurs as an isolated phenomenon or with Albright's syndrome in which the melanocyte count and the melanocyte pigment granules are normal. It has been said that five or more café au lait spots are suggestive of neurofibromatosis. No treatment is required.

Fibrous Molluscum

This is a circumscribed violaceous dome-shaped lesion of a few millimeters to a few centimeters in size. Histologically it is formed by whorls of Schwann cells and nerve axons within the dermis and upper portion of the subcutaneous tissue.

Plexiform Neurofibroma

The lesions are of greater size than the molluscum; indeed, they may be as large as an extremity. They have a light tan color with a slightly irregular pachydermatous appearance. On occasion they are quite extensive, involving the subcutaneous tissue and bone, and they may be associated with hemihypertrophy.

Nevi

The incidence of large nevi in neurofibromatosis is approximately 2 to 10 percent as compared to the incidence of 1:10,000 in the general population. This is not surprising considering that nevi are formed from neural crest, as are the Schwann cells in neurofibromatosis.

Rarely, malignant tumors are associated with neurofibromatosis either as a neurofibrosarcoma, pheochromocytoma, or medullary thyroid carcinoma. The incidence of malignancy has been estimated at between 2 and 10 percent.

Complications from neurofibromatosis are numerous in that the lesion can involve any bone or nerve in the body. The incidence of bony lesions has been estimated at 25 to 50 percent, with scoliosis being the most common problem, and the incidence of neurological problems is judged to be 10 to 25 percent. Seizures, blindness, or any neurological symptom can be associated with neurofibromatosis.

Hemihypertrophy is a rare complication, but when it is found, the most likely cause is a neurofibromatosis. It is thought that the hemihypertrophy is related to release of neurotropic factor, the invasion of the periosteum of the long bones by the highly vascular neurofibromas, or a common genetic aberration. Hemihypertrophies can also be associated with the other hamartomas (lymphangiomas or hemangiomas), and frequently no specific etiology can be identified although Wilms' tumor of the kidney and pheochromocytomas may accompany hemihypertrophy.

MELANOCYTIC NEVI

The term *nevus* implies a circumscribed cluster of hamartomatous tissues within the skin. In the broadest sense, *nevus* could be used interchangeably with *cutaneous hamartoma*; but in practice it has been commonly associated with a relatively few malformations. The nevus flammeus (port wine capillary hemangioma), the epidermal nevus (nevus unius lateris), and sebaceous nevus are malformations that have been associated with the term *nevus*, but ordinarily the word is used for the melanocytic nevus and its more dramatic and larger form, the giant hairy nevus (bathing trunk nevus, nevus pilosus, pigmented nevus) [12, 15, 21, 30, 32].

The melanocytic nevus is formed by the clustering of melanocytic cells within the skin. Variations in the cytological appearance of the individual cells, their level in the skin, and their regional distribution determine the specific clinical and pathological diagnosis. Junctional nevi, intradermal (nevoid) nevi, neural nevi, blue nevi, and lentigo are the five common histological patterns.

Embryologically it is believed that melanocytes are derived from the neural crests and represent a hamartoma of neural ectodermal tissues. The close resemblance to Schwann-cell tumors and neurofibromatosis and histochemical studies is additional evidence of the neural crest theory of nevus formation.

Small Acquired Nevi

Clinically, melanocytic nevus can present itself as the small pigmented "moles" that almost all individuals have; they do not normally appear until approximately 1 to 3 years of age [35]. The delayed appearance of the small pigmented nevi has been attributed to the delay in the development of the central nervous system and the associated delay of the capability of melanocytes to produce melanin pigment. It has been generally assumed, but not proved, that the melanocytes in small moles are clustered within the skin at birth but are not clinically apparent until they are capable of pigment production.

Large Congenital Nevi

The extreme form of this hamartoma is the giant pigmented nevus, which may cover the entire trunk or extremity. Coincident with the massive size of the giant nevus are many other abnormalities of neural crest maturation and neural crest maldistribution. The presence of benign melanocytes in the meninges has been called *leptomeningeal melanocytosis*. Since the meninges are developed in part from neural crest, it is not surprising to find an anomalous development of melanocytes in the meninges associated with giant nevi. Meningeal melanocytosis can interfere with the absorption of cerebrospinal fluid and lead to hydrocephalus and seizures.

The melanocytic nevus will enlarge proportionally to the adjacent structures. Hairiness, a dermatome distribution, mesenchymal tumors (fibromas, lipomas), and café au lait spots are often, but not necessarily, a part of the clinical picture. The condition is sporadic, and no family history has been identified.

There is now considerable documentation that malignancy can arise within congenital nevi and probably with even greater frequency in giant nevi. Although the incidence of malignancy cannot be precisely determined, it has been reported as being between 2 and 42 percent with an overall average of 14 percent. There is no established reason for the high frequency of malignancy but it is probably due to one of two factors: First, on account of the immense total area of the hamartomatous melanocytes there is a greater probability that a melanocyte will undergo a degenerative change leading to

melanoma. The alternative explanation is that hamartomatous melanocytes are inherently premalignant because they represent a more primitive form of the melanocyte, or because whatever teratogenic factor produced the malformation persists and acts as a carcinogen.

MESODERMAL HAMARTOMAS

Hemangiomas

Hemangiomas are hamartomas formed by endothelial cells, although certain hemangiomas could be considered neoplasms [5, 20, 24, 31, 38]. The clinical presentation and histopathology are quite variable, so that many specific clinical diagnoses and pathological descriptions permeate the literature. Hemangiomas can be classified on the basis of the histology of the individual endothelial cells, the resemblance of the vascular space to arteries, veins, and capillaries, and the level of the endothelial hamartoma within the skin.

One of the major distinctions of clinical importance is the maturity of the individual endothelial cells. Cells that are histologically immature are called *embryonal* or *angioblastic*. Those hemangiomas (usually the strawberry-capillary type) that enlarge during the first year of life will spontaneously involute. This enlargement and actual cellular multiplication does not represent neoplasia. Remember that the primitive embryonic vascular system is characterized by islands of vascular endothelium that coalesce to form a functional circulatory system (six dorsal arches, cardinal artery and vein, etc.), then subsequently undergo necrosis. The life-death cycle of embryonic endothelial cells is part of an orderly genetic program. It is my belief that strawberry hemangiomas are analogous hamartomas of embryonic vascular endothelium that are genetically programmed to multiply, then die. Certainly the growth pattern can be modified by radiation, steroids, or trauma.

On the other hand, the endothelial cells may have the characteristics of adult endothelium. In that case they have little or no tendency toward spontaneous regression. The port wine stain and the cavernous hemangioma exemplify the mature histological type of hemangioma that does not involute.

Although hemangiomas are described in their pure form, it is most common to find various mixtures of all types of hemangiomas. That is, a hemangioma may be part port wine stain, part strawberry-capillary hemangioma, and part cavernous hemangioma. Furthermore, hemangiomas may be associated with other mesenchyme hamartomas (lymphangiomas, fibromas, lipomas) and may involve an entire extremity. In this situation the lesion is usually described as a mixed hemangioma or a vascular hamartoma.

One of the major complications of hemangiomas is hypertrophy of adjacent tissues. A true gigantism can be associated with vascular hamartomas, and although the exact reason for this generalized tissue hyperplasia is not known, it is suspected that an increased vascularization, particularly when associated with arteriovenous fistulas of the periosteum, is the cause. Entire extremities, digits, or facial parts may be involved by the hypertrophy. Occasionally distortion of tissues because of the pressure exerted by the mass may mimic a hypertrophy, but careful examination and radiological measurements can clarify the nature of the growth disturbance. The Klippel-Trenaunay syndrome is the syndrome of lower limb hypertrophy, venous varicosities, and port wine hemangiomas associated with a mixed vascular hamartoma. The hamartoma component is port wine hemangioma, along with cavernous hemangioma, and frequently there are lymphangioma and lipoma. Hemangiomas are not associated with an increased rate of malignancy or frequent infections.

Port Wine Hemangioma

The port wine hemangioma, or nevus flammeus, is composed of adult-type endothelium with a capillary-like structure located within the dermis. It often follows a dermatome distribution. When it is located in the distribution of the ophthalmic division of the trigeminal nerve and associated with intracranial hemangioma or calcification and mental retardation, this whole complex is called the *Sturge-Weber syndrome.* Port wine hemangiomas do not become hyperplastic and do not undergo spontaneous regression, but grow proportionally with the adjacent tissues. They may however elevate above the skin surface and develop small nodules.

Strawberry Hemangioma

Strawberry hemangiomas are made up of angioblastic capillary-type endothelium which is aggregated in large masses with relatively few vascular spaces. The hemangioma is often flat at birth but during the first year of life can enlarge significantly. The enlargement may be due to engorgement of the capillary spaces with blood or to actual increase in the number of endothelial cells. Gradual resolution of the hemangioma follows this initial enlargement, so that by age 4 or 5 it has usually completely disappeared and left only the atrophic, stretched-out skin.

Capillary hemangiomas are also found within the parotid gland and within the muscle, where they are often described as hemangioendotheliomas because of the predominant cellularity. The large, deep-seated strawberry-capillary hemangiomas are occasionally associated with a vascular coagulopathy called the *Kasabach-Merritt syndrome* [22]. Trauma may incite the trapping of platelets within the hemangioma and secondarily leads to thrombocytopenic hemorrhagic diathesis. Platelet transfusion, radiotherapy, cortisone, and, in some circumstances, heparin have been used for treatment of this coagulopathy.

Cavernous Hemangioma

Cavernous hemangiomas are composed of adult endothelium organized into large venous or sinusoidal vascular spaces in the dermis and subcutaneous tissue. They do not spontaneously regress and are not usually associated with Kasabach-Merritt syndrome. Cavernous hemangiomas are more likely to be deep in subcutaneous tissue or muscle, but this is not invariably the case. Maffucci's syndrome is characterized by cavernous hemangiomas and dyschondroplastic nodules of the fingers or toes.

Lymphangioma

Lymphangiomas are hamartomas of endothelium associated with lymphatic vasoformative tissue [4, 9, 10, 11, 18, 29, 33]. It is difficult to distinguish the individual endothelial cell of a lymphangioma from that of a hemangioma, but the contents of the vascular spaces, distribution, and natural history of the lesion will make the diagnosis apparent. Although many theories have been proposed regarding the origin of lymphangiomas, the most generally accepted is the "centrifugal" theory of Sabin, who stated that the lymphatic system results from sprouting buds from the venous system at five sites. These embryonic anlagen of the lymphatic system are called *lymphatic buds* and are located bilaterally in the axillary-supraclavicular region and the groin and unilaterally in the mesentery. Failure of the lymphatic buds to connect with each other or maintain the connection with the venous system results in isolation and overgrowth of that lymphatic endothelium. Dowd proposed a "centripetal" theory that islands of mesenchyme coalesce to form peripheral lymphatics, then connect to veins [10]. Lymphangiomas result when the islands of mesenchyme are sequestered.

Most lymphangiomas are anatomically related to the five embryonic lymph buds but may be found in any part of the body. Lymphangiomas may slowly enlarge during childhood because of accumulation of lymphatic fluids in large cystic spaces [33]. These lymphangiomas with large cysts are also called *cystic hygromas* and occur most commonly in the neck and lower face. Rarely, there may be proliferation of lymphatic endothelium and

true neoplastic growth. Lymphangiomas may not become clinically apparent until early childhood or adult life (10 percent), at which time the lymphatic spaces are distended. Lymphangiomas do not spontaneously regress during early childhood but do tend to diminish in size during adulthood—although they may persist throughout life. Their growth pattern is similar to that of the lymph glands. Hypertrophy of tonsils, adenoids, and lymph glands is expected during early childhood, but in the prepubertal years lymphatic tissues slowly begin to diminish in size. Perhaps that same biological control is inherent in lymphatic hamartomas.

The major complication of lymphangiomas is the extreme susceptibility to infection. An early review by Dowd reported a 43 percent mortality in all cases [10]. In the antibiotic era, the mortality has been quite low. Lymphangiomas of the floor of the mouth, tongue, and neck and mediastinum are still of particular concern because rapid enlargement associated with upper respiratory infections may cause acute airway obstruction. Malignancy and bleeding diathesis have not been reported in association with pure lymphangiomas. Regional growth disturbances in the form of either a true hyperplasia or distortion by pressure are occasional complications.

MIXED HAMARTOMAS

Teratomas

The teratoma can be considered a hamartoma but perhaps is more appropriately regarded as a neoplasm formed by an embryonic rest of totipotential cells derived from all of the embryonic germ layers [3, 14, 17, 36]. Because of the frequent finding of various organs and tissue, including teeth, hair, endocrine glands, and skin, such a lesion was considered a remnant of a twin.

Teratomas usually occur in the ovaries, sacrococcygeal region, and thyroid but can occur in almost any site in the body. There is a specific predilection toward a midline location except for the orbits and the ovaries. Teratomas have an extremely high incidence of malignancy, estimated at 15 to 50 percent. The sacrococcygeal lesions in particular have a high risk of malignancy.

Dermoids

Dermoids are inclusion remnants at the site of embryonic fusion [28, 42]. During embryogenesis, fusion of adjacent parts takes place at various sites. If there is a failure of the normal fusion process, a cyst (or sinus) may occur at that site of incomplete fusion.

The dermoid cyst is an inclusion cyst of epithelial tissues and the associated dermal stroma (skin, hair follicles, sweat glands). Common sites are at the midline of the nose, the lateral supraorbital ridge, and the midline of the neck and mandible. The lesions do not contain elements of endoderm or mesoderm (other than the connective tissues which are normally associated with the skin). They do not have the malignancy potential of the teratoma and seem to enlarge as a result of the accumulation of epithelial debris within the cyst, rather than because of a true hyperplasia or neoplasia of the cells.

Branchial Cleft Cysts (Sinuses or Fistulas)

Branchial cleft cysts form at the site of the branchial clefts and pouches separating the branchial arches [11, 44]. The branchial cleft may have an endodermal lining that resembles respiratory epithelium or may have ectodermal lining of stratified or squamous epithelium. The epithelial lining is surrounded by lymphocytes and supportive connective tissue. The most common site of the branchial cleft cyst is the second branchial cleft between the second and third branchial arches. The cyst occurs along the anterior border of the sternocleidomastoid muscle and may communicate with the oropharynx in the region of the posterior tonsillar pillar. The first branchial cleft cyst is usually found along the margin of the mandible and may have a common communication with the ex-ternal auditory canal. Cysts of the second branchial arch are six times as common as cysts of the first branchial arch. The major complication is infection. Malignancy is an extremely rare occurrence.

Thyroglossal duct cysts are the result of retained remnant of the thyroid gland along the embryonic pathway of the descent of the thyroid gland from the base of the tongue (foramen caecum linguae) to the trachea [8, 23, 26, 37]. The sinus tract can pass through or adjacent to the hyoid bone. The entire thyroid gland may fail to descend and remain as an ectopic thyroid (20 percent of the cases). Therefore, a thyroid scan is essential before excision of midline lesions that are suspected of being thyroglossal duct cysts. Carcinoma is a rare occurrence.

REFERENCES

1. Ballantyne, J. W. *Manual of Antenatal Pathology and Hygiene.* Edinburgh: Green, 1904.
2. Baxter, H., and Fraser, F. C. Production of congenital defects in offspring of female mice treated with cortisone. *McGill Med. J.* 19:245, 1950.
3. Berry, C. L., Keeling, J., and Hilton, C. Teratoma in infancy and childhood: A review of 91 cases. *J. Pathol.* 98:241, 1969.
4. Bill, A. H., and Sumner, D. S. A unified concept of lymphangioma and cystic hygroma. *Surg. Gynecol. Obstet.* 120:79, 1965.
5. Blackfield, H. M., Torrey, F. A., Morris, W. J., and Low-Beer, B. V. A. The management of visible hemangiomas. *Am. J. Surg.* 94:313, 1957.
6. Cheng, D. W., and Thomas, B. H. Relationship of time of therapy to teratogeny in maternal avitaminosis E. *Proc. Iowa Acad. Sci.* 60:290, 1953.
7. Crowe, F. W., Schull, W. J., and Neel, J. V. *A Clinical, Pathological, and Genetic Study of Neurofibromatosis.* Springfield, Ill.: Thomas, 1956.
8. Dalgaard, J. B., and Wettesland, P. Thyroglossal anomalies. *Acta Chir. Scand.* 111:444, 1956.

9. Dingman, R. O., and Grabb, W. C. Lymphangioma of the tongue. *Plast. Reconstr. Surg.* 27:214, 1961.
10. Dowd, C. N. Hygroma cysticum colli. *Ann. Surg.* 58:112, 1913.
11. Drinker, C., and Field, M. *Lymphatics, Lymph, and Tissue Fluid.* Baltimore: Williams & Wilkins, 1933. P. 1.
12. Fish, J., Smith, E. B., and Canby, J. P. Malignant melanoma in childhood. *Surgery* 59:309, 1966.
13. Fitzpatrick, T. B., Arndt, K. A., Clark, W. H., Jr., Eisen, A. Z., Van Scott, E. J., and Vaughn, J. A. *Dermatology in General Medicine.* New York: McGraw-Hill, 1971.
14. Gifford, G. H., and MacCollum, D. W. Facial teratoma in the newborn: Report of 5 cases. *Plast. Reconstr. Surg.* 49:616, 1972.
15. Greeley, P. W., Middleton, A. G., and Curtin, J. W. Incidence of malignancy in giant pigmented nevi. *Plast. Reconstr. Surg.* 36:26, 1965.
16. Griffith, B. H., McKinney, P., Monroe, C. W., and Howell, A. Von Recklinghausen's disease in children. *Plast. Reconstr. Surg.* 49:647, 1972.
17. Gross, R. E., Clatworthy, H. W., Jr., and Meeker, I. A., Jr. Sacrococcygeal teratomas in infants and children. *Surg. Gynecol. Obstet.* 92:341, 1951.
18. Harkins, G. A., and Sabiston, D. C. Lymphangioma in infancy and childhood. *Surgery* 47:811, 1960.
19. Hicks, S. P. Developmental malformations produced by radiation. *Am. J. Roentgenol.* 69:272, 1953.
20. Jacobs, A. H. Strawberry hemangiomas—the natural history of the untreated lesion. *Calif. Med.* 86:8, 1957.
21. Kaplan, E. N. The risk of malignancy in large congenital nevi. *Plast. Reconstr. Surg.* 53:421, 1974.
22. Kasabach, H. H., and Merritt, K. K. Capillary hemangioma with extensive purpura: Report of a case. *Am. J. Dis. Child.* 59:1063, 1940.
23. Klopp, C. T., and Kirson, S. M. Therapeutic problems with ectopic noncancerous follicular thyroid tissue in the neck: 18 case reports according to etiologic factors. *Ann. Surg.* 163:653, 1966.
24. Matthews, D. N. Treatment of haemangiomata. *Br. J. Plast. Surg.* 6:83, 1953.
25. McBride, W. G. Thalidomide and congenital abnormalities. *Lancet* 2:1358, 1961.
26. Meyerowitz, B. R., and Buchholz, R. B. Midline cervical ectopic thyroid tissue. *Surgery* 65:358, 1969.
27. Nelson, M. M. Mammalian Fetal Development and Antimetabolites. In Rhoads, E. P. (Ed.), *Antimetabolites and Cancer.* Washington: American Association for the Advancement of Science, 1955. (Monograph.)
28. New, G. B., and Erich, J. B. Dermoid cysts of the head and neck. *Surg. Gynecol. Obstet.* 65:48, 1937.
29. Paletta, F. X. Lymphangioma. *Plast. Reconstr. Surg.* 37:269, 1966.
30. Pers, M. Naevus pigmentosus giganticus. *Ugeskr. Laeger* 125:613, 1963.
31. Reed, R. J., and O'Quinn, S. E. Neoplasms and Tumor-like Conditions of Neural and Supporting Tissue Origin. In Fitzpatrick, T. B., et al. (Eds.), *Dermatology in General Medicine.* New York: McGraw-Hill, 1971.
32. Reed, W. B., Becker, W., Becker, W. S., and Nickel, W. R. Giant pigmented nevi, melanoma, and leptomeningeal melanocytosis. *Arch. Dermatol.* 91:100, 1965.
33. Singleton, A. O. Congenital lymphatic diseases—lymphangiomata. *Ann. Surg.* 105:952, 1937.
34. Smith, D. W. *Recognizable Patterns of Human Malformation.* Vol. VII, Major Problems in Clinical Pediatrics series. Philadelphia: Saunders, 1970.
35. Spitz, S. Melanomas of childhood. *Am. J. Pathol.* 24:591, 1948.
36. Stone, H. H., Henderson, D., and Guidio, F. A. Teratomas of the neck. *Am. J. Dis. Child.* 113:222, 1967.
37. Ward, G. E., Hendrick, J. W., and Chambers, R. G. Thyroglossal tract abnormalities, cysts, and fistulas. *Surg. Gynecol. Obstet.* 89:727, 1949.
38. Warkany, J. *Congenital Malformations.* Chicago: Year Book, 1972.

39. Warkany, J., Roth, C. B., and Wilson, J. G. Multiple congenital malformations: A consideration of etiologic factors. *Pediatrics* 1:462, 1948.

40. Warkany, J., and Schraffenberger, E. Congenital malformations induced in rats by maternal nutritional deficiency: V. Effects of a purified diet lacking riboflavin. *Proc. Soc. Exp. Biol. Med.* 54:92, 1943.

41. Warkany, J., and Schraffenberger, E. Congenital malformations induced in rats by maternal nutritional deficiency: VI. The preventive factor. *J. Nutr.* 27:477, 1944.

42. Weisman, P. A., and Johnson, G. F. Concealed extensions of dermoid cysts of the nose: How can the surgeon be forewarned? *Plast. Reconstr. Surg.* 34:373, 1964.

43. Willis, P. A. *The Borderland of Embryology and Pathology.* Washington: Butterworth, 1962.

44. Wilson, C. P. Lateral cysts and fistulae of the neck of developmental origin. *Ann. R. Coll. Surg. Engl.* 17:1, 1955.

45. Wilson, J. G., Roth, C. B., and Warkany, J. An analysis of the syndrome of malformations induced by maternal vitamin A deficiency. Effects of restoration of vitamin A at various times during gestation. *Am. J. Anat.* 92:189, 1953.

14

Growth and Aging
Desmond A. Kernahan

The scope of plastic surgery is such that its practitioners are forced to appreciate not only the form and proportions of the body at any one time but also the progressive changes in these characteristics from birth to old age. Changes occurring with aging of the skin, particularly in the facial region, are the basis of the practice of much aesthetic surgery. Growth is not a uniform process in which all organs of the body proceed from size at birth to adult size at a steady rate. For instance, the changes in the proportions of the head, limbs, and trunk are obvious and are of importance in assessing the percentage of body surface involved in burns.

Some background knowledge of the development of the facial skeleton and the facial organs is needed both for the planning and timing of surgery and for understanding the effects on growth of the face of such deformities as cleft lip and palate, first branchial arch syndrome, and craniofacial abnormalities. Many of the facial structures reach adult or nearly adult size relatively early in life—for instance, the ear and globe of the eye—whereas others, such as the nose and dental structures, achieve full growth at a

much later date. The present chapter, therefore, considers some of the changes from birth to old age more particularly as they apply to the skin and the face and indicates how these changes are measured and their importance in an understanding of the way they affect surgical decisions.

THICKNESS OF THE SKIN

The thickness of the skin changes with age and also differs in any one individual in different areas of the body. The thickness of the skin also varies between male and female and with race. These are important facts in the problem of selecting donor sites for split-skin grafting and of selecting the appropriate thickness of skin grafts in different areas.

Southward carried out an investigation of the thickness of the epidermis and dermis in the skin of cadavers from the commonly used donor sites of abdomen, thighs, and buttocks [17]. He cut specimens around a circular template and measured the skin thickness with the skin pinned out under normal tension. The epidermis was relatively thin at birth and in childhood, he found, but thickened during puberty and thereafter remained constant in thickness until the fifth or sixth decade, at which time it again became thinner. The thickness of epidermis between the ages of 1 and 5 years in most of the usual donor sites was about 25 microns, increasing to 53 microns in adolescence and remaining at about that figure until the age of 65 and over. The thinning process at that age was accompanied by reduction in the size of the papillae. In general, the epidermis proved to be thicker in males than in females.

Similar changes were noted in the thickness of the dermis, with it being relatively thin in childhood and reaching its maximum thickness in the fourth or fifth decade. Thinning occurred with the onset of old age until final thickness approximated that of childhood. The thickness of the dermis in the 1- to 5-year-old age group was approximately 600 microns, increasing to a maximum of 1200 microns in adult life and then decreasing to childhood thickness. Again, the dermis was significantly thicker in men than in women and in any one individual was thickest on the trunk. Southward also found that in the limbs the dermis tended to be thicker on the extensor than on the flexor aspect.

THE EFFECTS OF AGING ON THE SKIN

Medawar has defined aging as a lowering of biological efficiency accompanied by a decreased rate of cellular turnover [6]. Plastic surgeons are familiar with the macroscopic changes that occur in the skin and skin appendages with advancing age. The principal facial creases—the smile line, the glabella lines, the transverse creases in the forehead and around the eyes—are scarcely noticeable at birth and in the infant but become progressively more marked with advancing age. These lines form where the skin is repeatedly creased or folded, particularly on the face, where they occur at right angles to the line of contraction of the facial muscles. Medawar speaks of the dermal fibrous skeleton to which are attached the muscles of expression and states that old people have acquired lined

faces for two reasons: because of "an innate deterioration of their skin which has made it more susceptible to the engravery of constant usage" and because they have smiled, frowned, or raised their eyebrows more often than their juniors. He indicates that the first of these factors—deterioration of the skin with age—far outweighs the latter in importance. Other commonly observed macroscopic changes are graying of the hair and loss of hair, particularly in the male. There is also a progressive loss of subcutaneous tissue beneath the skin accompanied by a decrease in skin elasticity so that when it is pulled into a fold the fold persists longer and the skin flattens less rapidly in the older person than in the young. The nasal vibrissae and the eyebrows both show increased length, and straggly hair appears on female skin.

In addition to the main creases described above, multiple fine lines develop all over the skin of the face and the dorsum of the hand, especially at the angle of the mouth and vertically across the upper and to a lesser extent the lower lips. Drooping of the eyebrows occurs so that they lie below the line of the bony supraorbital ridge, and the skin of the eyelids becomes creased and relaxed, with the formation of pouches. Jowls appear along the inferior border of the mandible, and single or double vertical folds of skin form in the submental region to give the characteristic "turkey-gobbler" look. The nails become irregular, grooved, and more brittle, and there is atrophy of the erector pili muscles. Skin color changes, with the appearance of "liver spots" and plaques of hyperkeratotic skin in some areas. The skin is drier because of partial atrophy of the sweat glands, and the activity of the sebaceous glands decreases, particularly in women following the menopause.

Microscopic Changes

Microscopic changes can be observed corresponding to the macroscopic changes just described. Thinning of both the epidermis and dermis has already been mentioned, and this is accompanied by a reduction in the number of cellular layers leading to thinning of the epithelium. There is also a marked flattening of the rete pegs. Changes observed within individual cells of the epidermis in aging skin include hypertrophy of the nucleoli and lobulation of the nucleus. In the dermis the total cell population of all fibroblasts and motile cells is reduced as compared with that in younger age groups. Atrophy of the erector pili muscles and the sweat and sebaceous glands is noted, and there will be both thickening and an increase in the number of the elastic fibers in the dermis and a change in their pattern to give the characteristic appearances of elastosis senilis. The areas of senile keratosis show marked epidermal atrophy accompanied by hypertrophy of the keratin layer.

Biochemical Changes

The dermis shows a decrease in the extractable collagen fraction and an increase in insoluble collagen due to increased crosslinkage of collagen fibers. There is an overall increase in collagen in the dermis and a decrease in the total acid mucopolysaccharides. The epidermis shows an overall decrease in enzymatic activity.

FACTORS AFFECTING THE AGING OF THE SKIN

Genetic factors determine the marked variations among individuals in the development of the skin changes accompanying age. There are also marked ethnic differences. The skin of the Mongolian and the Negro races shows fewer signs and slower onset of aging than does that of Caucasians. Constant exposure to ultraviolet rays in sunlight and to ionizing radiation hastens the aging process. While the tanned, pigmented, and wrinkled skin of people who have lived most of their life outdoors may resemble that of the aged person, quite different biochemical changes are in fact involved in the exposure of the skin to actinic radiation. Exposure to the sunlight is well recognized as a predisposing factor in the development of skin malignancy, and there is a definite genetic predisposition to actinic damage in certain ethnic groups.

Other factors that may affect the speed of aging of the skin include illnesses such as alcoholism, anorexia nervosa, and progeria. Excessive weight loss can also give the effect of increased skin aging.

NORMAL GROWTH AND DEVELOPMENT

It is as important for the plastic surgeon caring for a child with a congenital abnormality as it is for the pediatrician to be able to assess the child's growth and development since delays are more common in such children and can influence the timing and chances of success of corrective surgical procedures.

Length, weight, and head circumference are the three main parameters of growth assessment in infants, and length, height, and weight in children from 2 to 13 years old. Comparisons are made with figures obtained by measurement of a series of normal children carried out at the Harvard School of Public Health, the findings being expressed in percentiles (Fig. 14-1).

CHANGES IN BODY PROPORTIONS

Changes in body proportions between the newborn infant and the adult vary markedly and are most visibly expressed in the comparison of head size to total body length (Fig. 14-2). At the second month of fetal life the face is 50 percent of total body length. In the newborn it is still 25 percent of the length of the infant. A progressive relative decrease continues into adult life, at which time the head represents only 10 percent of body height. These changes in body proportion find their main application in the assessment of the percentage of body surface burned in infants compared with adults. Figure 14-3 indicates how the relative percentages of body area are affected by growth between birth and 5 years of age.

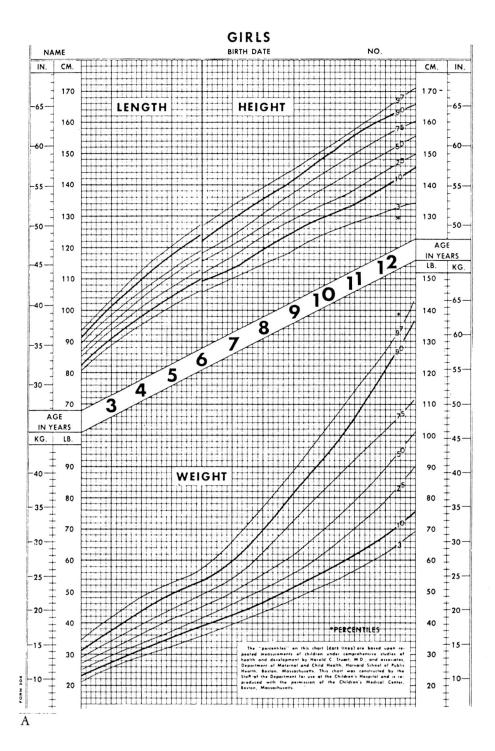

A

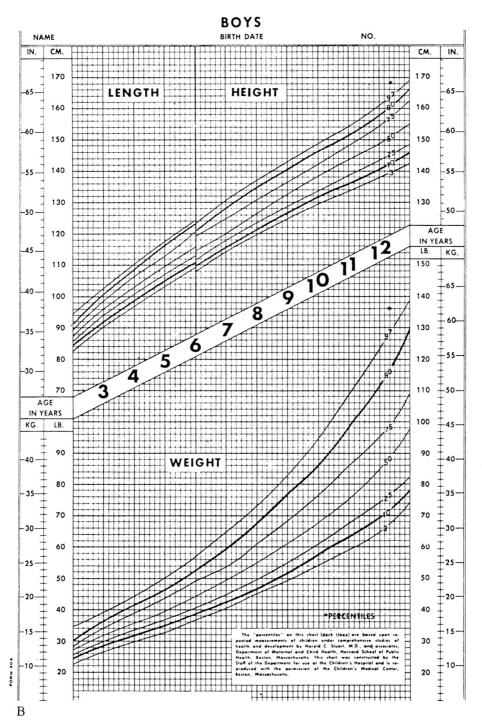

FIGURE 14-1. *Graphs of height and weight in childhood from 2 to 13 years. (From the Children's Medical Center, Boston.)*

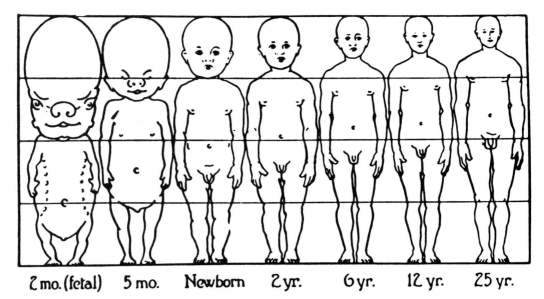

2 mo. (fetal)   5 mo.   Newborn   2 yr.   6 yr.   12 yr.   25 yr.

FIGURE 14-2.   *Changes in body proportions from second fetal month to adulthood. (From C. M. Jackson [Ed.], Morris's Human Anatomy [5th ed.]. Philadelphia: P. Blakiston's Son and Co., 1914. Published by permission of McGraw-Hill Book Co., successors to Blakiston's.)*

GROWTH AND DEVELOPMENT OF THE FACE

Since a considerable amount of the plastic surgeon's time is given to the treatment of children with congenital anomalies involving the facial skeleton, an outline of current concepts of normal facial growth and development is appropriate.

Several approaches to the development of the face from birth to maturity are possible, but the plastic surgeon will probably find it most valuable to consider facial development as occurring in a series of functional cranial components as established by van der Klaauw [4]. A similar approach has been used by Scott, who described the skull as consisting of a series of craniofacial regions, each one related to a particular function [15]. Moss accepted the importance of these functional areas but in addition introduced the concept of the "functional matrix," by which he meant the soft tissues related to each functional area and which he believed to be the governing factor in their growth rate and development [7]. Moss pointed out that the functions of

the skull are digestion, respiration, vision, olfaction, audition, equilibrium, speech, and neural integration. It was possible, he felt, rather than thinking in terms of the individual bones of the facial skeleton, to think of composites of bony structure related to each of these functions and of the individual bones of the skull as being commonly involved in more than one functional area.

CRANIOFACIAL REGIONS

Scott described nine craniofacial regions, each one related to a distinct function [15]. He designates the combination of soft and skeletal tissue in each such structure a "functional unit." These regions are shown diagrammatically in Figure 14-4. They are (1) the cranial vault, (2) the cranial base, (3) the auditory capsule, (4) the nasal region, (5) the orbital cavities, (6) the alveolopalatal region, (7) the facial buttress system, (8) the oral region, and (9) the pharyngeal region. It is apparent that these are readily related to the specific functions of brain cover, forward and downward growth of the face, hearing and

FLUID REPLACEMENT IN BURNT CHILDREN

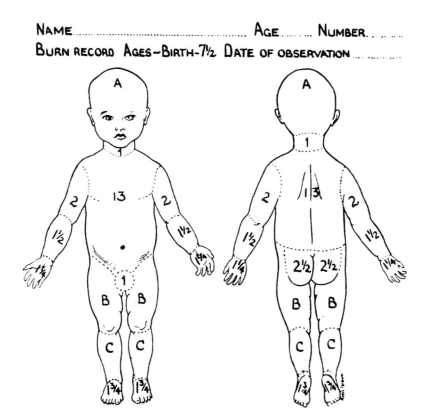

NAME.. AGE......... NUMBER..........

BURN RECORD AGES-BIRTH-7½ DATE OF OBSERVATION...............

RELATIVE PERCENTAGES OF AREAS AFFECTED BY GROWTH

AREA	AGE 0	1	5
A = ½ OF HEAD	9½	8½	6½
B = ½ OF ONE THIGH	2¾	3¼	4
C = ½ OF ONE LEG	2½	2½	2¾

PERCENTAGE BURN BY AREAS

PROBABLE HEAD.......   NECK   BODY   UP. ARM
DEEP BURN FOREARM   HANDS   GENITALS

FIGURE 14-3. *Relative percentage of areas affected by growth. (From M. J. Kyle, and A. B. Wallace, Fluid replacement in burned children.* Br. J. Plast. Surg. 3:194, 1950–1951.)

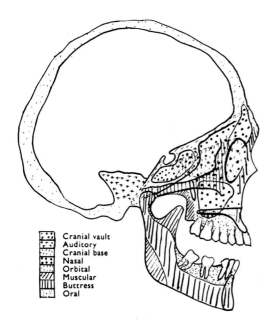

	Cranial vault
	Auditory
	Cranial base
	Nasal
	Orbital
	Muscular
	Buttress
	Oral

FIGURE 14-4.   *The craniofacial regions. (From J. H. Scott, Craniofacial regions—a contribution to the study of facial growth.* Dent. Pract. *5:208, 1955.)*

balance, respiration, sight, dentition, protection, mastication, and speech and swallowing.

The Cranial Vault

Increase in size of the cranial vault is contingent upon growth of the developing brain. It is large at birth, continues to grow rapidly until the third year of life, and is almost complete by the seventh year. It is affected by abnormalities in the developing brain and is small in microcephalus, enlarged in hydrocephalus, and asymmetrical if there is absence of one of the cerebral hemispheres. Thus development of the cranial vault is dependent upon the growth of the brain rather than the size of the brain's being dependent on the growth of the cranial vault.

The Cranial Base

The cranial base lies between the foramen magnum and the foramen caecum and at birth is an entirely cartilaginous structure. Even

when ossification develops in the basioccipital bone and in the body of the sphenoid, the spheno-occipital synchondrosis persists, dividing the cranial base into an anterior and a posterior segment. The presence of the spheno-occipital synchondrosis permits an increase in the length of the cranial base to accommodate downward and forward growth of the middle third of the face and of the pharyngeal region. Its size is not related to that of the cranial vault, being within normal limits in microcephaly and hydrocephaly. Growth continues in both segments until early adult life; the anterior portion is related to the size of the frontal sinus and the posterior to facial and pharyngeal growth.

The Auditory Region

In fetal life the developing inner ear complex becomes surrounded by the cartilaginous auditory capsule, which in turn becomes ossified to form the petrous temporal bone. The growth of the auditory capsule is rapid during late fetal life and is complete by the age of 7 years. Similarly, the external ear shows rapid development early in life; 85 percent of external ear development has been achieved at the age of 3 years, and the ear then continues to grow slowly into adulthood. The width of the ear does not increase after the age of 10 years, and the height of the ear increases very gradually with age. Since this rate of growth is so much more rapid than that of the height and width of the face, the deformity of congenital prominent ears is much more marked in children than in adults. These observations on the normal growth of the external ear provide useful guidelines in reconstruction of the congenital microtic ear as regards timing of the procedure and the size of the cartilaginous implant to be employed relative to the size of the opposite normal ear.

The Nasal Region

The nasal region consists of an upper ethmoidal portion between the orbits related to olfaction and a lower portion between the maxillas related to respiration. Growth of the upper area occurs early and is complete by the seventh year. Growth of the lower portion, however—the external nose and the airways—is dependent upon the requirements of respiration of the growing body and continues until the end of adolescence. The importance of the integrity of the cartilaginous nasal septum in the development of at least the external nose has been substantiated by the experiments of Sarnat and Wexler [12], who studied the growth of the face and jaws after resection of the septal cartilage in young rabbits. Their findings showed that damage to the nasal septum early in life led to severe attenuation of the developing snout of the animal with secondary overeruption of the lower incisor teeth. This is confirmation of the common clinical observation that early trauma to the nasal septum leads to subsequent defects of the dorsum of the nose.

Increase in size of the airways occurs in conjunction with the descent of the hard palate. The process, accomplished by deposition of bone on the oral surface and its resorption on the nasal side, continues until early adult life.

The Orbital Region

The size and growth of the orbit is dependent on the presence and growth of the orbital contents, much as growth of the cranial vault responds to the increasing size of the brain. If the eye is absent or microphthalmic, normal development of the orbit does not occur. Like the other special sense organs, the globe of the eye is large at birth and shows early progression toward adult size. Rapid growth occurs until the age of 3, particularly in the first year. Thereafter, growth progresses more slowly until the age of 14, when adult size has been reached. The orbit then remains constant in size until death, showing no tendency to shrinkage with advancing age [3]. The cornea is 10 mm in diameter at birth and reaches the full adult size of 12 mm by the

age of 1 year. Orbital volume increases somewhat less rapidly than the globe, being only 44 percent of adult size at age 1 and reaching adult volume at 16.

The Alveolopalatal Region

This region consists of the upper and lower alveolar arches and the hard palate. It is the area of principal interest to the orthodontist since it contains the teeth and the alveolar bone in which he moves them. The alveolar bone depends upon the presence of the teeth for its existence and responds readily by resorption and deposition to the application of pressure on the teeth by tongue thrust, thumb-sucking, or the application of orthodontic appliances. Progression in size of the alveolar bone from infancy to adult life is contingent on the presence of the teeth, and it therefore grows as the primary and secondary dentition occurs and reaches full development with the appearance of the last molar teeth. When teeth are lost or removed, involution of the alveolar bone takes place and in the edentulous and those of advanced years resorbs completely, leaving only the basal bone of the maxilla and mandible from which it must be distinguished. Growth of the remainder of this region occurs by the process of bone resorption and deposition. Growth is permitted by the midline suture system in the palate and the symphysis of the mandible during the first year of life and thereafter by deposition on the oral surface of the palate and anterior surface of the maxilla and resorption on the opposite surface.

The Facial Buttress System

This system contains the principal buttresses of the face and consists of the mandible excluding the alveolar bone and coronoid process, the frontal and temporal processes of the zygoma, the frontal process of the maxilla, and the pterygomaxillary articulation. In the mandible and maxilla it forms the basal bone immediately beneath the alveolar bone and is not altered in size or shape by orthodontic procedures. The strength of the facial buttress system is related to the presence and development of the muscles of mastication.

The Muscular Process

The pterygoid plates, the lateral and medial surfaces of the ramus of the mandible, the coronoid process of the mandible, and the zygomatic arches make up the area of attachment of the muscles of mastication. The development of these parts of the facial region depends upon the presence and activity of the corresponding muscle. Washburn has shown experimentally that development of the coronoid process of the mandible does not take place if the temporalis muscle is detached from it early in life [18].

The Pharyngeal Region

Growth in the pharyngeal region is progressive from infancy to adult life. The nasal and oral cavities grow anteriorly, the cervical vertebrae posteriorly. Increase in the anteroposterior dimension of the pharynx corresponds to growth at the spheno-occipital synchondrosis. The oral, nasal, and pharyngeal spaces are regarded by Moss as functional units within the concept of his functional matrix theory of growth control [7]. He feels that the size of the spaces themselves and the relationship of their size to their functions of respiration, mastication, and swallowing qualify them for this consideration equally with more obvious functional units such as the eye and ear.

GROWTH OF THE SKULL

While it is recognized that genetic factors play a basic part in the form of the skull, controversy has existed regarding the control and sites of growth of the skull and the importance and role of various tissues. Growth at sutures, growth occurring secondarily to the growth of cartilage (Scott) [14], and growth occuring in response to the presence of specialized soft tissues (the functional matrix of Moss) [7] are the three principal concepts that have been studied. In order to understand the differences among them and their application to facial skeletal growth, a distinction must be drawn between the growth center, described by Baume as a "place of endochondral ossification with tissue separation force," and a growth site, which is a region of "periosteal or sutural bone formation and modeling resorption adaptive to environmental influences" [1].

Growth at Sutures

The question of whether there are in fact any true growth centers in the cranium has been extensively reviewed by Koski [5]. The classic growth center may be considered an epiphyseal growth plate. When an epiphysis is transplanted to the brain, the bone continues to hold its characteristic form and to grow by endochondral ossification—and hence demonstrates a true tissue separation force. On the other hand, cranial sutures similarly transplanted have been found not to grow, indicating that sutures do not have an innate growth potential by virtue of their structure and are not capable of exerting a tissue separation force comparable to that of the transplanted epiphyseal plate. Thus they fail the definition of a growth center and must fall into the more passive definition of a growth site. They appear to be areas that allow for adjustment and deposition of bone, permitting growth in a passive manner secondary to the influence of other developing tissues rather than demonstrating an intrinsic ability to grow alone. They cannot, therefore, be considered to control craniofacial growth. However, they are nonetheless important because they allow growth to take place. This attribute is shown by the fact that premature suture closure such as occurs in craniosynostosis leads to increased intracranial pressure as the brain increases in size and is unable to be accommodated by a correspondingly larger cranial size on account of the early sutural fusion.

As with sutures, it has been suggested that the synchondroses of the cranial base are growth centers. Although the spheno-occipital synchondrosis is undoubtedly the site of endochondral ossification, the presence of a tissue separation force as would be required for the true definition of a growth center has not been established. As with cranial sutures, when the synchondrosis is transplanted to a soft tissue site, it does not evidence any independent growth potential, as does the transplanted epiphysis. One might more accurately regard the spheno-occipital synchondrosis, then, as a growth site comparable to a suture rather than a growth center comparable to an epiphysis.

Cartilaginous Growth

Scott has been the major protagonist of the view that the cartilage of the nasal septum is a primary craniofacial growth center [13]. Scott describes two facial suture systems: (1) posterior, lying behind the maxilla and separating it from the palatine, lacrimal, vomer, and zygomatic bones, and (2) anterior, separating the premaxilla from the maxilla, nasal bones, and vomer. He points out that at birth the cartilage of the nasal septum is extremely extensive, reaching back to the cranial base, and that its growth is the force that pushes the facial skeleton downward and forward and is responsible for growth at both posterior and anterior suture systems.

Scott's concept of the septal cartilage as an active growth center has been challenged by Koski and by Moss. Koski states that, while excision of the nasal septum severely affects the growth of the nose, this outcome does not prove that the nasal septum is an active force in growth but shows only what occurs when it is absent [5]. Moss et al. described two clinical cases of agenesis of the nasal septum in which the resulting growth defect was confined to the dorsum of the nose and reinforced the clinical observation by studying the effect of complete removal of the nasal septum in young rats [9]. The experiment showed that

while dorsal collapse of the nose occurred growth of the midfacial skeleton was essentially normal in both vertical and anteroposterior dimensions, indicating at best a local and limited role in growth for the cartilaginous nasal septum.

The Functional Matrix

If neither the suture system nor the nasal septum can be conclusively shown to be an active growth center, some other explanation must be found for the growth of the craniofacial skeleton. This has been supplied by Moss with his concept of the functional matrix. Like van der Klaauw [4], Moss [7] considers the facial skeleton to be made up of units each related to a specific function and each growing in a semi-independent manner and at different rates from the others. Examples of functions are respiration, hearing, and vision. The functional matrix is the soft tissue associated with each of these areas of function, and it is the soft tissues that determine the presence, rate of growth, and size of the bones related to each functional area in much the same way the growth of the cranial vault is related to the growth of the brain. Moss includes in this concept the growth not only of areas such as the orbit and auditory mechanism but also the increase in size of the spaces in the facial skeleton required for respiration, mastication, and deglutition. He points out the effect on skeletal growth of absence of the soft tissue matrix, as, for instance, in the case of microphthalmia and anodontia, in which the associated skeletal elements either do not appear at all or are markedly abnormal.

Ross and Johnston consider that including only the soft tissue in the functional matrix is too restrictive and that there must be times when skeletal tissues also have a determinant role to play [11]. They feel that bone should be included with the soft tissues in the functional matrix.

Certainly from the point of view of the plastic surgeon interested in the observation and treatment of facial anomalies the concept of the face as consisting of a series of functional units is an attractive and a simplifying one. It may be of help in a detailed classification of the anomalies existing in specific craniofacial abnormalities.

REFERENCES

1. Baume, L. J. The principles of cephalofacial development revealed by experimental biology. *Aust. J. Orthod.* 47:881, 1961.
2. Broadbent, B. H. A new x-ray technique and its application to orthodonture. *Angle Orthod.* 1:45, 1931.
3. Duke-Elder, S. *System of Ophthalmology.* St. Louis: Mosby, 1963. Vol. 3, p. 310.
4. Klaauw, C. J. van der. Cerebral skull and facial skull. *Arch. Neurol. Zool.* 7:16, 1945.
5. Koski, K. Cranial growth centers—facts or fallacies. *Am. J. Orthod.* 54:566, 1968.
6. Medawar, P. B. The Definition and Measurement of Senescence. In *Aging—General Aspects.* Boston: Little, Brown, 1955. Vol. 3.
7. Moss, M. L. The Functional Matrix. In Kraus, B. S., and Reidel, R. A. (Eds.), *Vistas in Orthodontics.* Philadelphia: Lea & Febiger, 1962. P. 85.
8. Moss, M. L. Vertical growth of the human face. *Am. J. Orthod.* 50:359, 1964.
9. Moss, M. L., Bromberg, B. E., Song, I. C., and Eisenman, J. The passive role of nasal septal cartilage in mid-facial growth. *Plast. Reconstr. Surg.* 41:536, 1968.
10. Pritchard, J. J., Scott, J. H., and Gergis, F. G. The structure and development of cranial and facial sutures. *J. Anat.* 90:73, 1956.
11. Ross, R. B., and Johnston, M. D. *Cleft Lip and Palate.* Baltimore: Williams & Wilkins, 1972. P. 106.
12. Sarnat, B. G., and Wexler, M. R. Growth of the face and jaws after resection of septal cartilage in the rabbit. *Am. J. Anat.* 118:755, 1966.
13. Scott, J. H. The cartilage of the nasal septum—a contribution to the study of facial growth. *Br. Dent. J.* 95:37, 1953.
14. Scott, J. H. The growth of the human face. *Proc. R. Soc. Med.* 47:91, 1954.
15. Scott, J. H. Craniofacial regions—a contribution to the study of facial growth. *Dent. Pract.* 5:208, 1955.
16. Scott, J. H. The analysis of facial growth: 1. The anteroposterior and vertical dimensions. *Am. J. Orthod.* 44:507, 1958.
17. Southward, W. F. W. The thickness of the skin. *Plast. Reconstr. Surg.* 15:423, 1955.
18. Washburn, S. L. The relation of the temporalis muscle to the form of the skull. *Anat. Rec.* 99:239, 1947.

V

Surgical Modification of Unfavorable Factors

INTRODUCTION

As has already been seen, whether unfavorable factors are congenital or acquired, internal or external, they will upset the well-being of the body if circumstances are such that they are against the organism.

Because an unfavorable outcome often leads to a tissue defect that the body itself cannot repair with the maintenance of function and/or cosmesis, surgical intervention may be resorted to. Much of the handicraft of the reconstructive surgeon is related to the use of various types of flaps and to knowledge of tissue tension, skin biomechanics, and surgical geometry.

Part V does not attempt to instruct the reader in how to design flaps and how to move tissue. Instead it examines why the surgeon succeeds (or does not succeed) when his skill is called upon to repair the injuries of various types of onslaught. The last chapter in the section should be a natural transition to a conventional textbook of plastic surgery, which does discuss actual methods of treatment rather than the broad principles outlined herein.

15

Flap Design:
The Anatomical and Physiological Bases

Ernest N. Kaplan and
Terry R. Knapp

ANATOMICAL PRINCIPLES

The successful transfer of a skin flap is one of the most exacting tests of the skilled reconstructive surgeon. To a great degree, this skill is acquired by long experience and the learning that comes from inevitable mistakes. However, certain rules have been quoted repeatedly to guide those who have yet to benefit from their own experience. The aim of the present chapter is to review the anatomical and physiological bases of these classic axioms and of new principles of flap surgery. The validity of their clinical application will also be considered.

Definitions and Classifications

John Staige Davis defined a pedicle flap as "a mass of tissue, usually the skin and subcutaneous fat, which is raised from its bed, but is left attached to the surrounding skin at a selected portion of its periphery" [17]. The flap is the portion of skin and subcutaneous tissue that has been raised from the underlying tissues. The pedicle is the area of continuity of the flap with the surrounding tissues through which the vascular supply to the flap is transmitted.

Various terms are used to describe the design of skin flaps. We have condensed these terms into eight specific categories which help describe all aspects of flap surgery. The outline categorizes the considerations inherent in the design of any flap:

I. Topographic location
   A. Forehead flap
   B. Groin flap
   C. Cross-leg flap
   D. Thoracoepigastric flap
   E. Pharyngeal flap

II. Shape
   A. Rectangular
   B. Triangular
   C. Circular
   D. Bipedicle
   E. Bilobed

III. Spatial relation of flap pedicle to recipient bed
   A. Distant (flap base to be transected and blood supply maintained from recipient bed)
   B. Local (flap to remain in continuity with its pedicle)

IV. Geometry and dynamics
    A. Rotation
    B. Advancement
    C. Transposition
    D. Interpolation
    E. Caterpillar
    F. Turnover
V. Spatial relation of pedicle base to the flap or to other anatomical landmarks
    A. Superiorly based
    B. Inferiorly based
    C. Medially based
    D. Laterally based
    E. Antegrade—i.e., the vascularization of the flap is in the same direction as normal arterial inflow and venous outflow
    F. Retrograde—i.e., the flow into the flap is not in the normal direction from which the arteries and veins would normally enter the skin segment
VI. Type of vascular pedicle
    A. Arterial (superficial temporal, superficial iliac, circumflex, etc.)
    B. Venous (thoracoepigastric)
    C. Dermal
    D. Subcutaneous
    E. Arterial island

VII. Management of raw undersurfaces
    A. Open (exposed)
    B. Closed
      1. Tubed
      2. Lined (graft or other flap)
VIII. Timing of transfer
    A. Delayed
    B. Nondelayed (immediate)

This chapter will focus on categories I, V, VI, VII, and VIII.

Anatomy of Skin Vascularization

A thorough knowledge of the anatomy of the vascular supply to the skin and subcutaneous tissues is a valuable aid to the accurate planning of the design, delay, and eventual successful transfer of skin flaps (Fig. 15-1).

Dermal Plexus

The skin is vascularized from an extensive, two-tiered web of interconnecting microvessels. The lower tier of vessels is in the subcutaneous tissue in the immediate subdermal area and is called the *subdermal plexus*. From these vessels, branches course upward through the reticular dermis into the papil-

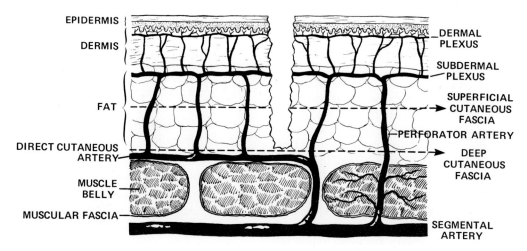

FIGURE 15-1. *Anatomy of arterial vasculature of the skin—perforator (musculocutaneous) arteries and axial (direct cutaneous) arteries.*

lary dermis where a more superficial arterial plexus arborizes into the basal layer of the epidermis and to the dermal appendages. When encountered at surgery, these vessels are referred to as "skin bleeders." A skin flap based only on these vessels is termed a *dermal*, or cutaneous, *flap*.

Segmental Patterns

The major segmental arterial trunks (femoral, brachial, etc.) have numerous branches that terminate in the subdermal plexus. There are two patterns of arterial distribution from the segmental vessels to the subdermal plexus: (1) *perforating*, or musculocutaneous, arteries and (2) *axial*, or direct, cutaneous arteries.

Perforating Musculocutaneous System

The perforators have a vertical course from the segmental arteries into the muscle where they nourish the muscle and then continue through the anterior muscular fascia into the subcutaneous tissue. Here they further arborize and eventually terminate in the dermal plexus.

The perforating musculocutaneous vessels are the major blood supply to the skin but, with few exceptions, are unnamed vessels. A flap designed in an area with a perforating vascular system may require transection of the principal blood supply to the skin. If the underlying perforator is transected when the flap is elevated, the flap is dependent on the collateral circulation in the subcutaneous tissues and dermis for its survival. As previously stated, such a flap is called a *cutaneous flap*. Examples are the cross-leg flap, the facial and neck flaps, and the deltoid portion of the Bakamjian deltopectoral flap.

In general, the perforating vessels can seldom be identified, but a few musculocutaneous arteries are quite constant in their site of perforation. Therefore, flaps can be designed to include perforating arteries to create an arterial flap in much the same manner as will be described for the direct cutaneous arteries. For example, the supraorbital or supra-trochlear arteries are the bases for forehead flaps. The sites of major perforating arteries throughout the body have been mapped by Manchot [35]. According to the maps, there is significant variation in the distance between perforators and few anatomical landmarks to identify their positions. Thus the surviving length of flaps of similar length-width ratio will be altered by the random chance that a major artery is incorporated. In part, this explains the difference between the reliability of flaps on the face and flaps on the lower extremity. Since there are many more and closer-placed perforators on the face than on the leg, there is greater probability that the facial flap will contain perforating vessels.

The Axial Direct Cutaneous System

An axial, or direct, cutaneous artery is also a branch of a major segmental artery; however, there are relatively few such vessels. The artery directly enters the subcutaneous tissue and follows a longitudinal course parallel to the plane of the skin. It does not perforate the muscle. A flap based on a direct cutaneous artery is called an *arterial flap*, and all the classic "named" flaps are of this type. For example, the superficial temporal artery gives rise to the forehead flap, the superficial iliac circumflex artery gives rise to the McGregor groin flap, and the intercostal branches of the internal mammary artery are the source for the Bakamjian deltopectoral flap. Any of these flaps can be converted to an island pedicle flap.

The longitudinal pathway of the artery is within the loose areolar tissue just above the anterior muscular fascia and deep to the cutaneous fascia. For example, the superficial iliac circumflex and superficial epigastric arteries lie above the fascia lata of the thigh and above the inguinal ligament just below the deepest layer of the superficial fascia (Scarpa's fascia). At variable intervals smaller cutaneous branches ascend vertically into the subdermal plexus. Skin flaps based on direct cutaneous arteries maintain an uninterrupted circulation. The design of these flaps is not determined by the classic length-width ratios but by the regional distribution of the direct cutaneous artery. Unfortunately, the patterns of regional distribution of cutaneous vessels are extremely inconsistent.

The distinction between perforating and axial vessels is not absolute because in certain areas the perforating vessel does not ascend vertically into the skin, but may follow a longitudinal course similar to that of an axial vessel. For example, the supratrochlear artery is a perforating artery that gives off muscular branches within the orbit, then continues onto the skin of the glabella and scalp. Furthermore, there are areas of overlap of autonomous regions. Certain skin areas have both a perforating and a direct cutaneous vascular pattern.

Mapping the Regional Vascular Distribution to the Skin

As previously stated, the pattern of blood vessel distribution to the skin was thoroughly investigated by Manchot [35] in 1889. From anatomical dissections he mapped the major perforating and direct cutaneous arteries and then plotted the regions that were dependent primarily upon those vessels for their arterial supply. Additional maps of the regional cutaneous vascular pattern were determined by Conway et al. [12], using arteriography, and by Kaplan et al. [28], using fluorescein dye injections. The perforating arteries of the neck and shoulder were identified by Walsh during surgical operative procedures in that region [56]. The area of skin deriving its vascularity from a specific musculocutaneous or axial artery is considered an autonomous skin region. Thus, it is possible to conceptualize the skin as a mosaic of island pedicle flaps (autonomous areas) (Fig. 15-2). Overlap of autonomous areas does occur because of the dermal collaterals. If the vascular pedicle is left in continuity with the flap, the skin needs no other dermal or vascular connection, but the subcutaneous and dermal plexuses provide a collateral circulation if the major cutaneous or perforating artery is injured or surgically interrupted.

If the flap designed extends beyond the autonomous region of the cutaneous vessel, the nonautonomous part of the flap is at risk and must survive through collateral channels. The clinical problem is the extreme variability of the autonomous skin regions and the lack of technique to determine their distribution in each individual patient. Although Manchot [35] showed consistent vascular autonomous regions, the studies by Kaplan et al. [28] revealed an extreme variability in the size and distribution of the autonomous regions of cutaneous vascularization. For example, injection studies have shown that the superficial iliac circumflex artery can vascularize a very small skin segment of 8 by 12 cm or a huge skin segment covering the entire anterior thigh and abdomen on one side of the body. At present there is no method for identification of the autonomous vascular regions other than subjecting the patient to dissection of major vessels and using direct injection techniques.

Not only should the design of skin flaps be influenced by the regional arterial distribution, but the need for, and the type of delay of, skin flap should also be influenced by regional vascular anatomy. In general, flaps that contain a major direct cutaneous artery do not require delay if the boundaries of the skin flap are within the distribution of that cutaneous artery. If for some reason delay is considered essential, a direct cutaneous arterial flap is minimally delayed by incision of the skin and elevation of the flap from its bed. Maximal delay is achieved by interruption of the cutaneous artery.

On the other hand, skin flaps in the region of perforating musculocutaneous arteries are maximally delayed by incision of the boundaries of the flap plus elevation of the flap from its bed so that the perforating vessels will be severed.

The Anatomical Basis for Flap Design

The concept has prevailed in plastic surgery that skin flaps should be designed on the basis of the ratio of length of the flap to width of the pedicle. For example, facial flaps can be designed with a length-width ratio of from 3:1 to 5:1. Flaps of the abdomen and chest reportedly require a length-width ratio of 2:1, and flaps of the lower extremity should have a length-width ratio of 1:1. In part, these concepts are correct and reflect long clinical experience. It should also be understood that these classic ratios are based on the specific design requirements and the limitations imposed by the location and size of the flap; to a lesser degree they reflect inherent differences in cutaneous circulation. Furthermore, these dogmatic length-width ratios are customarily applied to all skin flaps that are randomly located within a specified area and tend to ignore the significant influence of the relation of the flaps to underlying cutaneous arteries and veins.

For example, the volume of flap tissue required for replacing the tip of the nose is small (design requirement). The width of the flap (say, a nasolabial flap) must be minimized so that the donor site (nasolabial crease) can be closed without distortion. As a result, many nasolabial flaps can have as much as a 5:1 ratio—with the length of the flap about 5 cm and the width about 1 cm. Does that mean that one can design a nasolabial flap 25 cm long and 5 cm wide, or 50 cm long and 10 cm wide? Of course not. It probably means that 5 cm is the length of tissue that can survive in that particular situation, regardless of the width of the flap base.

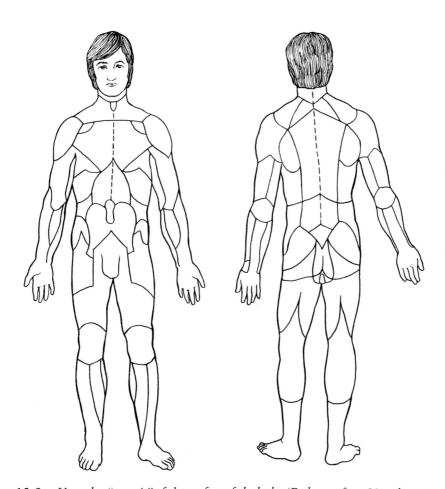

FIGURE 15-2.   *Vascular "mosaic" of the surface of the body. (Redrawn from Manchot, 1889 [35]).*

Another example is the cross-leg flap. The axiom is that cross-leg flaps must be of a 1:1 length-width ratio. Otherwise they should be delayed. Most cross-leg flaps require a width of 10 to 20 cm to cover defects on the opposite leg. Moreover, because the flap is a distant one and must bridge the gap between the legs as well as provide tissue for the defect, a length of tissue of 10 to 20 cm is also necessary. Such design requirements, demanding a 10- to 20-cm length and a 10- to 20-cm width, ostensibly call for a 1:1 flap.

From Manchot's map and from our own anatomical studies we know that the areas of skin from which a cross-leg flap is taken are supplied by a perforating musculocutaneous vascular system, and when the flap is elevated most of the musculocutaneous arteries are transected. The flap must survive on collaterals in the dermal plexus. Care must be taken that the flap is designed with a major perforating artery and vein as close to the base as possible so that collaterals can perfuse the 10- to 20-cm length of the flap.

Hypothetically, a flap 50 cm long and 50 cm wide designed in the same area is a 1:1 flap and should survive (according to the classic axiom). But it will not survive beyond the 10- to 20-cm length which is predicated by the limited distance the collateral vessels can perfuse.

On the other hand, a flap 15 cm long and only 5 cm wide on the leg is a 3:1 flap and should not fully survive. But it will survive because the collaterals can perfuse the length of the flap (assuming one can identify the site of the perforating vessel so that it is located at the flap base).

Milton proposed and proved a new hypothesis: "Flaps made under the same conditions of blood supply survive to the same length, *regardless of width.* The only effect of decreasing the width is to reduce the chance of the pedicle containing a large vessel" [41]. Support for this hypothesis came from several observations. The surviving length of very wide-based flaps of 24 to 35 cm was the same as the surviving length of comparably designed flaps with only 1- to 8-cm width pedicles (Fig. 15-3). The occasional occurrence of a flap with a longer surviving length coincided with the random chance that the skin pedicle contained a major artery and adjacent pedicles did not. The occurrence of a shorter surviving length coincided with the absence of a major artery when adjacent pedicles did incorporate a major artery. Furthermore, if the very wide-based pedicles of 24- to 35-cm width had deliberate transection of the major segmental vessels, their surviving length was comparable to the surviving length of the narrow-based flaps that did not contain a segmental vessel. Milton concluded, "The surviving length of vascular pedicled flaps is about 50 percent greater

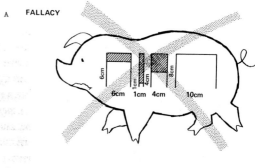

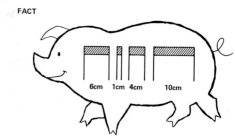

FIGURE 15-3. *Fallacy of the length-width ratio in flap design. A. Fallacy. Flaps constructed with varying lengths and widths, according to traditional concept, should all survive with approximately a 1:1 length-width ratio. B. Fact. "Flaps made under the same conditions of blood supply survive to the same length,* regardless of *width. The only effect of decreasing width is to reduce the chance of the pedicle containing a large vessel"* (S. H. Milton [41]).

than that of cutaneous flaps which are not based on specific vessels" [41].

The long-held axiom of a fixed length-width ratio appears to have been based on the concept that increasing width will allow a greater blood supply and therefore support a proportionally greater length of flap. This assumption is not true. If, for example, the width of a flap is doubled from 4 to 8 cm and the length of the flap is similarly doubled from 8 to 16 cm, the basic length-width ratio is maintained at 2:1. However, the metabolic demands of the flap are proportional to the area of the flap and not the length; thus, doubling the length and width of the flap will quadruple the metabolic requirements. (A 4 by 8 cm flap has an area of 32 cm² and an 8 by 16 cm² flap has an area of 128 cm².) In fact, doubling the width of the flap provides only for a *proportional* (doubling) increase in blood supply to satisfy the metabolic requirement (unless a major cutaneous artery is included by chance). Therefore, as Milton [41] has shown, for the supply to remain proportional to the demand, the length of the flap must remain constant.

Additional confirmation of the fallacy of the universal application of the length-width ratio axiom is seen in the island pedicle flap. The island flap can be considered to have a pedicle of "no width." Thus, a 1 mm artery and vein will allow the survival of the same length of a skin segment as could be achieved with the cutaneous pedicle of infinite width. The island pedicle emphasizes the importance of vascular anatomy and supports the concept of autonomous areas of skin vascularization.

In summary, there is practical value in the length-width ratio concept of flap design, but one must realize that the concept is valid for the specific clinical situations in which experience has determined the safe limits of *actual* length and width of the flap as well as the ratio. However, the *principle* upon which the length-width concept has been based is not valid. Rather, the concept of surviving length appears to be a more acceptable prin-ciple. The maximum surviving length of the flap is primarily a function of the anatomical distribution of blood vessels of the skin.

THE DELAY PHENOMENON

Definition

The delay phenomenon as applied to skin flaps is the beneficial effect of a preliminary operation, or series of operations, which, because of anatomical and/or physiological adjustments of the flap tissues, enhances the chance for survival of the flap at the time of final transfer.

Introduction

In the middle of the fifteenth century, five members of the Vianeo family in Italy performed rhinoplasties with arm flaps that were undercut from each side, separated by medicated linen, and allowed to mature for a month before transfer to the nose [40]. This method was later perfected and publicized by Gasparo Tagliacozzi during the latter part of the sixteenth century. Since that time, generations of surgeons have observed that partially interrupting the blood supply to a skin flap, without further manipulation, subsequently enhances the survival of the flap when it is subject to the manipulations of transfer.

The mechanism by which pedicled tissue adjusts itself to a decreased blood flow and is able to resist further compromise remains incompletely understood. Many workers have observed the vascular reorientation of the small vessels of such delayed flaps. However, controversy has arisen among different investigators attempting to explain the delay phenomenon on a physiological basis. Some maintain that the delay phenomenon is based on the ability of the compromised tissue to become "conditioned" to the ischemia imposed. Others assert that, as a result of the initial compromise, a rebound phenomenon occurs by which the blood supply is actually increased to the tissues. Still others feel that the ischemia produced at the time of the delay operation causes the tissues to release toxic substances that have many and varied physiological effects, leading to the observed anatomical changes. As one perhaps would expect, the complex physiological changes observed in the alteration of blood supply to pedicled skin flaps are not readily explained by the answers called for in the individual suppositions stated above [50].

Skin Metabolism and Blood Supply

There is little doubt that average blood flow to skin is far in excess of its metabolic requirements. Goetz showed that the average flow of blood through the skin and subcutaneous tissue was approximately 15 ml per minute per 100 cc of tissue [21]. However, he also demonstrated that skin can survive on as little as 2 ml of blood flow per minute per 100 cc of tissue. The superfluous blood flow, in terms of nutrition, functions to dissipate the heat generated by the body's metabolic engine. Furthermore, this heat-dissipating and temperature-regulating function of the skin can be aided by a blood flow in excess of 90 ml per minute per 100 cc of tissue.

Anatomical Changes in Delayed Skin Flaps

Gillies (1920) noted that an axial orientation of vessels seemed to occur in tube flaps (i.e., parallel to the incisions) [20]. In 1933 German and his co-workers utilized dye injection techniques to study vascular changes occurring within pedicled tissue [19]. Working with tubed abdominal flaps on experimental animals, these authors showed that, as soon as 24 hours after construction of the flap, reorientation of the small arteries took place so that these vessels were arranged parallel with the long axis of the tube. Concomitantly, the number of macroscopically identifiable arteries within the flap increased, although there was no direct evidence of neovascular formation. The changes took place over the first week postoperatively;

thereafter little additional change was seen in the vascular pattern.

Braithwaite et al. (1951–1952) studied the changes in venous circulation occurring in experimental tubed pedicle flaps [6, 8]. They found that the many fine arborizations of the subdermal venous plexus were replaced with fewer but larger endothelium-lined sinusoidal venous spaces. Referring to Poiseuille's law (the amount of flow through a vessel is proportional to the fourth power of the radius of the vessel), Braithwaite postulated that the augmentation of flow produced by the increased caliber of the vessels of the flap would much more than offset any decrease in the number of venous channels. For example, if the dermal-venous channels were reduced in number by half but doubled in caliber, flow would be augmented by eight times the original potential for venous blood flow.

In the same series of experiments, Braithwaite also postulated that the survival of skin flap tissue was related to the endothelial surface available for absorption of nutrients and the diffusion of metabolic wastes. He noted that the absorption of radioactive sodium from tube flaps tended to parallel the vascular reorientation and dilation.

In summary, the anatomical changes observed in pedicle flaps consist of a reorientation in the direction of the small arteries of the flap to correspond to the long axis of the pedicled tissue and an increase in the number of macroscopically observed small arteries. Venous channels of the flap, however, are reduced in overall number and undergo a corresponding increase in size to make up for the absorptive endothelial surface lost by the numerical reduction, and at the same time allow for an overall augmentation of venous outflow.

Physiological Changes in Delayed Skin Flaps

Several physiological mechanisms have been proposed to account for the delay phenomenon. There is still controversy over actual mechanisms, however. Some researchers believe that the vascular changes occur as a result of altered local sympathetic nervous system control; others maintain that the toxic products of anaerobic metabolism account for the phenomenon, or that the tissues of the flap are "conditioned" to hypoxia; and still others propose that an actual circulatory enhancement beyond the normal takes place with time in delayed flaps. Most recently, investigators have been less speculative and have studied the simple effects of graded ischemia on skin flaps and the subsequent enhancement of the survival at transfer. The concept of arteriovenous shunts being responsible, as recently proposed, is intriguing, indeed.

Sympathetic Theory

In 1950 Hynes demonstrated the absence of sympathetic control on the distal portions of pedicle flaps [26]. Observing, also, that blood flowed with reduced pressure in denervated vessels in comparison to surrounding areas which retained sympathetic control, Hynes proposed that the vascular changes observed in flaps were due to localized sympathectomy. He gave no direct evidence that sympathectomy per se was responsible for the vascular changes observed, and his theories were largely speculative.

Subsequently, Braithwaite pointed out that in areas previously sympathectomized and denervated by nerve injury pedicle flaps underwent identical vascular changes when compared to those flaps raised in normally innervated areas in the same individual [6]. Moreover, Lutz et al. noted that certain fibers of sympathetic nervous system are vasodilating, and the denervation of local areas can result in vasoconstriction rather than vasodilatation [34].

Metabolites of Hypoxic Tissue Theory

A rather complex theory was advanced by Braithwaite et al. in 1959 to explain the vasodilating and enhanced flow characteristics in delayed skin flaps [7]. Braithwaite recalled the observation by Lewis, in 1927, who proposed that a histamine-like substance was released in injured and hypoxic tissues [33]. The substance was believed to cause secondary vascular changes consisting of an increase in number of identifiable vessels and vasodilatation, resulting in an overall increase in blood supply to the affected area.

Using isotope clearance methods, Braithwaite et al. studied the extracellular tissue fluid turnover (circulatory efficiency) of upper limbs that had been subject to tourniquet-induced ischemia [7]. After the expected period of reactive hyperemia had subsided, they observed a secondary rise in blood flow. In order to explain this phenomenon they proposed that, in response to the period of hypoxia, the affected tissues released a substance (substance A) which caused relaxation of the precapillary sphincters and was responsible for the initial reactive hyperemia. Then, as the tissue oxygenation improved, substance A was converted to substance B, which caused dilatation of preexisting arteriovenous shunts that precede the precapillary sphincters. Since these channels bypass a large portion of the capillary bed, their dilatation results in an overall decrease of peripheral resistance producing a secondary rise in blood flow. The continued enhancement of clearance of fluid from the capillary bed, as measured by isotope studies, was then postulated to occur by Venturi suction effect as shunted blood coursed by the capillary orifices. Braithwaite theorized that substance B is the product of ischemic but viable tissue, causes dilatation and hypertrophy of arterioles, and is the mediator of the vascular augmentation occurring with the delay of skin flaps.

Circulatory Enhancement Theory

In 1957 Hoffmeister determined the circulatory efficiency (extracellular tissue fluid turnover) of flaps by means of the dermal clearance of sodium 22; he also determined the optimum interval between delay and transfer [24]. The operations for delay were carried out by two different methods. In the first, two parallel skin incisions were made, with undermining of the flap. In the second, incisions were utilized from three sides, with undermining of the flap.

The results were consistent. There was a decrease in the circulatory efficiency in the immediate postoperative period. The drop in circulatory efficiency, as expected, was much greater in the flaps that had been incised on three sides and undermined. Following the initial decline, circulatory efficiency increased, with a maximum value surpassing that of the control state. Again, the maximum overall circulatory efficiency beyond control levels was achieved in the flaps in which blood supply had been most severely compromised in the delay operation. The interval between the delay and the circulatory peak was, on the average, approximately three weeks after the delay operation. Following the postdelay circulatory maximum, circulatory efficiency rapidly declined. Normal values were

reached in three to five days after peak flow (Fig. 15-4). Flaps that had been delayed three weeks previously were again raised, and circulatory efficiency was compared with the equivalent nondelayed flaps. The circulatory efficiency of the delayed flaps was significantly higher than that of nondelayed flaps.

The flaps incised on two sides and undermined achieved a circulatory peak at 10 to 21 days after the delay operation. The flaps incised on three sides and undermined achieved their circulatory peak at 17 to 63 days. Despite the fact that Hoffmeister's flaps were on dogs, the physiological changes regarding timing for transfer correlated very well with the traditional axiom, previously unsupported except by clinical judgment, that three weeks was the optimum time between delay and transfer.

From Hoffmeister's presentation one is left to assume that the flaps constructed by incision on two sides and undermining as opposed to those constructed by incision on three sides and undermining were of equal length. Flaps so constructed would relegate

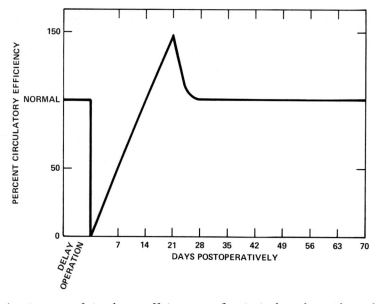

FIGURE 15-4. *Recovery of circulatory efficiency to a flap incised on three sides and undermined. Note initial drop to 0 and subsequent recovery to greater than "normal" circulatory efficiency. (Data from Hoffmeister* [24].)

the flap delayed with two parallel incisions to a better overall blood supply. One is then led to believe, solely on the basis of Hoffmeister's data, that the rebound circulatory enhancement to delayed flaps is in some way proportional to the degree of ischemia created by the delay operation.

Tissue Acclimatization to Hypoxia Theory

In 1965 McFarlane et al. conducted a series of experiments on skin flaps on rats [36]. Using methyl methacrylate casts to examine the small arteries of the flaps, they showed that the previously described vascular changes (reorientation and dilatation) were of only a transient nature, lasting about three weeks in their bipedicled undermined flaps. However, the changes were not reversed if the flaps were tubed. Nevertheless, the delay was equally effective whether the flaps were tubed or not.

To further elucidate the true nature of the delay phenomenon, these authors examined the uptake of radioactive rubidium by delayed and undelayed raised flaps. Rubidium is a nontoxic cation. Like potassium, it is an intracellular cation and following injection is cleared rapidly from the blood and occupies an intracellular position. If the tissues are hypoxic, however, the cells will not take up the rubidium as expected and resulting counts will be low.

Utilizing this information, McFarlane injected rubidium 86 into the bloodstream of rats at various intervals after raising previously delayed flaps. He then measured the uptake of the rubidium in the flap tissue. Similar tests were conducted on flaps that were raised primarily without benefit of delay. Both delayed and undelayed flaps had low uptake of rubidium—thus indicating hypoxia. Despite statistically equivalent findings of low rubidium uptake, the delayed flaps survived and the undelayed flaps necrosed. "Therefore," McFarlane concluded, "the delay conditioned the tissues at the distal end of the flap to withstand a state of hypoxia which was otherwise lethal."

No Ischemia–No Delay Theory

In 1969 Myers and Cherry constructed paired experimental delayed pedicles on groups of rabbits [45]. The flaps were identical in size and design, but different in the amount of blood supply remaining after operation. The results revealed that for a delay procedure to improve the survival of the flap at transfer, the blood flow must be diminished at the delay operation. The authors concluded that "the stimulus for delay is ischemia." Moreover, they showed that the beneficial effects of delay began within 48 hours after surgery, maximal effects being achieved in eight days. A subsequent set of experiments by the same authors revealed species differences regarding the time after surgery necessary to achieve maximum benefit from the delay operation [46].

In a review article in 1969 Stuart Milton stated, "Unless it can be shown that the preliminary raising of a bipedicle tubed flap doubles the length which is viable on one pedicle, the value of the procedure is in question" [39]. He then went on to perform a series of experiments to assess the value of delayed bipedicled tube flaps. In a subsequent article later the same year he reported on the effects of four methods and three durations of delay on the surviving length of experimental flaps in the pig [40]. He found that undermined bipedicle flaps were most effective and flaps in which margins were incised but not undermined least effective in promoting ultimate survival—"suggesting that the best form of delay is the one which divides most vessels short of causing necrosis." A maximum increase of 60 percent of surviving flap length was observed, and the optimal timing for transfer was about two weeks after delay in his porcine model.

The Arteriovenous Shunt Concept

An imaginative correlation of many of the previously cited observations—together with his own investigations—has led Reinisch to propose that the delay phenomenon is due to the existence of arteriovenous shunts in the microcirculation to the skin which are activated by a sympathectomy effect [49].

Reinisch initially showed in experimental flaps in pigs that fluorescein (injected intravenously) would suffuse the flap to a point corresponding to the surviving length. However, the surface temperature of these flaps was much higher at the most distal end even though the portion eventually necrosed. Furthermore, fluorescein was not identified in the dermal capillary circulation in distal portions of a flap in which the temperature was normal. This finding was interpreted to mean that blood flowed through arteriovenous (A-V) shunts to give the distal flap warmth but bypassed the dermal capillary bed to that distal area. There are, Reinisch postulated, A-V shunts that allow blood to bypass the capillary bed and that are opened or activated by a sudden decrease in the sympathetic neural tone.

In order to test his hypothesis, Reinisch performed the following experiments:

1. ^{51}Cr-labeled red cells were administered at varying intervals after skin flaps were raised in pigs. Results of counts from different portions of the flap were correlated with the level of an injection of fluorescein dye.

2. [85]Sr-labeled 15 micron diameter microspheres were also injected into the animal and the flaps assayed for their presence. Flaps delayed for two weeks were also studied.

3. Several pig flaps were scanned with a gamma camera after the flap had been raised (and in some instances delayed for two weeks) and the animal was injected with technetium 99.

The results of these experiments indicated that (1) blood indeed circulated in the eventually necrotic acral portions of the skin flaps—as determined by the presence of substantial amounts of ^{51}Cr-tagged red cells; (2) A-V shunts existed in these areas—as determined by failure to trap the larger-than-capillary-diameter microspheres; and (3) technetium entered and cleared the acral portions of the flaps faster than one would expect

with a normal capillary circulation—but at a rate compatible with the existence of A-V shunts. However, delayed flaps, when tested in the same manner, were more like skin areas having a normal capillary bed and not having A-V shunts.

Reinisch's explanation for the delay phenomenon based on his investigations tends to tie together many of the observations summarized earlier in this chapter. When a bipedicle flap is raised, the tissue is denervated. The resulting sympathectomy allows multiple arteriovenous shunts in the skin circulation to become patent. But the blood supply from each end of the pedicle flap prevents skin necrosis. After 10 to 14 days of denervation the A-V shunts again regain resting tone, and a more normal capillary flow is reestablished. Division of one end of the bipedicle flap no longer then causes the shunts to open, and the blood supply to the capillary bed is not diverted. Thus the delayed flap survives even in its acral portions.

Reinisch has utilized this view of the delay phenomenon in an attempt to produce a "delayed" flap by electrical and chemical means. He used direct current across skin electrodes to effectively "denervate" the skin area and subsequently elevated flaps with a surviving length significantly increased over that of control flaps. The use of injected 6-hydroxydopamine and dilute epinephrine solutions also produced some promising preliminary results. These initial trials may herald a new era for the manipulation of flaps and enhancement of their survival.

Other Observations and Thoughts for the Future

Recent advances in microsurgical vessel anastomosis have resulted in successful transfer of large portions of skin and subcutaneous tissues as composite grafts with immediate revascularization [13, 14]. In addition, methods have been suggested to enable the mapping of areas of skin supplied by discrete vessels amenable to microsurgical anastomosis [28]. The delay of many flaps may be made obsolete by wide use of such methods.

In fact, Milton has shown that flaps raised without delay on a single vascular pedicle can withstand double the total ischemia time without undergoing subsequent necrosis when compared to similar island flaps that had previously been delayed [42]. This observation, while seeming to be paradoxical at first glance, is consistent with the premise that delay does not enhance survival of tissues fed by a single major vessel, for the blood supply is never compromised to the degree necessary for the physiology of delay to be manifest.

Practical Considerations

Many pitfalls line the path of the surgeon attempting to carry out the successful transfer of a delayed pedicle flap. In the design of the flap to fill a specific recipient defect, one must take into consideration not only the size and configuration of the donor tissue and the tension and torsion to which it may be subject, but also the induration, stiffness, and edema the delay process itself will produce in the flap. Since the delayed tissue is stiffer, more indurated, and harder to handle than flaps constructed by primary transfer, one must pay special attention to minimize such changes. For example, skin flaps vascularized by axial vessels (temporal artery, superficial iliac circumflex, etc.) should not, and need not, be delayed. Great care must be taken to dissect tissues along naturally occurring tissue (fascial) planes and not through subcutaneous fat. Milton also stresses that, if a flap is to be tubed, the width must be 17 times the thickness to allow for subsequent edema and to avert subsequent tamponade of vessels [39]. Thus, tubed flaps are sometimes impossible to construct in obese persons without endangering the subcutaneous vascular integrity.

From the experimental studies cited heretofore, the bipedicle flap, devoid of an axial artery, raised, undermined, and replaced in its bed, would appear to be the optimum form of delay. Such a procedure can nearly double the surviving length of a single pedicle raised and transferred in a single operation. However, one must always be aware that the clinical circumstances may warrant variations in the delay operation. Effective forms of delay are often achieved by tubing the bipedicle flap, incising the flap on three sides, undermining and replacing it in its bed, incising the flap and undermining it only partially, or not at all, and subsequently performing an additional one or two delay operations before final transfer. Unfortunately, only long experience and precise clinical judgment can dictate the exact type of delay operation called for in a difficult clinical case.

Conclusions

The true physiological mechanisms underlying the delay phenomenon have yet to be fully elucidated. From the studies to date, the following assumptions seem valid:

1. There is at least a transient morphological reorientation of afferent and efferent limbs of circulation in delayed flaps—with more macroscopically identifiable arteries reoriented in an axial direction and fewer but much larger venous elements.
2. The stimulus for the vascular changes may be chemically mediated by increase in toxic products of metabolism in an ischemic environment.
3. The buildup of such products can be assumed from experimental studies showing an initial decrease in circulatory efficiency and an increase in cellular hypoxia.
4. Short of a critical point of irreversible ischemia resulting in tissue death, the greater the compromise in blood supply, the greater the enhancement of the subsequent survival of the delayed tissue. Alternatively, the delay phenomenon occurs to a greater extent in a flap not containing an axial artery in the pedicle.

TIMING OF TRANSFER AND PROGNOSTIC TESTS FOR FLAP SURVIVAL

The practicing surgeon appreciates explanations of physiological mechanisms involved in vascular augmentation and prolongation of survival of the skin flaps with which he deals. Of more immediate concern, however, for one engaged in some stage of reconstruction utilizing skin flaps, is estimating accurately the timing involved in various flap maneuvers. One wishes to transfer or manipulate the flap when chances are best for its survival, yet avoid undue delays that may cause awkward immobilization of the patient or prolonged hospitalization. Toward this end, many investigators have searched for objective methods and criteria that would allow the novice as well as the experienced surgeon to proceed as rapidly as possible and with confidence of a good result in the manipulation of skin flaps. Such noble attempts have by and large failed to ultimately supersede sound clinical judgment based on long experience—reflecting the inadequacy of a simple test to give information concerning a large number of parameters, many of which are critical to the survival of the flap tissue. Such tests as have been devised fall into several broad categories: *indirect measurements* of the total metabolism of flap tissues, *indices* only of the *arterial limb* of flap circulation, and *indices* of the *efficiency* of tissue fluid turnover within flap tissues.

Indirect Indices of Flap Viability and Suitability for Transfer

Temperature Measurements

In 1943 Douglas and Buchholz attempted to evaluate the "circulatory efficiency" of tubed flaps by a "temperature return test" [17]. Tourniquets were placed around the pedicles of the flaps, thus inducing a temperature drop within the tube. The tourniquets were then released, and, by means of a thermocouple placed subcutaneously, rewarming rates were observed. As the vascularity of the flap improved, the temperature changes utilizing the testing format became more pronounced (i.e., the *rate* of rewarming of the flap increased). The authors reported that bipedicled tube flaps regained circulatory efficiency after seven days and were, therefore, ready for transfer.

In 1961 Winsten et al. utilized much the same format as Douglas and Buchholz to correlate skin temperature as an index of circulation [57]. After a series of well-documented experiments, they stated that "the method described for testing circulation by skin temperature is still too imprecise to be relied upon as a diagnostic test for any individual flap."

In 1968 Bloomenstein used an infrared thermometer to predict flap viability [5]. This device relied upon surface temperature measurements of the flap as compared with other body areas in which the blood supply was found to be "normal." Laboratory studies were carried out in experimental flaps on rats, and clinical studies on patients were also performed. It was felt by the author, in conclusion, that the method was a useful, noninvasive adjunct to clinical judgment in predicting flap viability. However, he has acknowledged that variations in room temperature and areas of the body make interpretation difficult.

Hair Growth as a Metabolic Index

Douglas and Buchholz studied the comparative rates of growth of hair on single pedicle flaps, double pedicle flaps, and adjacent skin sites [17]. They concluded that the growth rate of hair on double pedicle flaps was only slightly retarded in comparison with that on adjacent skin from which the flaps were formed. The rate of hair growth on a single pedicle flap was definitely retarded in comparison with the hair on adjacent skin. As a rule, however, though the rate of hair growth is disturbed in flap tissues, the measurement of relative rates of hair growth as a prognostic test of flap survival at transfer is too imprecise for general clinical use.

Assessment of the Arterial Limb of Flap Circulation

Measurement of Arterial Pressure

Douglas and Buchholz measured the blood pressure in tubed flaps by means of a pneumatic cuff [17]. The pedicle of the flap was occluded by the cuff, and a sudden color change was observed as the cuff was deflated.

The point at which the color change took place was considered to be the systolic pressure of the arteries within the tubed flap. These authors found that arterial pressure in bipedicled flaps reached 90 to 95 percent of normal at one month. Single pedicle flaps, however, required nearly two months to regain only 50 percent of their "normal" arterial pressure. Clinical judgment has dictated that flaps may be transferred successfully much sooner than one might infer from the data presented with the mentioned arterial measurements. This would seem to reflect the previously discussed "excess" in blood flow to skin and subcutaneous tissue beyond basic metabolic needs.

The Fluorescein Test

Several authors, including Dingwall and Lord [16] in 1943 and Conway et al. [10] in 1949, have adapted the fluorescein test to the study of the suitability of a flap for transfer. Ten milliliters of sodium fluorescein solution injected intravenously will cause vascularized skin to glow bright yellow-green under ultraviolet illumination. In newly formed tubed flaps, however, the acral portions remain dark while the bases glow brightly. Subsequently, over a period of days to weeks, the entire area of the flap begins to glow following the fluorescein injection. By Conway's method the "circulatory efficiency" in bipedicle flaps is equal to that in control areas by the twelfth day. Moreover, Conway has demonstrated that between 16 and 24 days following formation of the tubed flap the fluorescein tests indicate the development of a greater degree of circulation than in the control areas. These data would appear to corroborate the previously discussed work of Hoffmeister [24]. The fluorescein, while seeming to be a good adjunct to clinical judgment regarding suitability for flap transfer, has been criticized on the ground that it gives only an index of the arterial limb of flap circulation and no indication of the integrity of venous drainage.

Nicotinic Acid–Epinephrine Test

In 1950 Olander induced a generalized cutaneous flush with nicotinic acid and then infiltrated the tissue about the base of a pedicle flap with a 1:30,000 solution of epinephrine [48]. He then evaluated circulatory adequacy on the basis of color changes in the skin of the flap and the surrounding "normal" tissues. He described detailed criteria for the interpretation of the results from this test. The time-consuming nature and subjective end point inherent in the testing method have precluded its wide general use.

Photoplethysmography

Thompson and Pollard [54] in 1968 and Thorne et al. [55] in 1969 described the use of the photoplethysmograph to help determine the viability of skin flaps. This small, simple, noninvasive device is used in nearly every modern operating room by the anesthesiologist as an aid in pulse monitoring. A beam of light is reflected by the underlying tissue and analyzed by a simple photoelectric transducer, which feeds its responses through an amplifier and onto an oscilloscope screen. Pulse amplitude and frequency in the microcirculation are therefore easily measured in this manner. The authors have correlated such readings with the ultimate viability of various skin flaps. The method is easy to use, causes no discomfort to the patient, and gives a precise indication of arterial flow. It does not, however, give any indication of venous outflow from the flap being tested and thus no real indication of total tissue fluid turnover, which is critical in most instances for flap survival.

Measurement of Tissue Fluid Turnover (Total Circulatory Efficiency)

Saline Wheal Test

One of the earliest tests for circulatory efficiency was presented in 1926 by Stern and Cohen: the saline wheal test [52]. An injection of 0.2 ml of saline solution was given intradermally into the test area. The time for disappearance of the wheal was then determined by inspection and palpation. *Inadequate* circulation was indicated if the wheal disappeared in less than one hour. The physiological mechanisms involved would seem to depend on the efficiency of both limbs of the circulation. However, the results appear somewhat paradoxical, and no adequate explanation of the mechanism was offered by the authors.

The Atropine Test

In 1948 Hynes introduced the atropine test, the predecessor of more recent and sophisticated clearance methods [25]. He injected 1/25 grain (2.6 mg) of atropine subcutaneously into the flap, then measured the rate of its absorption by three separate end points requiring systemic dispersion of the drug. These end points were tachycardia, cycloplegia (inability of the patient to focus on newsprint), and dryness of the mouth. Time of onset for these phenomena was measured after injection into the subcutaneous tissue of flaps and compared with the time of onset after injection into the undisturbed control sites. Hynes stresses that the doses of atropine used are quite safe and that the three specific actions act as a check of one against the other. The atropine, of course, may be dangerous in patients with incipient glaucoma. Hynes has shown by the atropine test method that safe transfer of the flap can be expected if the time of onset for the specified end points approaches that for the control sites.

The Histamine Wheal Test

In 1951, Conway and coauthors described the application of the cutaneous histamine reaction, which had been previously used as a test of collateral circulation in peripheral vascular disease of the extremities, to the evaluation of circulation in tubed pedicles and flaps prior to their division and surgical transplantation [11]. After needle scarification of a small area of the cutaneous surface to be tested, a drop of histamine (1:1000) was applied. This procedure was followed in a number of places over the tissue being considered as well as at control sites. Formation of a wheal at the test site in eight minutes or less was thought to be an indication of the integrity of both limbs of the underlying cutaneous dermal circulation. If the eight-minute end point was achieved, it was felt that further manipulations of the flap could be carried out successfully.

The "Congestion" Test

In 1955 Barron described a test that assessed by mechanical means the arterial and venous elements of intermediate-stage tubed flaps with a forearm carrier [2]. First, a rubber tourniquet was used to occlude the abdominal pedicle of the flap close to its base. A blood pressure cuff was then placed around the upper aspect of the carrier arm and inflated to midway between systolic and diastolic pressure. After a few minutes the forearm and, if the arterial circulation was intact, the tubed flap became congested with venous blood. A second tourniquet was then placed upon the flap a few inches closer to the forearm. The arm cuff was then deflated. If there were adequate venous return across the arm suture line, the tubed flap would become decongested as the forearm did. When the congestion is cleared, there should be a marked color differential between the forearm of the tubed flap and the adjacent area trapped between the tourniquets. The second tourniquet (the one nearest the arm) is then removed, and the rate of decongestion of the previously trapped segment of flap is timed. A 10-second clearance time is considered rapid; a time of 20 to 30 seconds is only fair. When a total of five minutes has elapsed after application of the first tourniquet, that tourniquet is released. If there is arterial insufficiency across the suture line from arm to flap, a reactive hyperemia will develop in the flap as a result of resurgence of blood flow from the abdominal pedicle. Barron considers this a contraindication to severing the abdominal pedicle. The method as described would seem to give good evidence of the integrity of both the arterial and the venous limbs of the circulation. The maneuver is readily performed, and the end points are well defined.

Isotope Clearance Methods

Various authors, including Kety [31], Barron et al. [3, 4], Conway et al. [9], and Braithwaite et al. [7, 8] have used radioactive isotopes of sodium to measure the clearance of this ion from flap tissues. They have correlated the rate of clearance relative to control sites with the circulatory efficiency or total tissue fluid turnover within the flap tissue. While these methods do not bear a direct relation to the traditional concept of "blood flow," they are probably a more realistic measure of the ability of the tissue to sustain its metabolism via the integrity of the microcirculation. Though the tests have given reproducible results in the hands of all the above-named authors, and have in general been accurate prognostications of flap viability and suitability for transfer, the expense and difficulty in control of the various parameters involved without special tools and assay methods confine their use to the laboratory at present.

Conclusion

The criteria for the ideal "test" to assess suitability for flap manipulation and transfer and to accurately predict the survival of the flap tissue are as follows:

1. The test must assess both arterial and venous components of circulation to the flap as well as its general metabolic state.

2. The test must be unaffected by environmental disturbances within the usual hospital or operating room.

3. The test should preferably be noninvasive and cause no patient discomfort.

4. The test should require minimal, readily available, and easy-to-operate equipment or tools.

5. The test should be inexpensive.

6. The test should be rapid.

7. The test should have well-defined objective end points.

8. The test should require minimum skill of the user—whether novice or seasoned surgeon.

Unfortunately, no such means is now available. The ones discussed in the preceding section all have drawbacks, some more than others. In the utilization of such measures to assess a particular flap, the limitations of the test should always be kept in mind, and sound clinical judgment should never be superseded.

PATHOPHYSIOLOGY OF FLAP DEATH

General Considerations

In no area of surgery are the factors enhancing tissue survival and those precipitating its demise so finely balanced as in flap construction. Indeed, the surgeon often chooses, as in the case of the delay procedure, to severely compromise the blood supply to the pedicle flap which he forms. In all instances a skin flap by its very nature does not possess the vascular reserve of undisturbed tissue and is, therefore, liable to necrose should it be forced to bear the burden of stress, torsion, tension, kinking, twisting, or heavy-handedness that a portion of tissue not subject to such predetermined vascular limitations could survive with some ease. Then, too, as in any form of surgery, bacterial infection can occur. However, in a relatively ischemic environment with poor resultant defenses of the host tissue, infection is both more easily established and harder to treat.

To be successful in flap surgery, the practitioner must not only have the foreknowledge of the possible complications but constantly keep them foremost in his thoughts in order to avert a subtle error which may be the deciding factor tipping the balance toward tissue slough. Once the error has occurred, be it one of omission or commission, the situation is seldom retrievable.

The "White" Flap

If a flap is cold and pale, it usually lacks arterial blood to nourish the tissue. Fortunately, this complication is often noted immediately and can be corrected by remedying the etiological factor, provided one has not severed a major vessel to the flap or irretrievably transected the base of the pedicle. The pathophysiology most often responsible for the "white" flap includes:

1. Lack of perfusion due to arterial tamponade
   a. By twisting or kinking of the base of the flap
   b. By tension of the pedicle over bony prominences
   c. By improper application of external splints or dressing
   d. By tight sutures that may occlude vascular supply to peripheral portions of the flap
2. Lack of perfusion due to irretrievable loss of arterial flow
   a. By designing a pedicle with an arterial component insufficient to supply the metabolic demands of the flap tissue
   b. By inadvertently cutting an essential feeding vessel
   c. By arterial thrombosis
3. Lack of perfusion due to systemic or constitutional factors
   a. Hypotension and/or shock
   b. Age and atherosclerotic cardiovascular disease or arteriosclerosis obliterans
   c. Diabetes mellitus
   d. Previous local radiation injury

The "Blue" Flap

An axiom of flap surgery is that more flaps die "blue" than die "white." In reality, probably *all* flaps die blue, for even though a flap may be initially pale and nonblanching, the compromised flap takes on a deep cyanotic color as the tissue progresses toward a nearly black-appearing necrosis.

To assume that a blue flap is due solely to venous insufficiency is probably erroneous in the majority of circumstances. Fujino demonstrated the importance of the venous drainage to flap survival and has shown that flaps *can* die from venous insufficiency [18]. In a series of experiments on dogs, he raised standard flaps of a 3:1 length-width ratio on the thighs of the animals. Five types of flaps were constructed: (1) perforators (artery and vein) severed; (2) perforators (artery and vein) and axial (saphenous) artery severed; (3) perforators (artery and vein) and axial (saphenous) vein severed; (4) perforators (artery and vein), axial vessels (artery and vein), and cutaneous artery and vein all severed; and (5) same as group 4, but perforators (artery and vein) preserved. Fujino then studied the severity of circulation disturbances in the five groups of flaps using sodium 22 clearance as an indicator of interstitial fluid exchange. Clinical patterns of survival were also noted. He found that the most severely compromised flaps were those in group 4 (all vessels cut) and group 5 (only perforators preserved). Next most severely compromised were flaps in which the perforators and axial (saphenous) *vein* were severed (group 3). Group 2 (perforators and axial *artery* severed) was less compromised, and least compromised were the flaps in which the perforators alone were severed (group 1). On the basis of these data, Fujino emphasized the importance of the axial vein as compared to the axial artery in flap survival.

Milton pointed out, however, that in experimental observations in pigs blue flaps survived to a significantly greater length than white flaps [39]. Moreover, dye injected systemically did not appear at the tips of nonviable blue flaps. It would seem that if blue flaps died a venous death, dye would have appeared in the flap tips and remained there. Milton also alludes to the basic notion of circulation accepted since the time of Harvey—that the propelling force in veins (the vis a tergo, or "force from behind") is derived from an intact arterial capillary flow. In many instances, therefore, one must assume that venous stasis depends on the stasis in the arterial system of the flap.

If venous stasis should be the factor compromising a flap, one can look to most of the same etiological factors that limit arterial inflow as outlined in the previous section. Moreover, in order to obstruct venous outflow, these detrimental elements need be present to a much lower degree.

Late Complications

Hematoma

Hematoma is rarely noted in the operating room and may take hours to become evident. Its appearance, however, is often disastrous in flap surgery. Not only can it be a source of pressure, which—though seldom compromising arterial inflow—is likely to obstruct venous outflow from a flap. It can also prolong healing by limiting revascularization of flap tissue by the recipient bed and act as an excellent medium for subsequent infection.

Infection

The basic mechanisms by which infection becomes established, spreads, and causes tissue necrosis are the same for flap tissue as for any other tissue so affected. However, resistance to or arrest of the process of infection in any tissue depends on (1) a sound metabolic state of the affected tissue, to enable optimum and appropriate cellular response to the invasion of microorganisms, and (2) an intact circulation to the affected area to facilitate circulating antibody and leukocyte deposition, and to deliver parenterally administered antibiotics. Unfortunately, flap tissues are often severely compromised on both counts, and the measures against infection should be preventive ones.

Regrettably, once infection is manifest in the flap, only local mechanical means are likely to be of real benefit (debridement, soaks, frequent dressing changes, etc.) until the infection is stopped and the tissue loss can be assessed.

MEASURES TO ENHANCE FLAP SURVIVAL

That many investigators have sought ways to prevent impending necrosis in previously constructed skin flaps is mute testimony to the hazards inherent in flap surgery. With few exceptions, one can say that if a flap appears severely compromised in its recipient site, the best chance for its survival lies in restoring it to its original bed—free of tension, torsion, kinking, etc. Occasionally, circumstances tend to prevent this course (exposed joints, nerves, etc., at the recipient site or a severed pedicle base at the donor site). Under such conditions surgeons have attempted to assess the primary factors tending to promote tissue death and to devise methods for effectively alleviating the situation.

Reducing Metabolic Demands of Flap Tissue

In an attempt to lower tissue metabolic requirements and buildup of toxic metabolic products in flap tissue prior to development of an adequate blood supply, Kiehn and Desprez used localized hypothermia on experimental flaps in rabbits [32]. The flaps were designed to necrose uniformly in their acral portions if left untreated. These authors found that cooling the flaps to a surface temperature of 15° to 20°C delayed the appearance of necrosis for several days and limited the overall severity of the expected slough. However, because of practical problems of equipment availability, sterility, and various other factors the application of this technique has limited clinical value. Moreover, there has been no statistical evidence that the cooling of flaps will be beneficial in humans.

Furnishing the Metabolic Requirement

Oxygenation

Kernahan et al. [29] and Gruber et al. [22, 23] explored the use of hyperbaric oxygen to prolong the survival of the severely ischemic experimental flap. No alteration of the ultimate surviving length of the flap was observed with the application of the hyperbaric oxygen. It was felt that the pinkness of the tissue seen during application of the oxygen merely represented oxygenated but stagnant hemoglobin, which contributed nothing to other parameters of tissue metabolic need.

Augmenting Arterial Inflow

DMSO (DIMETHYL SULFOXIDE) AND DEX-TRAN. In an attempt to utilize the histamine-like effects of DMSO to increase blood flow to the skin in areas of local application, Adamson et al. applied the chemical to compromised experimental flaps in rats [1]. They reported significant increase in surviving length of flaps that had received the benefit of the DMSO. However, McFarlane et al. used DMSO and dextran to enhance survival of similar flaps but could show no data substantiating its use in a clinical situation [37].

Dextran alone was tried for its rheostatic properties in areas of sluggish blood flow in experimental flaps by Myers and Cherry [44]. No data to support the efficacy of this treatment were presented.

HISTAMINE IONTOPHORESIS AND HYPER-TENSION. In 1967 Ketchum et al. reported significant increases in the surviving lengths of experimental pedicle flaps on rabbits when histamine iontophoresis was used to dilate local blood vessels and hypertensive perfusion was used to take advantage of the vessel dilatation [30]. In their paper, however, they did not make clear how the hypertensive state was established.

Milton and Corbett challenged the premise of Ketchum et al. by repeating the experiments utilizing renally induced systemic hypertension [43]. The title of their subsequent paper testifies to the results: "Failure to Increase the Survival of Experimental Flaps by Histamine and Hypertension."

Enhancement of Venous Outflow

Alternating Pressure Methods

In 1951 Hynes described the use of an "intermittent venous occluder" to transmit pressure to a sphygmomanometer cuff around a congested flap to actively express the blood at 2-minute intervals at a pressure of 30 to 40 mm Hg [27]. He reported the use of this device in several case studies and cited its efficacy in preventing necrosis in the blue flap.

Sturman et al. in 1964 also described successful prevention of necrosis in congested experimental tubed flaps on rabbits via an alternating pressure device much like that used by Hynes [53]. They stated that alternating pressures to 50 cm of water resulted in prevention of necrosis in 50 percent of flaps which, by the experimental method, would otherwise have sloughed. No protection was afforded at higher pressures.

On the other hand, other authors have condemned the use of such manipulation of flaps on the grounds that the additional trauma may be harmful. McGregor flatly states, "One can say that interference with massage to help the circulation is positively harmful" [38].

Gravity and Positioning

Myers and coauthors challenged the long-held belief that gravity alone promotes venous drainage from congested flap tissues [47]. In experimental flaps on rabbits and on pigs, constructed so as to provide for marked venous congestion of the acral portions of the flaps, positioning, regardless of whether the base of the flap was dependent or elevated, had no effect on either the blood supply or the surviving lengths of the flap tissue.

This study resulted also in the unexpected but interesting finding that "the blood supply of tubed flaps frequently decreased after 48 hours, and that this increase in the amount of necrosis was accompanied by the growth of anaerobic bacteria in the ischemic pedicle."

Anticoagulants

HEPARIN. The edema and color of the congested flap presuppose prolonged venous stasis. Venous thrombosis in such conditions has been regarded as a natural consequence. Under these circumstances one might assume that anticoagulants would influence the ultimate survival of the congested flaps. Sturman and coauthors investigated the use of heparin in treating congested skin flaps on experimental animals [53]. A continuous intravenous infusion of heparin during the period in which pressure was applied to the base of the pedicle to limit venous outflow was felt to be efficacious in promoting ultimate flap survival as compared to the control situation. The authors note, however, that in the clinical situation the use of anticoagulation in the immediate postoperative period may be fraught with the complications of bleeding, and with hematoma formation. Also, while heparin may reduce the incidence of venous thrombosis, it has no effect on tissue fluid turnover.

LEECHES.   Derganc and Zdradvic advocated the use of *Hirudo medicinalis* (medicinal leech) in the treatment of the flap compromised by venous congestion [15]. The action exerted by the leech is twofold. There is a mechanical removal of stagnant blood in the flap by the sucking action of the leech, and the leech excretes from its salivary glands hirudin—a powerful anticoagulant enzyme. The authors cited 20 clinical cases in which leeches were used to advantage in preventing necrosis in congested flaps. They concluded that "the use of leeches in the treatment of venous congestion represents an effective method based on a mechanical action by removing the stagnant blood and a biological action due to hirudin, preventing local clotting in the vessels." As a temporizing measure prior to the establishment of patent venous channels to provide for flap drainage, the use of the medicinal leech may be a sound practice and probably bears further investigation.

REFERENCES

1. Adamson, J. E., Horton, C. E., Crawford, H. H., and Ayers, W. T.   The effects of dimethyl sulfoxide on the experimental pedicle flap: A preliminary report. *Plast. Reconstr. Surg.* 37:105, 1966.
2. Barron, J. N.   The congestion test—a method of estimating the circulation in tubed pedicles. *Br. J. Plast. Surg.* 8:114, 1955.
3. Barron, J. N., Laing, J. E., and Colbert, J. G.   Observations on the circulation of tubed skin pedicles using the local clearance of radio-active sodium. *Br. J. Plast. Surg.* 5:171, 1952.
4. Barron, J. N., Veall, N., and Arnott, D. G.   The measurement of the local clearance of radio-active sodium in tubed skin pedicles. *Br. J. Plast. Surg.* 4:16, 1951.
5. Bloomenstein, R. B.   Viability prediction in pedicle flaps by infrared thermometry. *Plast. Reconstr. Surg.* 42:252, 1968.
6. Braithwaite, F.   Some observations on the vascular channels in tubed pedicles—II. *Br. J. Plast. Surg.* 4:28, 1951–52.
7. Braithwaite, F., Farmer, F. T., Edwards, J. R. G., and Inkster, J. S.   Simultaneous measurements of blood flow in sodium^{24} clearance in the skin. *Br. J. Plast. Surg.* 12:189, 1959.
8. Braithwaite, F., Farmer, F. T., and Herbert, F. I.   Observations on the vascular channels of tubed pedicles using radio-active sodium—III. *Br. J. Plast. Surg.* 4:38, 1951–52.
9. Conway, H., Roswit, B., Stark, R. B., and Yalow, R.   Radio-active sodium clearance as a test of circulatory efficiency of tubed pedicles and flaps. *Proc. Soc. Exp. Biol. Med.* 77:348, 1951.
10. Conway, H., Stark, R. B., and Doktor, J. P.   Vascularization of tubed pedicles. *Plast. Reconstr. Surg.* 4:133, 1949.
11. Conway, H., Stark, R. B., and Joslin, D.   Cutaneous histamine reaction as a test of circulatory efficiency of tubed pedicles and flaps. *Surg. Gynecol. Obstet.* 93:185, 1951.
12. Conway, H., Stark, R. B., and Nieto-Cano, G.   The arterial vascularization of pedicles. *Plast. Reconstr. Surg.* 12:348, 1953.

13. Daniel, R. K., and Taylor, G. I.   Distant transfer of an island flap by microvascular anastomoses. *Plast. Reconstr. Surg.* 52:111, 1973.

14. Daniel, R. K., and Williams, H. B.   The free transfer of skin flaps by microvascular anastomoses. *Plast. Reconstr. Surg.* 52:16, 1973.

15. Derganc, M., and Zdradvic, F.   Venous congestion of flaps treated by application of leeches. *Br. J. Plast. Surg.* 13:187, 1960.

16. Dingwall, J. A., and Lord, J. W., Jr.   The fluorescein test in the management of tubed (pedicle) flaps. *Bull. Johns Hopkins Hosp.* 73:129, 1943.

17. Douglas, B., and Buchholz, R. R.   The blood circulation in pedicle flaps—an accurate method for determining its efficiency. *Ann. Surg.* 117:692, 1943.

18. Fujino, T.   Contribution of the axial and perforator vasculature to circulation in flaps. *Plast. Reconstr. Surg.* 39:125, 1967.

19. German, W., Finesilver, E. M., and Davis, J. S.   Establishment of circulation in tubed skin flaps: Experimental study. *Arch. Surg.* 26:27, 1933.

20. Gillies, H. D.   The tubed pedicle in plastic surgery. *N.Y. J. Med.* 111:1, 1920.

21. Goetz, R. H.   The diagnosis and treatment of vascular diseases with special consideration of clinical plethysmography and the surgical physiology of the autonomic nervous system. *Br. J. Surg.* 37:165, 1950.

22. Gruber, R. P., Billy, L. I., Heitkamp, D. H., and Amato, J. J.   Hyperbaric oxygenation of pedicle flaps without oxygen toxicity. *Plast. Reconstr. Surg.* 46:477, 1970.

23. Gruber, R. P., Brinkley, F. B., Amato, J. J., and Mendelson, J. A.   Hyperbaric oxygen in pedicle flaps, skin grafts, and burns. *Plast. Reconstr. Surg.* 45:24, 1970.

24. Hoffmeister, F. S.   Studies on timing of tissue transfer in reconstructive surgery: I. Effect of delay on circulation in flaps. *Plast. Reconstr. Surg.* 19:283, 1957.

25. Hynes, W.   A simple method for estimating blood flow with special reference to the circulation in pedicled skin flaps and tubes. *Br. J. Plast. Surg.* 1:159, 1948.

26. Hynes, W.   The blood vessels in skin tubes and flaps. *Br. J. Plast. Surg.* 3:165, 1950.

27. Hynes, W.   The "blue flap": A method of treatment. *Br. J. Plast. Surg.* 4:166, 1951.

28. Kaplan, E. N., Buncke, H. J., and Murray, D. E.   Distant transfer of cutaneous island flaps in humans by microvascular anastomoses. *Plast. Reconstr. Surg.* 52:301, 1973.

29. Kernahan, D. A., Zingg, W., and Kay, C. W.   The effect of hyperbaric oxygen on the survival of experimental skin flaps. *Plast. Reconstr. Surg.* 36:19, 1965.

30. Ketchum, L. D., Ellis, S. S., Robinson, D. W., and Masters, F.   Vascular augmentation of pedicled tissue by combined histamine iontophoresis and hypertensive perfusion. *Plast. Reconstr. Surg.* 39:138, 1967.

31. Kety, S. S.   Measurement of regional circulation by the local clearance of radio-active sodium. *Am. Heart J.* 38:321, 1949.

32. Kiehn, C. L., and Desprez, J. D.   Effects of local hypothermia on pedicle flap tissue. *Plast. Reconstr. Surg.* 25:349, 1960.

33. Lewis, T.   *The Blood Vessels of the Human Skin and Their Responses.* London: Shaw & Shaw, 1927.

34. Lutz, B. R., Fulton, G. P., and Akers, R. P.   Neuromotor mechanism of all blood vessels in membranes of frog (*Rana pipiens*) and hamster (*Mesocricetus auratus*) with reference to normal and pathological conditions of blood flow. *Exp. Med. Surg.* 8:258, 1958.

35. Manchot, C.   *Die Hautarterien des Menschlichen Korpers.* Leipzig: Vogel, 1889.

36. McFarlane, R. M., Heagy, F. C., Radin, S., Aust, J. C., and Wermuth, R. E.   A study of the delay phenomenon in experimental pedicle flaps. *Plast. Reconstr. Surg.* 35:245, 1965.

37. McFarlane, R. M., Laird, J. J., Lamon, R., Finlayson, J. R., and Johnson, R.   Evaluation of dextran and DMSO to

prevent necrosis in experimental pedicle flaps. *Plast. Reconstr. Surg.* 41:64, 1968.

38. McGregor, I. A. Flaps. In Goldwyn, R. M. (Ed.), *The Unfavorable Result in Plastic Surgery.* Boston: Little, Brown, 1972.

39. Milton, S. H. The tubed pedicle flap. *Br. J. Plast. Surg.* 22:53, 1969.

40. Milton, S. H. The effects of "delay" on the survival of experimental pedicled skin flaps. *Br. J. Plast. Surg.* 22:244, 1969.

41. Milton, S. H. Pedicled skin flaps, the fallacy of the length-width ratio. *Br. J. Surg.* 51:502, 1970.

42. Milton, S. H. Experimental studies on island flaps: II. Ischemia and delay. *Plast. Reconstr. Surg.* 49:444, 1972.

43. Milton, S. H., and Corbett, J. L. Failure to increase the survival of experimental flaps by histamine and hypertension. *Plast. Reconstr. Surg.* 43:235, 1969.

44. Myers, M. B., and Cherry, G. Design of skin flaps to study vascular insufficiency—failure of Dextran 40 to improve tissue survival in devascularized skin. *J. Surg. Res.* 7:399, 1967.

45. Myers, M. B., and Cherry, G. Mechanism of the delay phenomenon. *Plast. Reconstr. Surg.* 44:52, 1969.

46. Myers, M. B., and Cherry, G. Differences in the delay phenomenon in the rabbit, rat, and pig. *Plast. Reconstr. Surg.* 47:73, 1971.

47. Myers, M. B., Cherry, G., and Bombet, R. On the lack of any effect of gravity on the survival of tubed flaps. *Plast. Reconstr. Surg.* 51:428, 1973.

48. Olander, G. A. The nicotinic acid and epinephrine test for determining the source of blood supply of delayed skin flap. *Plast. Reconstr. Surg.* 5:58, 1950.

49. Reinisch, J. F. The pathophysiology of skin flap circulation—the delay phenomenon. *Plast. Reconstr. Surg.* 54:585, 1974.

50. Seitchik, M. W., and Kahn, S. The effects of delay on the circulatory efficiency of pedicled tissue—a review. *Plast. Reconstr. Surg.* 33:16, 1964.

51. Spalteholz, W. *Handatlas der Anatomie des Menschen.* Leipzig: Hirael, 1917.

52. Stern, W. G., and Cohen, M. B. Intracutaneous salt solution wheal test: Its value in disturbances of circulation in extremities. *J.A.M.A.* 87:1355, 1926.

53. Sturman, M. J., Terry, J. L., Biggs, J. A., and Bennett, J. E. The prevention of necrosis in congested tubed pedicles. *Plast. Reconstr. Surg.* 34:555, 1964.

54. Thompson, L. K., and Pollard, J. A. A method for determining blood flow in pedicle flaps. *Plast. Reconstr. Surg.* 42:39, 1968.

55. Thorne, F. L., Georgiade, N. G., Wheeler, W. F., and Mladick, R. A. Photoplethysmography as an aid in determining the viability of pedicle flaps. *Plast. Reconstr. Surg.* 44:279, 1969.

56. Walsh, T. S. The dermal arteries of the neck and shoulders. *Plast. Reconstr. Surg.* 32:455, 1963.

57. Winsten, J., Manalo, P. D., and Barsky, A. J. Studies on the circulation of tubed flaps. *Plast. Reconstr. Surg.* 28:619, 1961.

58. Zbylski, J. R., Order, S. E., Walker, H. L., and Moncrief, J. A. The vascular structure of tubed pedicle flaps and the influence of surgical trauma. *Plast. Reconstr. Surg.* 36:420, 1965.

16

Tissue Dynamics and Surgical Geometry

Mark Gorney

In every discipline there is a block of "core" knowledge so basic that it literally constitutes the foundation for future progress. In reconstructive surgery, failure to comprehend thoroughly the nature of tissue dynamics and surgical geometry can have only disastrous consequences. Unfortunately, much of this core knowledge must be gained at the operating table or, worse yet, through bitter experience. It is patently impossible to teach the effects of stress, strain, and torsion in elastic three-dimensional tissues on stiff two-dimensional paper. Only principles can be outlined and explained in terms of physical effects. However, what can or cannot be done within the bounds of physiological limits often lies as much in the elasticity of the surgeon's imagination as it does in the patient's tissues.

It is easy to become lost in complex physical and mathematical formulas. It is also unnecessary. For the purposes of this chapter we are searching merely for an understanding of basic concepts. What follows, then, is essentially a framework which underlies most reconstructive surgical procedures.

STRESS AND STRAIN

When elastic tissues are put under traction, the force applied can be referred to as *stress*. The resulting physical changes within the tissue are called *strain*. Without entering into complex mathematical equations, we can best present these terms as pictured in Figure 16-1. The concept can be applied clinically in the following examples.

Skin Grafts

A newly applied free graft is essentially a section of tissue temporarily devoid of life which takes on new circulation and new life from its recipient site. The microphysiological process involved is discussed elsewhere in this book. It is generally agreed that, to survive in the first 24 to 48 hours, a free graft must depend on two factors: its low metabolic requirement and adequate oxygenated plasmatic transudate from the recipient site.

Imagine the free graft as a stack of fishing nets lying in the surf. Each net represents a microscopic layer of dermal tissue. The network itself represents the intercellular fibroelastic tissue; the spaces in it represent the

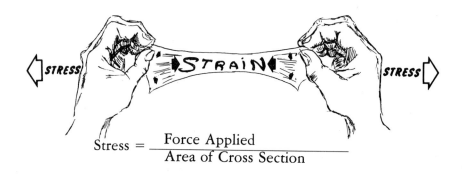

$$\text{Stress} = \frac{\text{Force Applied}}{\text{Area of Cross Section}}$$

$$\text{Strain} = \frac{\text{Elongation}}{\text{Original Length}}$$

FIGURE 16-1.   *Stress-strain relationships.*

cellular substance and its immediate environment. If one were to exert great stress in one direction, the strain within the network would create distortion, increasing the length in one direction while narrowing in the other. This distorting effect in each net would then result in a general narrowing of the spaces. It follows, then, that the water would be less likely to reach the topmost layers of the stack (Fig. 16-2).

If one transfers this image to the skin graft, it is understandable that when a graft is sutured into place under great tension the

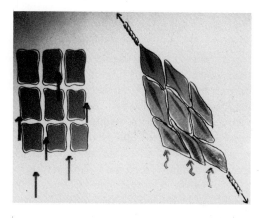

FIGURE 16-2.   *Tension or torsion narrows and distorts cellular spaces interfering with mechanical or osmotic fluid transfers across tissue layers.*

mechanical factor alone may account for failure of "take" of part or all of the graft. It was Rees's theory in designing his dermatome that, the closer to "normotension" one obtains and places the skin graft, the better the chance of "take."

Flaps

If one pulls firmly on a flap, it turns pale. Obviously arterial insufficiency caused by strain within the tissues narrows and limits the circulatory input. If the stress is maintained, the color will rapidly turn to violet. Through the same mechanical effect one is witnessing tissue anoxia and, beyond a period of time, irreversible changes and tissue death. Ordinarily, however, the violet color will not be a result of arterial insufficiency. Arterial blood, after all, perfuses all tissues under a much greater pressure gradient than does venous blood; unless the strain is very great, it will perfuse the flap. The question is, Can the venous network get it out? Any additional narrowing of venous outflow caused by tissue strain will compound the physiological problems with mechanical ones. If torsion stress is also added and gravity drainage not allowed for in the preoperative planning, the stage is set for the classic triad which is a prescription for disaster: strain, torsion, and gravity. Proper preoperative planning, then, must include considerations of design, proportion, and direction of venous outflow. We can summarize as follows:

Physical Problem	Planning Objective
1. Strain	
a. Arterial supply partly re-stricted	Correct proportions and design
b. Venous supply very re-stricted	
2. Gravity	Proper direction of venous outflow
3. Torsion stress	Correct planning

VECTORS

Whole books are devoted to vector analysis in mathematics and engineering. No complex definition is needed, but a comprehension of the underlying principles is indispensable in the application of surgical geometry.

A *vector* is a force having magnitude and direction. For our purposes it is sufficient to say that, when two lines of stress (vectors) pull in diverging directions from a given point, the stress applied at that point will pull it in a direction somewhere between the two original lines of force. The ultimate direction is determined by a combination of the two original vectors. This resulting direction of stress can be called the *net vector*. If the diverging stresses are equal in magnitude, the net vector will fall exactly between them. If one stress is significantly greater than the other, the net vector will be influenced by the stronger of the two pulls (Fig. 16-3).

Human tissues are inherently elastic. When a stress is applied to a section of tissue, the resultant strain produces a counterforce; that is, it tends to resist the deforming stress and pulls back. Thus, if a flap is rotated, its own "pulling back" strain represents one basic vector direction. The tissue to which the flap is sutured represents another. The net vector resulting from these actions depends on the nature of the tissue and the magnitude of the strain. Nevertheless, the net vector pull will be in a direction somewhere in between. If, on the other hand, the vector forces

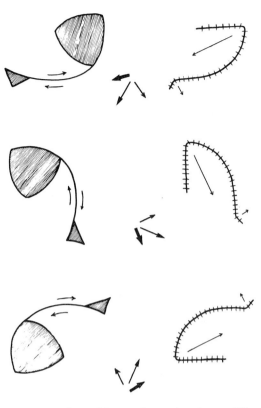

FIGURE 16-3. *Vector forces in tissue. The heavy arrow represents the stronger force; the longest arrow the net direction of pull.*

are equal in strength but in exactly opposing directions, they will cancel each other.

Examples:

1. A simple elliptical excision and closure will set up two divergent but equal stresses from both sides of the wound. The strain is greatest at the center where the ellipse is widest and least at either end. But if both stresses are equal, there should be no shift in position of the scar since the forces neutralize each other.

2. A flap is elevated and rotated under stress and attached to an area of loose tissue, such as the eyelid. The result is a net vector that can either help us or have a disastrous effect if not planned accurately (Fig. 16-4).

Almost universally, all flap procedures

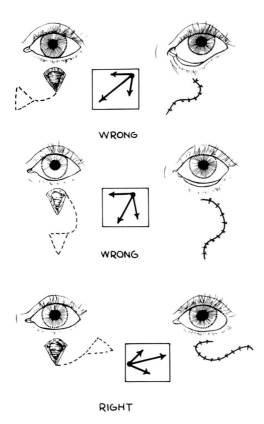

WRONG

WRONG

RIGHT

FIGURE 16-4. *Properly analyzed vectors can spell the difference between success and failure.*

should be planned with net vector effects in mind, tempered by circulatory and local anatomical considerations.

Stresses applied to elastic tissue will diffuse across that tissue in geometric proportion. The farther the stress from the desired target area, the greater the excision and the stronger the pull must be to achieve the same effect as a much smaller excision and pull nearer the target area (Fig. 16-5). The desirability of avoiding obvious scars must be the deciding factor.

TRANSMITTED STRESS OF CONTRACTURE

Scar tissue is composed mostly of contracting collagenous fibers. Since skin is an elastic membrane, it follows that when the scar tissue matures (and inevitably contracts) it will transmit certain stresses on normal surrounding skin. David Ju, in a masterful essay, has cleverly worked out the dynamics of this transmitted contracture [1]. From this study we can conclude that the transmitted stress is greatest at the line of contracture and diminishes rapidly with distance away on either side of it (Fig. 16-6A, B, C). If these forces are

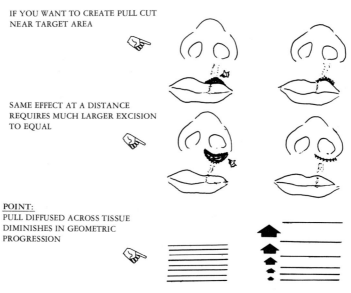

IF YOU WANT TO CREATE PULL CUT NEAR TARGET AREA

SAME EFFECT AT A DISTANCE REQUIRES MUCH LARGER EXCISION TO EQUAL

POINT:
PULL DIFFUSED ACROSS TISSUE DIMINISHES IN GEOMETRIC PROGRESSION

FIGURE 16-5. *The closer you work to the area of intended effect, the greater is your mechanical advantage.*

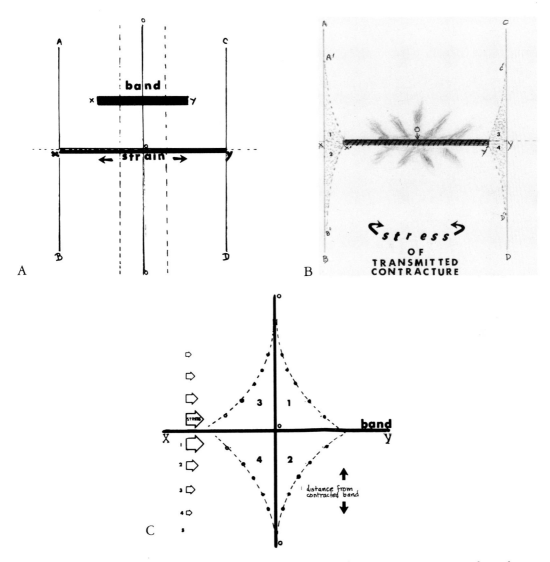

FIGURE 16-6. *Transmitted force of scar contracture (according to D. Ju [1]). A. If an elastic band X–Y is placed under stress and glued to an elastic sheet, the strain in the band will be transmitted to its underlying sheet. B. The transmitted stress of the stretched band will displace the underlying sheet medially (triangles 1, 2, 3, 4) and throw the tissues immediately adjacent to it into folds. C. The degree of displacement can be plotted. It is greatest directly at the line of contracture and diffuses rapidly as one moves away on either side. The magnitude of transmitted stress is represented by the diminishing arrows. Thus the displacement takes the graphic form of triangles 1, 2, 3, and 4.*

plotted as vectors on graph paper, a roughly isosceles triangle pattern emerges, the longest arrows representing the greatest force of pull directly at the band (or base of the triangle) and the smallest arrows representing the lesser force at the tip.

Ju also proved that a contracture band exerts transmitted stress on an elastic membrane (skin) in reverse proportion to the tension of the latter; that is, the less contractile the tissues, the less the contracture of the band and the less the effects of transmitted stress. The clinical application is obvious. A shrinking scar band will much more easily create deformity in the neck or axilla or eyelid, for example, than in the scalp or the sole of the foot. Ju's work also explains the mechanism of semicircular scar contracture and the effects of the Z-plasty operation, as we shall see.

THE GEOMETRY OF ELECTIVE INCISIONS

Since Langer in 1861 first noted the natural lines of tension of the skin, it has been recognized that elective incisions designed parallel to these lines make much better scars. Nonetheless, Langer's work was done on cadaver skin. While his observations are entirely valid, in the living human face natural "expression lines" must also be considered. Generally speaking, these lines are always at right angles to underlying musculature. In most cases they are created precisely by the intimate relationship between the underlying muscle and the skin above it; the horizontal forehead furrows over the vertical frontalis muscle or the radiating mouth wrinkles over the circular orbicularis oris.

The additional stress of that muscular action will work against the surgeon instead of in his favor if the wound is not placed parallel to the tension lines in general and facial expression lines in particular. Furthermore, a simple elliptical excision and closure will create two planes of stress (or two vectors of force). The sutures produce the stress while tissue elasticity produces strain. The maximum stress will always occur in the center (or widest point) of the ellipse. The greatest laxity is at either end of the wound. As a rule, then, elective excision where possible should be made in a proportion of at least three in length to one of width. If less than three to one, the effect of the closure will be to produce great tension in the center and forced laxity at either end. Viewed in profile such a wound will be depressed in the center and excessively full in the ends (Fig. 16-7).

Sometimes one is faced with a lesion whose principal axis is at right angles to Langer's

If proportion of wound is greater than 3 x 1:

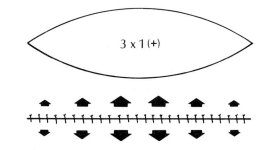

① tension better distributed
② dog-ear less

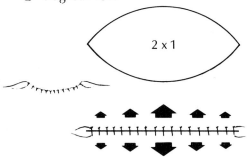

FIGURE 16-7.   *Tension represented by heaviness of arrows. Ratio of 3 × 1 (or better) in the excisional proportions results in better distribution of tension. Inset represents schematic of profile of poorly proportioned wound.*

lines. In this case, to follow the preceding dictum one would have to make a tremendously wide and long excision in order to stay within the lines of tension. There is a useful compromise. A sigma (or "cloverleaf") excision and closure (Fig. 16-8) will place the resulting scar at least two-thirds within the proper direction and only one-third against it and will not necessarily lengthen the total scar.

Occasionally a semilunar excision leaves wound edges one of which is distinctly longer than the other. Three solutions are possible: (1) Lengthen the short side. (2) Shorten the long side. (3) "Fudge." These solutions are illustrated in Figure 16-9.

Despite the great variety of flap designs

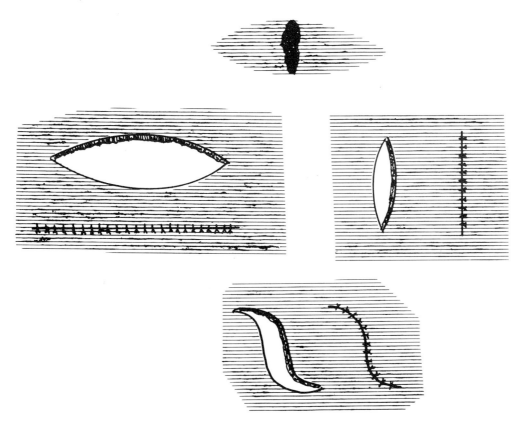

FIGURE 16-8. *Sigma, or "clover leaf," compromise for situations in which the long axis of the lesion is at right angles to elective incision lines.*

and names, they fall into three basic types: advancement, rotation, and transposition.

ADVANCEMENT FLAPS

An advancement flap is one that is partially detached from its underlying tissue carrying its own blood supply and is stretched along a single principal axis or plane. A simple elliptical excision and closure of the two wound edges after undermining constitutes two advancement flaps moving toward each other.

Relaxing incisions and the V-to-Y maneuver are other variants. The V-to-Y maneuver is an advancement flap in reverse. It is a procedure of secondary choice, however, and should be reserved for areas of no aesthetic importance, such as the inside of the mouth. We are asking a flap of x dimensions to crowd itself into a space of one-half x size. We are also creating a three-point junction and inevitable fullness or "dog ears" at the upper ends of the Y. If this maneuver must be used, it is far better to create two side cuts at the upper end of the divergent arms of the Y. When the V portion of the flap moves upward, these will then convert to diamond-shaped defects that can now be sutured side to side, thus adding needed length.

"Relaxing incisions" are mentioned only to be condemned. Anyone with a basic understanding of the principles of reconstructive surgery surely should be able to come up with a better solution than the addition of unnecessary scars.

ROTATION FLAPS

A rotation flap is a section of skin carrying its own blood supply which is detached from

PROBLEM:
Discrepancy in length of wound edges

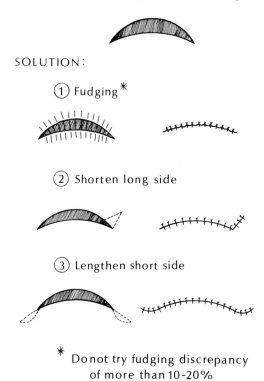

SOLUTION:

① Fudging*

② Shorten long side

③ Lengthen short side

* Do not try fudging discrepancy
of more than 10-20%

FIGURE 16-9. *Solutions for a semilunar incision with one side longer than the other.*

its underlying tissues and stretched in an arcing direction to cover a defect contiguous to it. It is one of the most frequently used and useful tissue transfer maneuvers in reconstructive surgery. A few key points will make its use easier.

1. The length of the arcing incision should generally be four to five times that of the desired rotation advancement. The differential will then be taken up easily by the elasticity of the flap tissue (Fig. 16-10).

2. As the flap rotates around its radius, a line of tension is created diagonally from the base of the flap to its point. The larger the flap, the more diffuse the distribution of tension. As it rotates, the flap shortens. Therefore extra tissue must always be taken in order to achieve adequate length. The greater the degree of rotation, the more the extra length is needed. The larger the radius of the arc along which the flap rotates, the easier the closure but the greater the "dog ear" at the base (Fig. 16-11).

3. When the flap is sutured into position, relative laxity will be encountered along the recipient side of the incision so that at the base the excess "dog ear" tissue will be evident. This can be corrected by one of the three solutions described above under The Geometry of Elective Incisions. If the surgeon elects to shorten the long side, he can do so by excising a triangle from the recipient side of the wound, but at the base of the flap. The base of this excisional triangle should be at least one-quarter of the distance that the flap must advance (Figs. 16-9, 16-10).

4. Another solution to the tight diagonal

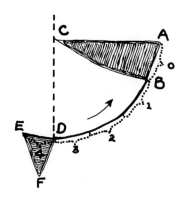

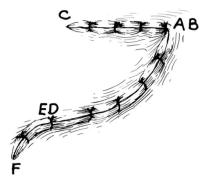

FIGURE 16-10. *Ideal proportions of the classic rotation flap maneuver. Excisional triangle base (E–D) should equal about one-half of desired advancement (A–B); this avoids dog ears.*

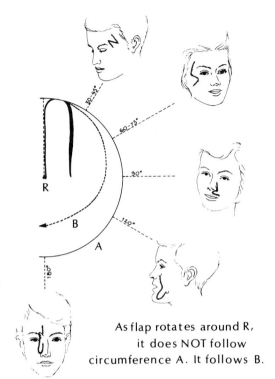

As flap rotates around R,
it does NOT follow
circumference A. It follows B.

FIGURE 16-11. *The need for greater flap
length with increased rotation is demonstrated in
examples in various areas of the face.*

line of tension across the flap is the "back cut"
across part of the base. This must be done
with the greatest caution lest one interfere
with vital circulation. A massive back cut
combined with undue diagonal tension spells
trouble. Additionally, a back cut will require
either a skin graft or additional maneuvers for
closure of the extra defect.

THE TRANSPOSITION FLAP

A transposition flap is a section of skin
carrying its own circulation which is partially
detached from its underlying tissue and
moved across normal skin to repair a defect
either contiguous or distant from the flap
donor site. Transposition flaps come in many
styles: open or closed, lined or unlined,
tubed, etc. A Z-plasty is a double transposition flap. A few key points will make its use
easier.

1. Generally, transposition flaps are
moved on a narrower circulatory base than
advancement or rotation flaps. For this reason
the dimensions of a flap are critically important. It is not the size that counts, but proportion. As a rule (but with certain exceptions), it
is unwise to design transposition flaps of proportions more than three in length to one of
width. This rule can be stretched (a) when the
flap is based on a known circulation (e.g., the
superficial circumflex vessels at the groin or
the temporals at the forehead) or (b) when
there have been adequate delays. The lower
down the body, the more stringently the rule
has to be applied since venous return, the sine
qua non of flap survival, becomes less favorable. When it becomes necessary to design a
flap that is retrograde to the main axis of
venous circulation, not only is delay mandatory but the rules of proportion should be
shortened; the flap should be less than three
to one.

2. Avoid "pointy" flaps. The circulatory
isolation of a section of tissue leads to increased arterial inflow, in turn leading to
greater venous outflow. Provided the arterial
inflow does not grossly exceed the venous
outflow, all is well. Beyond the point where
inflow balances outflow there is rapidly increasing chance of tissue necrosis from venous congestion. If the long flap designed
comes to a sharp point instead of a gentle
taper, the likelihood of necrosis at the tip
rises precipitously (Fig. 16-12).

3. A transposition flap involves a certain
inevitable amount of torsion, or twist, at the
base—in some cases as much as 180 degrees.
Naturally, the less the torsion, the less the
chances of circulatory problems. Where the
angle of transposition is to some extent elective, it should be made as small as possible.
The greater the angle of transposition, the
more the strain at the base of the flap on
closure. This in turn increases venous congestion at the tip (Fig. 16-13).

4. As the transposition flap rotates from 0
degrees to 180 degrees it undergoes several
important changes: (a) It changes shape. (b) It
shortens (in effect). (c) Tension and torsion at

Do Not Make Pointy Flaps

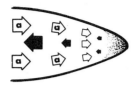 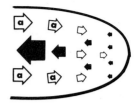

If Sympathectomized Arterial Inflow Grossly Exceeds
Number of Veins Carrying It Out, Tissue Will "Choke" to
Death Beyond Equilibrium Point

FIGURE 16-12.   *A rounded tip provides a flap more likely to survive than one with a pointed tip.*

the base increase. (d) The "dog ear" grows. Hence the flap should be planned backward. One should start with the area of desired coverage and transpose backward, making the fulcrum of the rotation on the tension edge of the flap and not in the middle of its base (Fig. 16-14). In a 180-degree rotation as much as 50 percent of the flap will be used as

PROBLEM:
Poor Planning Causes Needless Tensions
TOO SHORT
NEEDLESS TORSION
BIG DOG EAR
BASE STRAIN
CLOSURE DONOR SITE
   AGGRAVATES
      WRONG

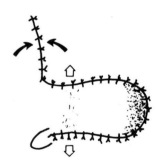

SOLUTION:
plan design so base has minimal tension; sluggish circulation at the end can use tension; base doesn't need it

RIGHT

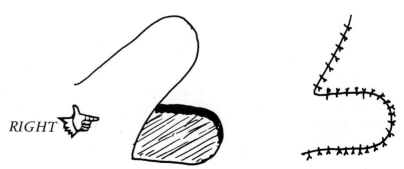

FIGURE 16-13.   *Proper planning and execution of a flap is the main key to survival.*

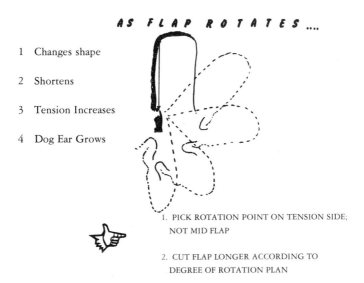

AS FLAP ROTATES ....

1 Changes shape

2 Shortens

3 Tension Increases

4 Dog Ear Grows

1. PICK ROTATION POINT ON TENSION SIDE;
NOT MID FLAP

2. CUT FLAP LONGER ACCORDING TO
DEGREE OF ROTATION PLAN

FIGURE 16-14. *Physical changes in the flap with progressively greater rotation.*

twisted base (dog ear) and this must be taken into consideration in the planning (Figs. 16-11, 16-14).

Z-PLASTY

A *Z-plasty* is an operation designed to gain length in one direction at the expense of width in another. It is essentially a double transposition flap. Clinically it is probably the most useful maneuver and one of the most widely applied in reconstructive surgery. Much has been written about it, so it will be reviewed here only briefly in order to emphasize its dynamic application. Figure 16-15 shows graphically how a Z-plasty works. Here again it is helpful to analyze a number of critical details.

1. There are in many cases a clearly right and a wrong way to lay out a Z-plasty (Fig. 16-16). It is evident that if applied incorrectly the Z-plasty can wind up with all three of its branches coursing contrary to the lines of tension. If it is applied correctly, two of the elements, at least, will be in the correct direction, the third in a nearly correct one.

2. Often the central element of a Z-plasty

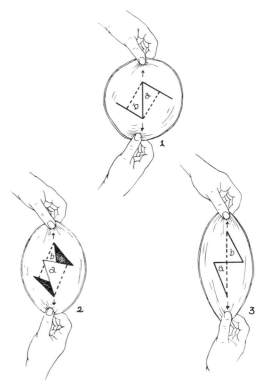

FIGURE 16-15. *How a Z-plasty works: De-crease in one dimension (width) results in in-crease in another (length). Flaps a and b trade places.*

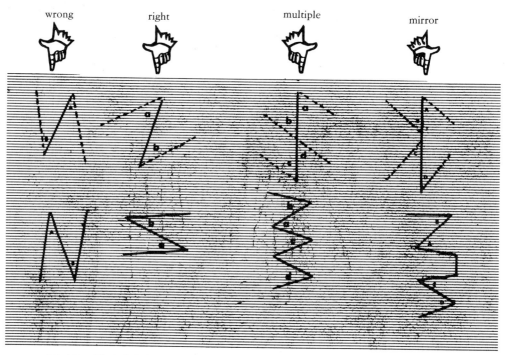

FIGURE 16-16.   *Think before you cut. The same central diagonal will not conform to the exact desired axis, but its two lateral legs can be made to fall exactly along the right lines or totally at right angles to them (and completely wrong). In the multiple Z illustrations resulting lines are better planned than in the mirror one; the former is a better choice.*

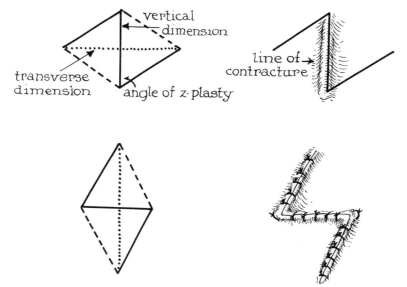

FIGURE 16-17.   *Gain in length in Z-plasty: If the Z is converted into a figurative rhomboid* (top left), *the central element is the vertical dimension represented by the solid line. The dotted line connecting the ends of the lines is the transverse dimension. The difference between those two distances is the expected gain. This is shown as the new vertical dimension represented by dotted line* (bottom left).

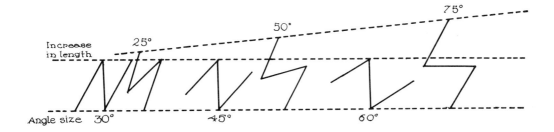

FIGURE 16-18. *Relationship of angles of Z to expected gain in length. (After I. McGregor [2].)*

has to be placed on the edge of a plane of contracted scar tissue or graft. One of the transposed triangles, then, has to be composed entirely of poor tissue. In this case the flap should be cut as thick as possible from the poor-quality tissue, but more important, the best venous outflow (in relation to the circulation gradient and gravity) should be given to the worst flap in order to assist its survival. This takes automatic precedence over choice of tension line directions in the finished Z.

3. The expected gain in length can easily be calculated and is shown in Figure 16-17.

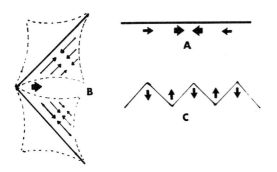

FIGURE 16-19. *Contrasting dynamics of straight-line contractures vs. triangle vs. "broken line." (After D. Ju [1].) A. Straight line (above) pulls toward center from each end, pulling with it neighboring loose tissue. B. Triangle (left) can be considered two diverging lines, each with its own straight-line characteristic behavior. The net result is a vector pulling apex of triangle toward its base. C. A broken line (bottom) consists of multiple triangles, each with its own characteristic behavior, each opposing pair canceling the other. Net result: no contracture.*

Obviously the angles of the flap have a good deal to do with the degree of actual length gained (Fig. 16-18). The more obtuse the angle, the greater the difference between the transverse and longitudinal axes of the rhomboid and thus the greater the gain in length [2]. This is self-limiting, however, since angles of more than about 60 degrees will make for almost rectangular rather than triangular flaps and they will consequently be mechanically much more difficult to switch.

4. The multiple Z-plasty can be laid out in a number of ways according to need. Is there more length to be gained by a multiplicity of Z's than a single large one? A careful mathematical analysis will show that the total gain is about the same. The choice should be made on other criteria. (a) What kind of tissue are we dealing with? (b) Is there normal circulation that will support two larger flaps or is it safer to do a number of smaller ones? (c) Will the final layout of scars meet the purposes better by one large Z (e.g., web neck or axilla) or a series of smaller multiple ones (e.g., mongolian eyelid folds)? (d) What is the anatomical location and what will be the total aesthetic result (if it is important at all)?

Why does a Z-plasty scar tend to prevent recontracture? Figure 16-19 shows once again that the contracture effect of a straight-line scar is that of both ends "pulling in" toward its center. This stress is transmitted to the surrounding tissues. Consider now the two sides of a triangular flap. If we return to Ju's concept of transmitted contracture [1], we can postulate that each side is "pulling in."

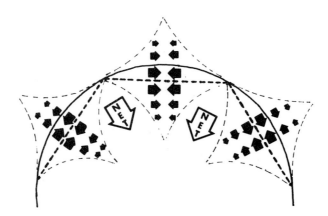

FIGURE 16-20.   *Extension of concept of previously explained dynamics applied to semicircular scars. The net vector forces are combined to create strong centripetal pull. A circular scar is essentially an infinite number of straight lines responding individually to forces of contracture.*

The net vector of stress at the point where they join (the apex of the triangle) is going to pull directly toward the baseline of the triangle. Z-plasty is, after all, two opposing triangles side by side. The obvious conclusion is: *The net vectors of each triangle cancel each other out.* Stated another way, the forces of contracture are then "broken up" in both the literal and the mathematical sense.

CIRCULAR SCARS

A common sequela of windshield trauma is the horseshoe-shaped or semicircular scar. The surgeon who spends hours meticulously suturing the trapdoor flaps often finds himself acutely disappointed in a result that looks like a boggy pincushion several weeks later. The traditional explanation of this phenomenon has always been trapped edema, scar barrier, and contracture of the flap base tending to hump up the tissues above it. Whereas these factors are valid, more careful analysis is in

order. Visualizing the semicircle as an infinite number of small straight lines, one sees that each line has its own tension contracture potential with its own "tension triangle." The cumulative effect is then an infinite number of net vectors all pulling centripetally. The net effect is circular or centripetal contracture (Fig. 16-20).

The solution is obvious. If we take each of these "straight lines" composing the semicircle in sections and convert each section into the central member of a Z-plasty, we immediately and effectively neutralize the centripetal pull and eliminate the tendency toward circular contracture.

REFERENCES
1. Ju, D. M. C.   Physical basis of scar contraction. *Plast. Reconstr. Surg.* 7:343, 1951.
2. McGregor, I. A.   *Fundamental Techniques in Plastic Surgery* (2nd ed.). Edinburgh: Livingstone, 1962.

VI

The Ultimate Modification

INTRODUCTION

In Part V the broad principles of conventional surgical procedures were discussed. Common to those procedures is the fact that they depend upon the rearrangement of existing tissue in some fashion, or, as has been otherwise stated, "Borrow from Peter to pay Paul"—to which should be added, "provided Peter can afford the loan."

Part VI discusses the principles of tissue transplantation—the ultimate modification of tissue response to unfavorable factors when conditions are such that "Peter" cannot "afford" the loan, or, to carry the metaphor further, when the bank is bankrupt.

This is not an easy topic to present in light of a current immense body of knowledge on the subject. The editors felt, along with the author, that a sketch would be meaningless and impossible. Thus it was elected to devote all of Part VI to it, in order to provide the reader with a comprehensive understanding of a complicated topic. Because so many of the basic items of information related to tissue transplantation were developed in relation to renal transplantation, many examples from this discipline are used for illustration although not directly related to reconstructive surgery per se. (But, lest we forget, a pioneer renal transplanter is a plastic surgeon: Dr. Joseph Murray.)

As a reward for absorbing the complicated material herein, the reader will be able to partake in one of the most exciting developments in the future of plastic surgery—the replacement of parts. The technique is known to all; only the question of rejection remains. With the background provided here, the reader will be prepared to be a frontiersperson.

17

Tissue Transplantation

Zoltan J. Lucas

Transplantation to replace diseased or functionless organs has long been a therapeutic dream. Yet, despite the emergence of the transplantation theme in antiquity, only within the last decade has the concept yielded clinical benefit.

Greek mythology, early Christian legends, and medieval folklore record transplantation of organs varying from noses to entire limbs, both from animals to man and from man to man [30]. Successful transplants of autogenous skin in sheep were sporadically done in Italy in 1804 [7]. The technique was not universally duplicated, however, until 1869, when Thiersch learned to consistently cover granulating surfaces with skin grafts [134]. He described the anatomical process of the "take" of a skin graft: adherence of the graft to the host bed, early connection of graft and host vessels, and ingrowth of host endothelium. Nevertheless, little benefit was derived because clinicians performing the skin grafting did not recognize the difference in the response to grafts originating from three genetically different sources: self, another human, or an animal.* Forty-seven

years later, Schöne, suggesting for the first time that allografting was usually *un*successful, coined the term *transplant immunity* [120].

In the next decade Emile Holman twice transplanted skin from a mother to a child, observing that the second graft was destroyed more rapidly than the first ("second set" rejection) while a simultaneous graft from another donor survived as long as the initial graft ("first set" rejection) [66]. He recognized that this finding supported Schöne's immune concept of graft rejection. However, the report went unnoticed until Gibson and Medawar, studying skin grafts between inbred strains of rabbits, established the immunological nature of homograft rejection [51].

Transplantation of organs with a discrete blood supply awaited Alexis Carrel's discovery in 1902 of a technique for anastomosing blood vessels [25]. In the following decade

---

*Duplicate terminology for the relationship of a donor to

a recipient exists. If the graft is from the recipient himself, it is *isogeneic*, or an *autograft*; from a genetically identical individual, *syngeneic*, or an *isograft*; from a member of the same species, *allogeneic*, or an *allograft* or a *homograft*; and if from another species, *xenogeneic*, or a *xenograft* or a *heterograft*.

renal transplants were performed on cats, dogs, and sheep.

By the outbreak of World War II, one tissue, blood, could be successfully transplanted. The genetic and chemical bases for blood compatibility (ABO blood groups), as well as simple serological tests for their determination (blood typing), had been developed during the 40 years following Landsteiner's description of the A and B blood groups. The war provided the impetus to set up large-scale blood banks; transfusions subsequently became routine.

The unsatisfactory results with burned patients in London following the Nazi air raids prompted the British government to subsidize Medawar's now classic work. The following view of skin graft rejection emerged [16, 100, 101]: In a latent period, when there is no obvious reaction from the host, allografts undergo the same primary healing as isografts. An inflammatory process begins around the sixth day and ultimately destroys the graft. It is characterized by vascular and lymphatic proliferation, massive monocytic invasion, and marked edema. Grafts exchanged between inbred strains always reject at a sharply defined time and in histologically identical fashion regardless of the anatomical location on the recipient. Grafts from noninbred lines reject at widely differing times; cellular reactions vary a great deal in intensity. Rejection is a *systemic*, not a local immune reaction; it makes little difference whether the second graft is placed in the bed of the first skin graft or in an entirely new site. Also, transplant immunity is not rigidly tissue specific, for intradermal immunization with foreign leukocytes confers a typical immune reaction toward later skin grafts from the leukocyte donor.

In the early 1950s the suspicion that lymphocytes play a role in graft rejection resulted in experimental attempts to prolong allograft survival with cortisone [17] and whole-body irradiation [34]. Thereafter, new knowledge accumulated at an exponential rate. Immunological tolerance was recognized [14];

radiation chimeras were induced (substitution of one blood or histocompatibility type by a previously incompatible type). Induction of second set rejection with cell-free extracts abolished the view that graft rejection could be elicited only by living cells. Transplant immunity was classified as a form of delayed hypersensitivity and equated with "cellular" rather than "humoral" immunity.

Clinical renal transplantation began in the early 1960s, following the demonstration that 6-mercaptopurine (6-MP) inhibited antibody production in rabbits [121]. In 1962 Starzl began his pioneering set of 64 transplants, obtaining a first-year survival rate of 67 percent for related and 33 percent for nonrelated donors [129].

Corticosteroids and antilymphocyte globulin (ALG) were added to the therapeutic regimen. Kidneys from cadaveric donors were salvaged for transplantation. Brain death replaced cardiac standstill as the criterion of legal death. Technical, surgical, or anatomical problems with the transplantation of other immediately vascularized organs—heart, liver, and lungs—were solved. The catastrophic effect of transplantation into a presensitized recipient was recognized, and preoperative tests to prevent such combinations evolved. Serological typing for HL-A antigens provided a basis for tissue matching, offering the same promise for success in transplants as ABO typing had provided for blood transfusions.

This chapter will summarize the current knowledge of transplant immunity, describe important factors in clinical renal transplantation, and project the areas of future investigation likely to provide a more nearly ideal replacement therapy.

GENETIC BASIS OF TRANSPLANT IMMUNITY

Operational Definitions of Transplant Antigens

The concept of *histocompatibility* is derived from the fate of tumor or skin grafts exchanged between inbred strains of animals. After brother-sister matings for 20 or more consecutive generations, a homogeneous strain showing permanent acceptance of grafts from each other may be obtained; the strain is then assumed to show complete *genetic identity*. Mating two inbred lines results in a first-generation offspring (F_1 hybrid) which accepts skin from either parental strain yet whose tissues are rejected by both parents. Figure 17-1 illustrates these relationships. Rejection represents the recipient's recognition that the graft is foreign. It is related to the presence of molecules on the transplanted cells which the recipient does not possess and recognizes as "nonself" [23]. The F_1 hybrid, possessing each parent's genes, cannot recognize either parental antigen as "nonself." Both parents, recognizing the foreignness of each other's genes, reject such graft combinations. The occurrence of histocompatibility phenomena presupposes

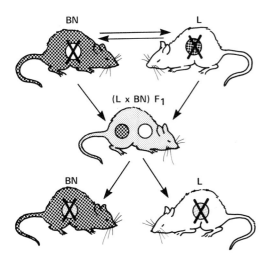

BN   L

(L x BN) F_1

BN   L

FIGURE 17-1. *Results of skin grafts exchanged between two different inbred strains of rats and their F_1 generation offspring. Grafts exchanged between the two strains are rejected. Parental grafts placed on the F_1 recipient are accepted. However, F_1 grafts placed on parental recipients are rejected. Such genetic data led to the concept of "self" and "nonself" as being the principle governing tissue acceptance.*

two factors: histocompatibility molecules or antigens on donor cells and recognition structures on recipient cells which perceive that these antigens are foreign.

Biologically Defined Antigens–Tissue or Organ Graft Survival

Antigens are considered histocompatibility antigens if they can be related to graft rejection. In its original definition, the term *histocompatibility* referred to the growth or failure of growth of tumor or tissue transplants [128]. Graft survival or growth is determined by H structures and is under the control of H genes or H loci.

It is estimated that a minimum of 29 to 32 histocompatibility loci are involved in the rejection of allogeneic skin in the mouse [3]. Inbred strains produced by brother-sister matings differ from one another in the number of H loci differences. The effects of individual H loci could be studied only after the breeding of congeneic resistant mouse strains—strains identical except for a single chromosomal segment. Different forms of a single segment or genetic locus are called *alleles*. Since each chromosomal segment is made up of two complementary DNA strands, two possible alleles may occur in one chromosome. If they are identical, the animal is homozygous for that gene; if different, heterozygous.

Studies with different single H gene mismatches report markedly different graft survival times. Mismatches at the H-2 locus result in rejection in 9.9 days. Mismatches at other H loci yield mean survival times (MST) varying from 21 to over 400 days. A "strong" antigen has been arbitrarily defined as bringing about rejection in 14 days. By this criterion the H-2 gene is the major histocompatibility gene in the mouse.

Fundamental laws governing histocompatibility were initially defined in mice because of the availability of inbred and congeneic strains with precisely known genetic disparity. Studies on graft survival established that:

1. Multiple H loci exist.

2. There are multiple allelic forms for each H locus. Where both alleles are present, both phenotypes are equally expressed; the alleles are codominant.

3. *Antigenic strength,* operationally defined as the speed or vigor of rejection of grafts mismatched at only that locus, varies markedly. It has not been determined whether molecular structure, cellular distribution of the antigen, or some other factor is responsible for antigenic strength.

4. Multiple histocompatibility differences exhibit additive effects only when the constituent antigens of the grafts are similar in strength [63]. Multiple weak incompatibilities can yield survival times similar to those of strong antigenic differences.

5. When a recipient exhibits its maximum response against a given antigenic disparity, adding more antigenic differences to that graft does not further accelerate graft rejection [54].

6. The weaker the histocompatibility, the later the time of onset of graft rejection and the greater the interval between onset and complete rejection.

Reports on kidney [65, 108] and skin [2] grafts in man show that their survival similarly depends on the genetic relationship between donor and recipient. These findings, not surprising considering the experimental evidence with animals, are of particular importance because genetic relationships in man cannot be controlled. Isografts in man occur only with monozygotic twins; there may be syngeneic grafts with certain sibling grafts, but the majority of sibling, almost all parent-child, and all nonrelated donor grafts are between nonidentical individuals. These allogeneic grafts have varying incompatibilities in the major H locus alleles and in the numbers and alleles of minor H loci.

Serologically Defined Antigens

Fortunately, histocompatibility antigens can be assayed by techniques other than observing the fate of skin or other grafts. Recipients of incompatible grafts or patients immunized with lymphocytes or other incompatible tissues (blood, multiple pregnancies) produce antibodies to transplantation antigens which can be detected in several ways. The sera agglutinate nucleated target cells (leukoagglutination assay), lyse them in the presence of excess complement (cytotoxicity assay), or, in the presence of a defined complement system, utilize a measurable amount of complement (complement fixation assay). In actual practice, the microcytotoxicity test is most often used. Serological analysis has proceeded most rapidly in the mouse system because the major histocompatibility antigens, H-2, occurred on red blood cells and permitted analysis by hemagglutination and hemolysis. Progress in humans awaited Dausset's demonstration that antigenic differences detected on leukocytes (human leukocyte antigens, HL-A) predict graft survival [32].

HL-A antigen typing is performed by reacting a panel of antisera of defined specificities with the patient's lymphocytes. If an antigen is present that is represented in the antibody specificities, cells are killed. Typing sera have been laboriously collected, analyzed, and rendered more or less monospecific by adsorption with cells of known HL-A phenotype. As of the 1972 HL-A Histocompatibility Workshop meeting, there were 27 defined HL-A antigenic specificities [142]. The serological analyses established that:

1. Immune sera define a major histocompatibility locus (serologically defined, SD) which has at least two subloci, the LA and the 4 subloci in the human HL-A system, and the H-2d and the H-2k subloci in the mouse H-2 system.

2. Each allele of every sublocus is phenotypically expressed; allelic genes are codominant.

3. Each sublocus has a large number of SD phenotypes (polymorphic alleles).

4. The LA and the 4 subloci in man and the H-2d and the H-2k subloci in mice, 0.5 per-

cent recombination units apart, are on the same chromosomes; at such low recombination frequency, the two genes are usually inherited together and constitute a *haplotype*. An individual inherits one haplotype from each parent. If the parents have different alleles at the two subloci, the offspring may have as many as four different SD antigens.

The possible genetic patterns of inheritance of the HL-A genes are illustrated in Table 17-1. Since a sibling may inherit only four haplotypes, there is a 25 percent chance that two siblings will be HL-A identical. Within siblings, HL-A compatibility can be classified as HL-A identical, one-haplotype difference, or two-haplotype difference. Recombination within the HL-A locus occurs in less than 0.5 percent of matings. This represents the frequency with which new haplotypes arise.

A positive correlation exists between inheritance of HL-A antigens and survival of both skin and kidney grafts exchanged within families. This relationship is illustrated in Table 17-2. Rejection of skin grafts between unrelated persons occurs in 12.11 days; between siblings with one allelic mismatch, 12.5 days; between parent and child (a one-haplotype difference), 13.75 days; and between HL-A identical siblings, 20.04 days [26]. Only with complete HL-A identity does graft prolongation occur. However, in the absence of immunosuppressive therapy, this has little clinical significance; rejection is delayed only eight days.

Renal grafts from HL-A identical siblings receive concurrent immunosuppressive drugs and have nearly 100 percent long-term survival; yet fully 50 percent of the patients experience rejection episodes of mild to marked severity [122]. Renal grafts between HL-A nonidentical donors, related or unrelated, show surprisingly little correlation be-

TABLE 17-1. *Segregation of Parental Alleles of a Simple Genetic Locus Made Up of 2 Subloci with a Low Recombination Frequency* [a]

	Father	x	*Mother*	
haplotype 1	a w		c y	haplotype 3
haplotype 2	b x	↓	d z	haplotype 4

Offspring

Usual Segregation (> 99.5%)				*Recombination* (< 0.5%)		
aw	aw	bx	bx	ax	new	haplotype 5
cy	dz	cy	dz	cw	new	haplotype 6

sublocus a . . . d   *sublocus w . . . z*

HL-A phenotypes of subloci [a]

LA locus			*4 locus*	
HL-A 1	HL-A 11		HL-A 5	W14
HL-A 2	W28		HL-A 7	W15
HL-A 3	W29		HL-A 8	W16
	W23		HL-A 12	W17
HL-A 9<	W30		HL-A 13	W18
	W31		W5	W21
	W24	W32	W10	W27
	W25			
HL-A 10<				
	W26			

[a]Terminology for defined antigens for the HL-A system from the Fifth International Histocompatibility Workshop, 1972 [142].

TABLE 17-2. *Skin Graft Survival and Genetic Relationship in Humans*

	n[a]	MST[b] (days)
Two-haplotype difference		
Unrelated	206	12.11 ± 1.55
One-haplotype difference		
Parent-child	30	13.75 ± 2.53
Siblings (1 HL-A allele difference)	10	13.80 ± 2.2
HL-A identical		
Sibling	12	20.04 ± 4.23

[a]Number of grafts performed.
[b]Mean survival time ± one standard deviation.
Source: Abridged from R. Ceppellini, P. L. Mattiuz, G. Scudellei, and M. Visetti, *Transplant. Proc.* 1:385, 1969.

tween survival and the number of HL-A incompatibilities [94, 102]. These observations become understandable with the realization that the HL-A system does not account for all the major determinants of histocompatibility.

Lymphocyte-Defined Antigens—Mixed Lymphocyte Culture

Another method of assessing genetic identity is the mixed lymphocyte culture (MLC) test [64]. The MLC test depends on the transformation of lymphocytes into DNA-synthesizing cells upon their contact with a foreign histocompatibility antigen. In practice, lymphocytes from two individuals, A and B, are mixed in tissue culture. One set of cells (stimulating cells) is treated with mitomycin (designated by *m*; e.g., Bm) so that they cannot synthesize DNA and respond to the other cells (one-way reaction). The other cells, A (responding cells), are not treated and in the presence of foreign antigens (A × Bm) transform, synthesize DNA, and divide. If the stimulating cells are not perceived as foreign, the rate of DNA synthesis measured by the incorporation of tritiated thymidine does not exceed that obtained in a culture of A cells mixed with other mitomycin-treated A cells (A × Am). Nonstimulatory combinations are MLC identical. Experiments with

lymphocytes from inbred rodent strains have established that a stimulatory response is a measure of the genetic disparity between the two lymphocyte populations [146].

Initial comparison of MLC tests and serological typing performed among siblings indicated a high degree of correlation. This led to the erroneous conclusion that MLC measured the same set of membrane antigens defined by the HL-A antisera. MLC analyses of HL-A identical, unrelated individuals, however, show the existence of differences causing transformation. Table 17-3 demonstrates that stimulation is the rule rather than the exception [149]. Skin graft survival in three of the four possible permutations of SD and LD identical matches varies only from 10 to 12 days in unrelated individuals [79] (Table 17-4). Not only do serological typing and MLC reactivity detect two sets of "strong" transplantation antigens, but other strong antigens still remain undetected. The frequent association of HL-A and MLC identities among siblings indicates that these genetic loci are usually inherited as a unit. Divergences with siblings occur as recombination events, frequencies varying between 0.5 and 1.5 percent. The increasing complexity of this chromosomal segment warrants the term *major histocompatibility complex* (MHC) rather than reference to individual subloci. An essentially identical situation exists in the mouse. The relative locations of the LD and SD genes in the MHC are summarized in the genetic map in Figure 17-2.

Further insight into the genetic control of the immune response comes from studies on antibody responses to simple polypeptide antigens [10]. Injecting a hapten conjugated to poly-L-lysine (PLL) into outbred guinea pigs does not consistently cause antibodies. If two responders are crossbred, the offspring yield 80 to 90 percent responders; crossbreeding two nonresponders yields 100 percent nonresponders. This finding suggests that responsiveness depends on a single autosomal dominant gene, christened the Ir gene (immune response gene). It is

TABLE 17-3. *Incorporation of ³H-Thymidine in Mixed Lymphocyte Culture in Unrelated HL-A Identical Individuals*[a]

Responding Cells	Stimulator Cells			
	Am	Bm	Cm	Xm
(a)				
A (1,8/3,7)	100	91,808	10,738	87,094
B (1,8/3,7)	70,372	926	51,329	66,491
C (1,8/3,7)	40,052	8,210	388	40,662
X (2,W28/8)	27,888	83,424	61,127	220
(b)				
A (1,8/2,12)	382	78,472	48,628	90,320
B (1,8/2,12)	113,981	1,894	117,893	64,879
C (1,8/2,12)	79,350	53,106	560	65,319
Z (1,3,7,Ao70)	110,791	66,993	67,716	319

[a]Counts per minute (cpm) ³H-thymidine incorporated.
Source: From E. J. Yunis and D. B. Amos, *Proc. Natl. Acad. Sci. U.S.A.* 68:3031, 1971.

confirmed with inbred strains of guinea pigs (and mice); animals are either responders or nonresponders. In all, some 30 examples of this type of genetic control of the immune response have been uncovered. The antigens are either synthetic polypeptides, with a small number of determinants, or isoantigens [97]. It was next shown that in mice the Ir gene is linked to the histocompatibility complex and that the Ir and MLC genes might be identical. Since the Ir-MLC genes are localized in the chromosomal segment coding for the HL-A antigens on cell surfaces, it is not an unlikely assumption that the Ir-MLC genes also code for surface antigens.

This section has shown that serological and cellular tests define certain genetic controls over graft survival. They represent major transplantation loci but not all loci. Skin grafts exchanged between both SD and LD identical pairs survive only a few days longer than completely mismatched grafts. HL-A identical renal grafts have almost 100 percent long-term success, but the patients experience rejection episodes despite the use of low-dose immunosuppressive therapy. Tissue matching for either SD or LD antigens offers major benefit with sibling donors because of the approximately 25 percent chance for histocompatible identity. The generally poor correlation between renal graft survival and the degree of incompatibility with non-HL-A identical donors is demonstrated at both limits of compatibility: Many poorly matched grafts have prolonged survival; some well-matched grafts have short or poor graft function.

TABLE 17-4. *Skin Graft Survival in Unrelated Individuals with HL-A and MLC Identities*

Relationship Between Donor and Recipient		n[a]	Graft Survival (days)
HL-A Phenotype	*MLC Reactivity*		
Nonidentical	+	4	9.7 ± .9
Identical	+	7	11.3 ± .7
Identical	−	2	12.0 ± 0

[a]Number of grafts between different individuals.
Source: From C. T. Koch, V. P. Eysvoogel, E. Fredericks, and J. J. van Rood, *Lancet* 2:1334, 1971.

General Characteristics of Transplantation Antigens

Transplantation antigens are products of histocompatibility genes. Knowledge of the

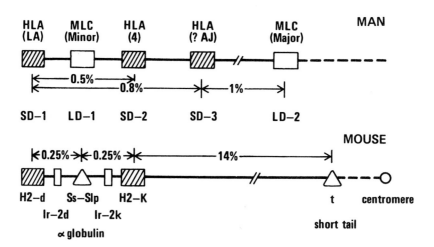

FIGURE 17-2. *Genetic map of the major histocompatibility complex of man and mouse. The percentages represent recombination frequencies between the two markers. The homology between the serologically defined antigens of man and mouse is readily seen. The apparent lack of homology of the lymphocyte-defined antigens may not be real and may represent insufficient data for precise localization.*

molecular nature of the antigens will provide answers to many current questions surrounding histocompatibility. An *antigen* is a molecule, usually of high molecular weight, which elicits an immune response. Antigen-recognition units such as the combining sites of antibodies recognize and react with only a fragment of the antigen, about 5-7 amino acids, or sugar residues in length. These structures are called *antigen determinants* or *antigenic sites.** Since the HL-A gene products are detected by reactions with antibodies, it is unclear whether various antisera detect different determinants on the same molecule or different molecules. To rephrase: Do the HL-A genes determine the primary amino acid structure of different proteins, or do they modify a basic backbone structure by attaching groups of amino acid or sugar residues as side chains?

A precedent for the latter structure is found in the organization of erythrocyte membrane antigens, ABO and Lewis groups. Interactions of several independent genetic loci which code for enzymes transferring sugar residues to side chains of a glycolipid precursor present on the erythrocyte surface determine the structure of these antigens.

Transplantation antigens are isolated from cells by a variety of methods. Purification with conventional biochemical techniques yields products that specifically inhibit the cytotoxic activity of monospecific antibodies on the same target from which the antigen was isolated. These studies establish that the transplantation antigens are lipoglycoproteins, that antigenicity is determined by the protein structure, that the products of the LA and 4 subloci in humans are on two different proteins, and that the various H-2d antigens differ in only about 10 percent of their resolvable peptides. Thus, the two SD subloci define two antigenic molecules located on surface membranes. It is not known whether the alleles of the subloci define different determinants on a basic backbone structure or entirely different molecules.

CELLULAR PARTICIPANTS IN THE IMMUNE RESPONSE

The remarkably complex immune system provides protection from assaults by viruses,

*If the antigenic determinant is experimentally added to the larger molecule, it is called a *hapten* (or haptenic determinant).

microbes, and the body's own transformed cancer cells. By several mechanisms, it destroys anything it recognizes as nonself. The immune response is generally divided into humoral and cellular reactions. The humoral response requires two and possibly three cell populations: B cells derived from bone marrow, T cells from the thymus, and macrophages. B cells make antibody upon contact with haptenic determinants on the antigen only if the T cells simultaneously recognize carrier-type determinants on the same antigen. Cellular immunity embraces a wide spectrum of reactions set in motion by T-cell recognition of the foreign antigen. This section describes the cellular events taking place during the elaboration of the immune response.

Functional Separation into T and B Cells

Since 1962 it has been possible to render animals uniquely deficient in either humoral or cellular immunity. In chickens, the removal of the bursa of Fabricius during early life increases susceptibility to infections with certain bacteria (streptococci, pneumococci, *Salmonella*) yet leaves the animal capable of rejecting allografts. Levels of circulating immunoglobulins are low. In contrast, mammals that have had neonatal thymectomy are capable of making antibodies, but tumor and organ allografts survive in them. Infections with viral, fungal, and mycobacterial organisms are usually lethal [89].

Certain genetic diseases of man constitute counterparts for these experimental manipulations. Congenital sex-linked agammaglobulinemia (Bruton type) and the DiGeorge's syndrome may represent failures to develop the "bursal," or B-lymphocyte, system and the thymus-dependent, or T-lymphocyte, system, respectively. The bursa, a saccular appendage in the fowl intestine, is composed of dense aggregates of lymphoid cells. This function in mammals has been ascribed to either Peyer's patches in the intestine or bone marrow.

Stem cells with multipotential capabilities

arise during early development from the embryonic yolk sac and the primitive blood islands in the fetus. They emigrate, forming hematopoietic colonies in the fetal liver and bone marrow. Further differentiation into unipotential progenitor cells of either lymphocytic or myeloid lines is induced in the microenvironment of different organs. Two primary fetal lymphoid organs develop; in the bird they are clearly identified as the bursa of Fabricius and the thymus. As fetal development proceeds, somewhere near birth, the two organs modulate nondifferentiated lymphocytes arising in the bone marrow to become B- or T-lymphocytes, respectively. These cells then migrate to lymph nodes and spleen. In mammals, the bone marrow appears to be the anatomical site where B function is generated, although it is also the origin of undifferentiated cells and an anatomical repository of low numbers of T cells.

Lymphoid cells have a unique pattern of circulation through the body. Lymphocytes in blood (90 percent T cells) transmigrate through endothelial cells of postvenule capillaries to the extracellular spaces in the various organs. They collect again as lymph fluid (80 to 85 percent T cells) in lymphatic channels, are transiently deposited in lymph nodes (75 percent T cells) located along the lymphatic channels, and ultimately discharge into the blood. The recirculating lymphoid cell pool, consisting mainly of T cells, forms the initial basis of contact with the immune system for most foreign antigens. This compartmentalization of the recirculating lymphoid cell pool is illustrated in Figure 17-3.

Stimulation of B Cells to Produce Antibody Requires T-Cell Function

Intensive study of the effects of neonatal thymectomy in mice reveals that the division between B- and T-cell functions is not absolute. In addition to having an impaired ability to reject allografts, the mice show a markedly decreased antibody response to certain antigens, notably heterologous erythrocytes and foreign serum proteins. In fact, the antibody response is normal to only a few bacterial

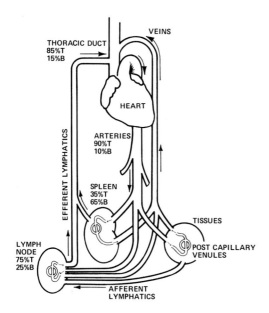

FIGURE 17-3. *Circulatory pathway of lymphocytes. Most lymphocytes enter lymph node or spleen parenchyma by transmigration through endothelial cells of postcapillary venules. Exit is through the efferent lymphatics, which ultimately empty via the thoracic duct into the left subclavian veins. Various lymphatic organs contain different proportions of T- and B-lymphocytes.*

and viral antigens. The above functions are restored by administering syngeneic T-lymphocytes, by grafting with a thymus, and, of greater significance in defining the mechanism of conferring T-cell functions, by adding a thymus enclosed in a millipore chamber. The latter suggests that the thymus functions as an endocrine organ. These antigens, however, have multiple antigenic determinants and constitute a complex experimental system.

Landsteiner, who devoted a lifetime to studying the chemical basis of antigen specificity, developed methods to conjugate simple organic molecules to complex protein carriers [84]. Such haptens are by themselves incapable of initiating an immune response, but complexing with a carrier molecule causes antibody to the hapten to be made.

The hapten specifically and avidly combines with antihapten antibody. Early study of the hapten-specific humoral response indicated that the haptens must be chemically linked to the carrier molecule, that optimum hapten-specific secondary responses require challenging immunization with the same hapten-carrier used for primary immunization, and that inducing tolerance to the carrier molecule causes a partial to total suppression of antibody formation to haptens on the tolerogenic protein carrier. There may be two recognition mechanisms in operation, one for the hapten, the other for carrier determinants.

Recent work (introduced in Lymphocyte-Defined Antigens—Mixed Lymphocyte Culture, above) establishes that two recognition systems occur separately in two different lymphocyte populations, the T and B cells, and that they may function independently. Thus, responsiveness to PLL is independent of the hapten conjugated to it. Hapten-PLL induces antihapten immunoglobulins in PLL-responsive animals as long as PLL is the carrier [9]. The animal's ability to respond to the carrier determines responsiveness. Three main lines of evidence establish the T-lymphocyte's role in recognizing the carrier. (1) Neonatally thymectomized mice do not make antibody to hapten-PLL; ability to make antibody is restored by thymus grafting or by infusion of "pure" T cells. (2) Adoptive transfer of pure T and B cells into syngeneic irradiated mice (presumably lacking either T or B cells capable of responding to hapten-PLL) requires T cells from PLL-responsive mice, but any B-cell population will suffice. (3) The in vitro formation of antihapten antibody is abrogated by selectively killing T cells with anti-T-cell serum and complement [117].

Experiments with mixed hapten-carrier conjugates further extend these views. An animal responsive to bovine serum albumin (BSA) but not to PLL will form hapten-reactive antibodies when immunized with BSA–hapten-PLL. Rendering the animal tolerant to BSA abolishes the response. The lack of cellular immunity to hapten-PLL demonstrated that immunization with BSA–hapten-PLL induced no T-cell response to PLL. Despite antihapten antibody synthesis, hapten-PLL could neither transform lymphocytes from those animals nor induce skin reactions, two parameters of cell-mediated immunity [76]. Thus, responders and nonresponders have the same genetic information for antihapten immunoglobulin synthesis, but nonresponders lack a recognition system for carrier determinants. This effect of T-cell activity on antibody formation is referred to as *T–B-cell cooperation* or *T-cell helper function.*

There is a class of thymus-independent antigens. "Pure" B-cell responses occur with such antigens as pneumococcal polysaccharide, purified polymerized flagella of *Salmonella,* and *Escherichia coli* lipopolysaccharide. They evoke strong primary responses even in neonatally thymectomized mice. The primary molecular structure of T-independent antigens is a linear repetitive structure.

Three possible explanations for T-cell helper function, currently under investigation, are illustrated in Figure 17-4. Two theories relate to the manner in which antigen is presented to the antigen-sensitive B cell. Mere physical interaction of the haptenic determinant and the B-cell receptor is considered insufficient to generate the signal activating B cells to replicate and/or differentiate into antibody-forming cells. Activation occurs with a secondary conformational change in the B-cell receptor, as when the antigen is itself a linear repetitive unit (T-independent antigen), when antigen receptors, possibly transferred to macrophages, linearly arrange several antigens (macrophage-processing of T-dependent antigen) [105], or possibly by the physical proximity of the T and B cells simultaneously binding to haptenic and carrier determinants on the same antigen. The third alternative proposes that activation of the T cell induces

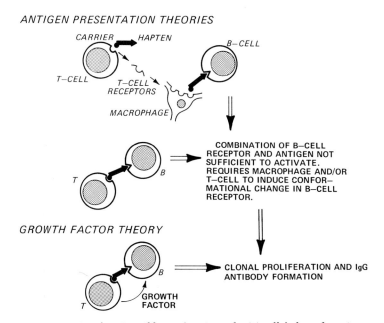

FIGURE 17-4. *Possible mechanisms for T-cell helper function.*

its release of a nonantigen-specific growth factor for B cells, stimulating only cells in close proximity, as occurs when T and B cells are bound to adjacent carrier and haptenic determinants.

Distinguishing Features of B and T Cells

The functional differences between B- and T-lymphocytes are currently not adequately explained by the known anatomical and biochemical differences. Table 17-5 summarizes their distinguishing features. Antigen recognition by B cells is mediated through an antigen receptor with the characteristics of IgM. This is based on the following: Sensitive tests of antigen binding, such as autoradiography with radio-labeled antigen,

are inhibited with anti-immunoglobulin antisera. Anti-immunoglobulin–coated glass bead columns remove potential antibody-forming cells. Lastly, fluorescein-labeled anti-immunoglobulin reagents bind strongly to B cells and hardly, if at all, to T cells. Quantitative immunofluorescence indicates that there are about 10^5 immunoglobulin receptors per B cell and 200 to 300 per T cell. Antibodies against IgG or IgM do not inhibit T-cell function although antibodies against Ig subunits do.

THE IMMUNE RESPONSE

The immune response is generally divided into three sequential phases: the *afferent*, in which antigen recognition occurs; the *central*, in which *cell* differentiation and clonal multi-

TABLE 17-5.   *Distinguishing Features of B- and T-Lymphocytes*

Parameters	B-Lymphocyte	T-Lymphocyte
1. Appearance on scanning electron microscopy	Multiple projections over entire surface	Relatively smooth surface
2. Specific surface antigens	B-lymphocyte antigens (mouse)	θ antigen (mouse) T antigen (human, rat)
3. Surface receptors	Specific antigen receptor (IgG or IgM) C3 receptor Receptor for Fc fragment of Ig Insulin receptor Growth hormone receptor	Specific antigen receptor (gene product of Ir and MLC genes?) Histamine receptor Heterologous erythrocyte antigens (human T-cell receptor for sheep RBC)
4. Surface immunoglobulin determinants	IgG or IgM in high density (10^5 molecules)	Zero or little IgG or IgM ($<10^3$ molecules)
5. Peripheral localization (as % of total lymphocytes)		
a. Blood	10% or less	90% or more
b. Thoracic duct	15–20%	80–85%
c. Lymph node	25%	75%
d. Spleen	60–65%	35–40%
6. Functional sensitivity		
a. X-ray	Sensitive to x-ray	Functionally resistant to x-ray (both helper and "effector" cell activity)
b. Corticosteroids	Resistant before leaving bone marrow; sensitive thereafter	Two populations of T cells—a sensitive population (95%) and a resistant population (5%); both populations perform all T-cell functions

Table 17-5 (continued).

Parameters	B-Lymphocyte	T-Lymphocyte
7. Response to antigens	a. Recognizes and binds antigen b. Differentiates into antibody-producing cells c. Appears to be effector cell in antibody-directed lymphocyte lysis (LDA phenomenon) d. Immunological memory for haptenic determinants e. Can be rendered specifically tolerant (by interaction with suppressor cell?)	a. Recognizes and binds antigen b. "Helper" cell in antibody formation c. "Effector" cell in cell-mediated immune reactions d. Immunological memory for carrier determinants e. Can be rendered specifically tolerant (suppressor cell?) f. Secretes a variety of factors (lymphokines) with a variety of biological effects
8. Experimental methods yielding a "pure" population	a. Incubates with anti-θ or anti-T serum and complement (kills T cells) b. Cell sorting machine with anti-IgG reagent	a. Effluent from anti-IgG–coated glass bead column b. Effluent from C3-coated column c. Effluent from Ag-Ab-C-complex–coated column d. Cell sorting machine with anti-θ reagent e. Sedimentation of human cells with sheep RBC (T cells remain with RBC)

plication for both immediate effector cells and replicating memory cells take place; and the *efferent*, in which the products of the differentiated immune cells neutralize or eliminate the foreign antigen. These divisions are schematized in Figure 17-5.

Afferent Phase—Antigen Recognition

Antigen-Sensitive Lymphocytes

Contact of antigenic determinants with antigen-sensitive cells (ASC) begins the immune response. The initial contact is mediated through surface receptors on the lymphocytes: immunoglobulin IgM for B cells and an undefined structure on T cells. A single antigenic determinant actually induces many different antibodies; these react with the determinant with different avidities, presumably due to different primary amino acid sequences. As the immune response progresses, the antibodies produced become more homogeneous. Ultimately only antibodies with the highest avidity for the antigen are left. A cell selection theory explaining the phenomenon is presented in the next section; briefly, it presumes the bone marrow's continuous production of *uncommitted* ASC, cells capable of reacting with a variety of antigenic determinants until "genetically locked in" or "programmed" by the initial contact with the antigen. Thereafter, these few types of cells multiply and produce a finite number of antigen-reacting clones.

Of particular import to transplantation biology is the relative number of ASC for various types of antigens. Unprimed animals usually have 0.1 to 0.5 percent splenic lym-

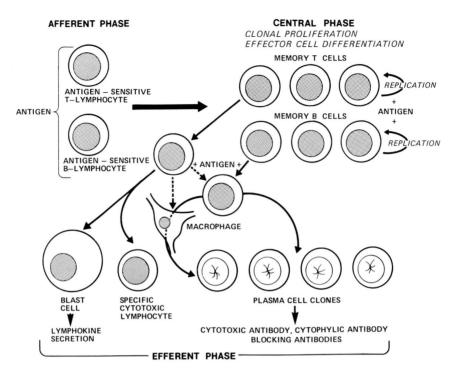

FIGURE 17-5.   *Sequential phases of the immune response.*

phocytes able to bind radio-labeled antigen. Hyperimmunization increases this amount 20- to 100-fold, in the maximum range of 6 to 10 percent of total spleen cells. In contrast, ASC reacting to histocompatibility antigens, as recognized by the MLC reaction, are usually about 10 percent in unprimed animals. Preimmunization with cells or by allogeneic grafting does not increase the number although it does alter the kinetics of the second set response.

Pathways of Graft-Induced Sensitization

Sensitization may occur peripherally (i.e., ASC migrate to the graft) or centrally (i.e., immunogen released from the graft into the venous or lymphatic circulation contacts ASC in spleen or lymph nodes, respectively). Strober and Gowans elegantly demonstrated the former route [133]. They showed allogeneic sensitization after one hour of recyclic perfusion of thoracic duct lymphocytes through a rat's kidney in situ. It is not clear

whether contact of the lymphocytes with the allogeneic endothelial cells is sufficient, or whether the lymphocytes have to enter the renal parenchymal interstitial space to effect sensitization.

Two mechanisms create central sensitization. In one, donor lymphocytes existing in the graft as passenger cells leave the graft and colonize in lymph nodes and spleen. The major route is via the venous effluent, happening mainly with vascularized organ grafts. Wrapping a grafted kidney in cellophane to prevent the reconstitution of lymphatic channels does not decrease the rate of rejection [70]. Removing passenger lymphocytes by irradiating skin or renal grafts delays rejection; however, rejection ultimately occurs. Data indicate that passenger lymphocytes are important only before vascular and lymphatic connections are established [82].

Graft antigens also reach host lymphoid organs by shedding antigen into veins or lymphatics. H antigens are not tightly bound to cells; HL-A antigens have been detected in the blood of healthy people [13] and in urine and blood of renal transplant recipients, increasing with rejection episodes [110].

All three routes of sensitization occur, differing in quantitative importance with various types of grafts. Release of shed antigen is greatest with skin grafts; elimination of passenger leukocytes has less effect on skin than on kidney grafts; prevention of early lymphatic reconnections in the recipient markedly prolongs skin graft survival [4].

Privileged Sites for Allografts

Placing grafts in areas of absent or insufficient vascular or lymphatic connections permits very long survivals. Such areas include the anterior chamber of the eye, meninges of brain, testes, or the cheek pouch of hamsters. Although primary grafts provide increased survival, these sites offer no advantage after presensitization. It has been assumed that these locations do not permit adequate primary sensitization. However, recent studies purporting to show lymphocytic infiltration of nonrejecting implants placed in the eye suggest the importance of other factors [118].

Central Phase—Clonal Proliferation Yields Memory Cells and Differentiated Effector Cells

The small lymphocyte is predominantly a metabolically inactive or resting cell. The conclusion that DNA, RNA, and protein syntheses are minimal is supported not only by little incorporation of labeled macromolecular precursors but also by its cytological appearance: a dense nucleus and scant cytoplasm containing few ribosomes or meager endoplasmic reticulum. A period of four to six days is required to mount an immunological response to antigen or homograft, a time during which the small numbers of specific antigen-sensitive T and B cells both undergo clonal proliferation. Some ultimately differentiate into effector T cells, ef-

fector B cells, or antibody-secreting plasma cells; the others "regress" into memory T or B cells.

The molecular process whereby a membrane event, the combination of the specific antigen with the specific membrane receptor, is translated into gene depression or activation remains a mystery despite voluminous biochemical data. This section on the central phase summarizes current information on lymphocyte transformation in vitro and clonal proliferation and differentiation in vivo.

Lymphocyte Activation in Vitro

In 1960 Nowell noted that lymphocytes incubated with phytohemagglutinin (PHA) transform into large blast cells after 48 to 72 hours in culture [111]. This cellular transformation is morphologically identical to the changes in lymph nodes following antigen stimulation. PHA, or any other mitogenic agent, combines with a receptor unique for each mitogen on the cell membrane.

The earliest biochemical changes (in less than two hours) include increased membrane fluidity, increased phosphorylation of phospholipids, and changes in the fatty acid moieties of lipopolysaccharides of membrane glycoproteins. Membrane permeability to amino acids and nucleoside precursors increases markedly, and, ultimately, decreased viscosity (i.e., increased fluidity) occurs in the cytoplasmic matrix [31, 90]. An apparently "programmed" process of sequential synthesis of enzymes critical for RNA and DNA synthesis [90] follows these events. Ribosomes, endoplasmic reticulum, lysosomes, and the Golgi's complex appear in the enlarging cell. New protein synthesis occurs early (2 to 6 hours), but DNA synthesis is delayed; cell divisions take place 30 to 60 hours after contact with PHA. Preliminary work suggests that the 30-hour variation in onset of cell division correlates with the number of PHA receptor sites on the lymphocyte membrane. A sequence of such changes is illustrated in Figure 17-6, a Wright's-stained

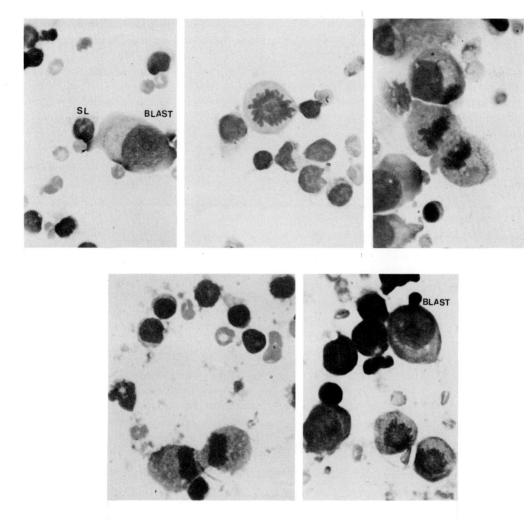

FIGURE 17-6.   *Blastogenic and mitogenic response of human lymphocytes to phytohemagglutinin. Smears of lymphocytes cultured in vitro for 36 to 72 hours were stained with Wright's stain. Stages represent enlargement of small lymphocytes to blast cells and the progressive stages of mitosis: early prophase, anaphase, cleavage plane, and separation of two daughter cells. (Microphotographs courtesy of Dr. Alan Coulson, Stanford University School of Medicine.)*

preparation of human lymphocytes various times after exposure to PHA.

Lymphocyte activation in vitro is induced by other means (Table 17-6). Both T and B cells are responsive in vitro and apparently undergo identical biochemical and morphological sequences of reactions. Most agents inducing blastogenesis require a discrete receptor on the lymphocyte membrane. Such reactions, of potentially great significance in vivo, include activation of in vivo–sensitized T and B cells by the specific antigen, activation of T-lymphocytes by allogeneic B-lymphocytes (the MLC test), and activation of B-lymphocytes by antigen-antibody-complement complexes. Other transforming agents include heterologous antilymphocyte globulin (reacting with undefined lympho-

TABLE 17-6. *Agents Inducing Lymphocyte Blastogenesis in Vitro*

Nonspecific	Specific	
	Noncellular	Cellular
Plant lectins	*Specific antigens*	*Histocompatibility antigens*
Phytohemagglutinin	Large number, including:	Allogeneic lymphocytes
Pokeweed mitogen	Smallpox vaccine	(mixed lymphocyte
Concanavalin A	Purified protein derivative	culture)
Other bean extracts	Tetanus toxoid	Allogeneic lymphatic
Trauma	Streptolysin O	lymphoma (of B-cell
Trypsin	Penicillin	derivation)
Chymotrypsin	Antigen-antibody	Allogeneic epithelial cell
Papain	conjugates	Any cell in monolayer
Hg^{2+}, Zn^{2+}	Protein-carrier-hapten	culture (in vitro
Peroxidase	conjugate	sensitization—fibroblasts,
Low-energy sonication	*Antisera*	tumor cells)
Microwave irradiation	Rabbit antihuman	*Self-antigens*
Supernatants of activated	leukocyte serum	Isogeneic cells in monolayer
lymphocytes (blastogenic or	Rabbit antirabbit	culture (in vitro
mitogenic factor)	immunoglobulin allotype	sensitization—reticulum
	sera	cells, fibroblasts)
	Sheep antirabbit	
	immunoglobulin sera	
	Monkey antihuman	
	immunoglobulin sera	

cyte surface antigens) and heterologous anti-IgG (reacting with surface IgG of presumably only B cells). In addition, certain forms of sublethal cellular injury can trigger blastogenesis.

The mechanism of triggering lymphocyte activation remains undiscovered. Interest in mitogen-induced pathways stems from belief that in vivo antigen-induced activation is similar.

Functional characteristics of lymphocytes activated in vitro have only recently aroused research interest. Supernatants of lymphocytes activated by most of the above methods contain nonimmunoglobulin factors that exert in vitro effects resembling cellular or delayed hypersensitivity reactions. These effector substances, generically called *lymphokines,* are assayed by the biological effect they produce: Lymphotoxin (LT) causes target cell death in vitro [137]; migration inhibitory factor (MIF) inhibits macrophage migration [33]; chemotactic factors cause local accumulation of polymorphonuclear (PMN) cells or macrophages [139]; inhibitor of DNA synthesis (IDS) inhibits proliferation of lymphocytes [69]; proliferation inhibitory factor (PIF) inhibits multiplication of HeLa cells [55]; blastogenic factor (BF) or mitogenic factor (MF) induces blastogenesis or mitosis in lymphocytes in vitro [58]; skin reactive factor (SRF) induces local erythema when injected intradermally [114]; lymph node permeability factor (LNPF) increases the influx and efflux of cells into lymph nodes, usually resulting in larger nodes [145]; osteoblastic factor (OF) activates osteoclasts [68]; and soluble T-cell factor(s) induces B cells to antibody production [41]. Lymphokines show no specificity in reacting with their targets; specificity is exerted at the initial triggering event, antigen or activator recognition.

Two additional factors are antigen specific: *transfer factor* (TF), which stimulates other lymphocytes to undergo clonal proliferation in response to a specific antigen [85]; and *specific macrophage arming factor* (SMAF), which confers specific macrophage-mediated cytotoxicity against the target cell used for immunization [37].

In vitro systems for inducing a primary antibody response have been described and partially characterized. The hemolytic response of mouse lymphocytes to sheep erythrocytes requires the participation of three cells, one a macrophage and the other two presumably T and B cells, and necessitates in vitro proliferation of the lymphoid cells [104]. Secondary in vitro responses to antigen are easier to induce, but again cell proliferation precedes antibody detection.

A major difficulty in investigating the activation process is the multiplicity of lymphocyte types and the diversity of their reactions. It is not clear whether an activator induces all the above changes directly, in all or most cells, or induces one reaction in one cell and a different reaction in another.

Lymphocyte Activation In Vivo

An animal immunized with antigen exhibits little evidence of an immune response for four to six days. Immediately thereafter, antibody-forming cells, serum antibody, and cytotoxic cells appear. These specific immune cells or antibody result from the proliferation and the differentiation of the few antigen-sensitive T and B cells initially reacting with the antigen.

The marked heterogeneity of antibodies to a single haptenic determinant and the fact that an antibody-producing cell makes only a single type of antibody molecule indicate that there are many different antigen-sensitive B and T cells capable of responding to a single hapten-carrier conjugate. B cells differ in the immunoglobulin class (IgM, IgG, IgA, IgD, or IgE), subclass (G_1, G_2, G_3, G_4), or avidity (strength of binding of antigen to antibody, a measure of the "molecular fit") of the antibodies produced.

Adoptive transfer experiments into irradiated syngeneic hosts show that an animal must be immunized for 48 hours before it can serve as a carrier-primed T-cell donor for antihapten production, suggesting that initially the number of carrier-specific T helper cells is rate limiting for B-cell stimulation of antibody synthesis. As the numbers of helper T cells become adequate, the diverse hapten-sensitive B cells undergo proliferation. After a few days, both antibody-forming cells and memory B cells appear. Once a cell has differentiated into the antibody-forming precursor stage, its life span is limited; it will undergo about three more divisions to form a plasmacyte, with a life span of about two weeks.

Williamson and Askonas traced the history of an antibody-producing clone of cells in vivo and established the existence of B memory cells [144]. The following characteristics of the B memory cell were inferred: Initial contact with antigen induces multiplication of several *different* clones of B cells, each producing antibodies of *differing* immunoglobulin class or avidity. In the absence of antigen, cells responsive to hapten remain viable for at least one month but no longer than 60 to 70 days. Cells can be passaged and stimulated with antigen about every 26 days for six months, during which time only those clones producing antibody of the highest avidity survive; the others are suppressed. The reason is presumably that the cells producing the most avidly binding antibodies sequester *all* the antigen, leaving none available to stimulate the other cells. The amount of antibody formed upon transfer finally declines and stops on the eighth passage. The ability to form monoclonal anti-DNP antibody dies out, a phenomenon interpreted as showing a finite life span, or in vivo senescence, of a single antibody-forming clone of cells. Further antibody response to the same antigen can come about only by the emergence of new, unprimed ASC from the bone marrow.

Knowledge about the clonal replication and functional characteristics of T cells is scant. Memory cells exist for T cells, but their proliferative characteristics and life span are unknown. Antigenic stimulation results in an initial proliferation (progeny restricted to memory cells?) and, after two or three days, the appearance of memory, helper, and effector functions. There is some evidence that an effector cytotoxic T cell has a limited life span, with no reproductive capacities, making it analogous to the plasmacyte.

Efferent Phase—The Expression of Immunity

The aim of the entire immune response is to dispose of a foreign substance. This task is accomplished by (1) clonal proliferation of specifically sensitized lymphoid cells that react with, or produce immunoglobulins that react with, the antigen, (2) recruiting a nonspecific cellular response (lymphoid, macrophage, or PMN) by lymphokines secreted by activated T cells, or (3) activating a general inflammatory response involving four cascading systems normally present in blood: coagulation, fibrinolysis, complement, and kinin generation. Each category will be discussed as it applies to tissue or cell death.

Specific Immune Cytotoxic Mechanisms

ANTIBODY-MEDIATED TYPES. An antibody is an immunoglobulin that reacts with an antigen. Its operational definition depends on the method of detecting its reaction with antigen. The reactions considered here will be limited to the mechanisms known to cause cell death. The five immunoglobulin classes are categorized according to differences in protein structure which determine the antibodies' ability to bind to various cells (B cells, mast cells, macrophages), complement, and secretory proteins. These variations profoundly affect their biological behavior. The biochemical and functional characteristics of the five major Ig classes are summarized in Table 17-7. IgD and IgA are not known to be involved in cytotoxicity.

1. IgG- and IgM-mediated mechanisms work as follows: Antibodies, mainly IgG and IgM, bind to cell surface antigens and cause

TABLE 17-7. *Chemical and Biological Characteristics of Major Immunoglobulin Classes*

Property	Human Ig Classes				
	IgG	IgM	IgA	IgE	IgD
Heavy chain	γ	μ	α	ϵ	δ
Light chain	κ or λ	κ or λ	κ or λ	κ or λ	κ or λ
Molecular formula	$(\gamma_2\ \kappa_2)$ or $(\gamma_2\ \lambda_2)$	$(\mu_2\ \kappa_2)_5$ or $(\mu_2\ \lambda_2)_5$	$(\alpha_2\ \kappa_2)$ or $(\alpha_2\ \lambda_2)$	$(\epsilon_2\ \kappa_2)$ or $(\epsilon_2\ \lambda_2)$	$(\delta_2\ \kappa_2)$ or $(\delta_2\ \lambda_2)$
Molecular weight $(\times 10^{-3})$	143–149	800–950	158–162	185–190	175–180
Secretory protein	No	No	Yes	No	No
Binds complement to Fc piece	Yes	Yes			
Cell type binding to Fc piece	Macrophage, PMN, B-lymphocyte	Macrophage, PMN	—	Mast cells	—
Physiological functions	Cytotoxicity, placental transfer, suppresses IgM formation	Cytotoxicity, cytophilic activator of phagocytosis	High in body secretions (tears, saliva)	Reagin activity (allergies, hay fever)	Unknown

cell death by *opsonic adherence* to phagocytes, *immune adherence* to macrophages, immune adherence to and activation of nonsensitized B-lymphocytes (*lymphocyte-dependent antibody* lysis phenomenon, LDA), and, finally, operation of the lytic complement sequence. These processes are schematically summarized in Figure 17-7. It is important to realize that the mere interaction of an antibody with a cell surface antigen does not cause cell death. Rather, it acts to link the target to the actual mediators of cytolysis: macrophages, PMN cells, B-lymphocytes, or the complete lytic sequence of complement factors.

Opsonic adherence, the major defense against bacterial invasion, is mediated through either IgG or IgM antibodies. Antibody adhering to the microbe alters its net surface electrical charge, permitting contact with phagocytes.

Immune adherence utilizes receptors on effector cells for antibody or complement to link to target cells. The Fc portions of IgG and IgM carry determinants that are specifically recognized by unique receptors (Fc receptor sites) on macrophages, PMN cells, and B-lymphocytes. Antibodies attach to the antigen by the opposite molecular end, the *Fab portion.* Not all immunoglobulins carry such Fc determinants; those that do are termed *cytophilic antibodies.* Cell destruction occurs either by digestion by lysozymal enzymes from macrophages and PMN or by an unknown mechanism with B-lymphocytes.

Macrophages and PMN cells adhere by still another specific method. These cells have membrane receptors for the C3 component of complement. The combination of IgG and IgM with the antigen induces a conformational change in the Fc portion so that certain serum factors, the complement sys-

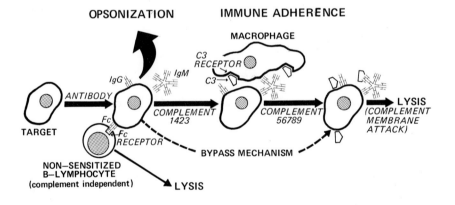

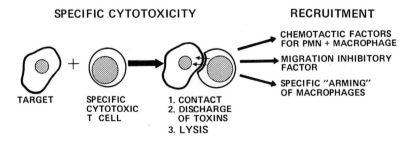

FIGURE 17-7.   *Cellular and humoral mechanisms of immune elimination of cells.*

tem, bind to both the Fc portion and the cellular antigen. Complement activation (Fig. 17-8) is a sequential cascading reaction of nine different components wherein each product acts enzymatically on the next component by peptide or ester bond cleavage. When C3 is added to the growing cellular-antibody-complement complex, macrophages bind to the C3 portion and cause lysis. These mechanisms are termed *immune complex–mediated.*

Continued sequential addition of complement ultimately results in the fixation and activation of the terminal component, an esterase with phospholipase activity causing "holes" visible by electron microscopy in the cell membrane [115]. IgM, having five Fc fragments, is more efficient than IgG in binding complement and hence in cytolysis.

2. Anaphylactic-type mechanisms operate in this way: The IgE class of antibody (IgG$_1$ in guinea pigs and possibly also IgG$_1$ in humans) binds to mast cells or circulating basophilic cells through another specialized region of the Fc fragment. Contact with antigen causes mast cell degranulation and release of vasoactive amines (histamine, serotonin) and the slow-reacting substance of anaphylaxis (SRS-A), which damage tissue by causing ischemia. These antibodies, termed *homocytotropic,* give rise to a variety of

anaphylactic, hay fever, and cutaneous allergic syndromes.

3. The antigen-antibody complex–mediated type takes a different course. By activating complement, immune complexes generate tissue-destroying factors in addition to facilitating macrophage binding. The major effect, the release of Hageman factor, causes localized thrombosis in areas of spasm secondary to bradykinin, anaphylatoxin, or platelet aggregation. The key role of complement in the triggering of the general inflammatory response is shown in Figure 17-9.

CELL-MEDIATED CYTOTOXICITY (T CELL). Histocompatibility-antigen-sensitive T-lymphocytes, upon contact with allogeneic cells, proliferate and differentiate into both memory and effector T cells. The MLC reaction is visualized as the in vitro counterpart of sensitization in vivo. MLC cultures generate cells that incorporate ^{3}H-thymidine (memory cells) and other cells that are cytotoxic to targets with the same histocompatibility antigens. The specific cytotoxic cells cause lysis in even a 10-minute contact with the target. T-cell–mediated cytotoxicity is the major immunopathic process during acute allograft rejection.

Methods for in vitro detection of cytotoxic

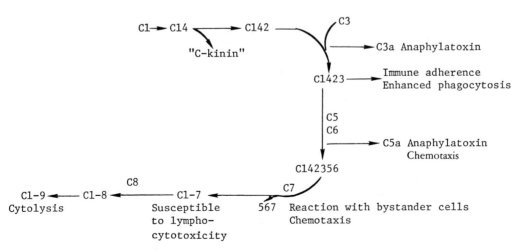

FIGURE 17-8. *Reaction sequence in complement activation.*

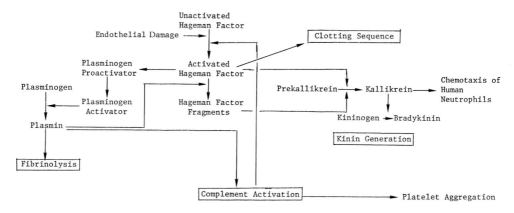

FIGURE 17-9. *Nonspecific humoral effector systems of acute inflammation.*

cells have only recently been developed [19, 60]. In vitro studies establish the sequence of cell lysis: specific contact between the receptors on T cells and cellular antigen, a process utilizing cyclic adenosine monophosphate (cAMP), and the creation of progressively enlarging "holes" in the cell membrane. The latter initially "leak" only low-molecular-weight substances (K^+ ions), but ultimately osmotic lysis occurs (Fig. 17-7, bottom portion). The mechanism of lysis is unclear. Demonstration that cAMP and protein synthesis are required suggests toxin secretion. A toxin has been detected in the supernatants of activated lymphocytes, lymphotoxin, but on in vitro testing it is able to kill *some*, but *not all*, mammalian cells [138]. The fate of cytotoxic lymphocytes is unknown; it is suggested that their half-life is only a few days, that they are consumed in the lytic reaction with target cells, and that they require antigen for continuous generation from memory cells.

Recruitment of Nonsensitized Effector Cells by Lymphokines Secreted by Sensitized T Cells

The histological hallmark of a rejecting graft is the dense mononuclear cell infiltrate; the cells are microscopically heterogeneous—mature antibody-secreting plasma cells, blast cells identical in appearance to mitogen-induced blast cells, monocytes, variable numbers of PMN cells,

and small lymphocytes with compact nuclei. The large numbers of mononuclear cells are several orders of magnitude greater than anticipated from the numbers of cells estimated to bear receptors for the transplantation antigens. The similarity between the sequential histological events during a delayed hypersensitivity skin reaction and during homograft rejection initially provided the basis for classifying homograft immunity as a cellular immune event.

As early as 1942 Landsteiner and Chase transferred contact sensitivity to picryl chloride by peritoneal cells. The skin reaction occurs in two phases: an initial wheal and flare in the area of an immunologically specific infiltrate of mononuclear cells (first 12 hours) followed by maximal induration (in 48 hours). The latter changes are nonspecific and of a secondary inflammatory response. Two decades later, the development of ^{3}H-thymidine labeling techniques of sensitized transferred cells demonstrated that over 90 percent of the cells at the site of a delayed skin reaction were nonspecific and host derived [96]. Antigen interactions with a small number of specifically sensitized cells led to the production of lymphokines that recruited unsensitized cells into the local infiltrate, ultimately causing tissue damage.

Unsensitized cells accumulate by the combined action of MIF and the various chemotactic factors for mononuclear, polymorphonuclear, and eosinophilic cells. In the local area, these cells are initially instructed by other lymphokines (SMAF, transfer factor) or locally produced immunoglobulin (cytophilic antibody, C3 activation) to kill the target specifically. Once activated, macrophages lose their specificity requirements and become cytotoxic for even normal cells in proximity [1, 81]. These substances, acting only over short distances, presumably in tissue extracellular fluids, have not yet been detected in blood.

Activation of the Host's General Inflammatory Response

Two pivotal reactions determine the direction, intensity, and speed with which inflammatory processes are superimposed on the immunological attack against a graft. One is the activation of complement; the other, the extent of vascular endothelial cell injury. The interrelations between complement activation and the clotting, fibrinolytic, and kinin-generating systems are summarized in Figures 17-8 and 17-9. The attachment of a component of complement to antigen-antibody complexes occurs by removal of polypeptides from the inactive form present in serum. The larger portion is incorporated into the growing complex; the smaller polypeptides also have biological activity. Thus, anaphylatoxins cause histamine release and local vascular permeability changes. Other complement split products act as chemotactic factors, leading to influx of PMN leukocytes. This process truly represents a marvelous example of the grand economic design with which various physiological functions are integrated by negative and positive feedback controls.

Such reactions at the endothelial interface between donor and recipient cause clotting via at least three mechanisms: (1) Anaphylatoxin, either directly or indirectly through vasospasm, activates Hageman factor present in endothelial cells; this activation permits thrombin synthesis and the conversion of fibrinogen to fibrin. (2) Massive en-dothelial cell damage directly activates Hageman factor. The result may be catastrophic, with total thrombosis and immediate infarction (see Hyperacute Rejection, below). (3) Immune complexes on the endothelial surface aggregate platelets, releasing vasoactive amines and forming microthrombi varying in platelets and fibrin content. In addition, activated Hageman factor induces kinin generation, which further decreases tissue perfusion and promotes tissue edema. Into this increased extracellular fluid space the chemotactic factors draw the mononuclear cells and PMN leukocytes from the locally slowed circulation.

The liberated Hageman factor simultaneously evokes a counterreaction, plasminogen activation. Plasmin has two major actions: inactivating Hageman factor, which stops further fibrin deposition, and enzymatically digesting the fibrin already deposited. In acute homograft rejection these events occur at a slow rate; thrombosis takes place only at a microscopic level, the fibrinolytic reaction keeping pace with the rate of fibrin deposition. This can be readily detected by the marked increase in fibrin split products in the urine of patients undergoing renal rejection.

We have described in a general way the induction of the immune reactions that cause cellular or tissue destruction. How these mechanisms respond to transplanted organs is of clinical importance. The next section will correlate the pathophysiological responses to both immediate and delayed vascularized grafts with histological and immunological events.

CORRELATION OF PATHOPHYSIOLOGICAL EVENTS WITH IMMUNOLOGICAL PROCESSES DURING REJECTION

Immediately Vascularized Grafts

The precise mechanism of organ graft destruction remains unknown. Only the initial events are immunological and specific; the final events culminating in organ failure constitute the inflammatory defenses against injury of any origin.

Acute Rejection

The earliest physiological change in organ allografts is blood flow alteration. There are variable degrees of afferent vascular spasm with patchy areas of decreased perfusion. These changes, appearing in both isografts and allografts, are attributed to reversible ischemic injury. But in allografts local and reversible perfusion defects continue. The earliest histologically recognized changes occur at the interface between the graft and the recipient's circulation—namely, at the vascular endothelium. Endothelial cells carry histocompatibility antigens and are susceptible to immune attack. Rarely, however, can one see either PMN or mononuclear cells attached to the endothelial cells. Instead, one observes the effects of injury: endothelial cell enlargement with withdrawal of the anchoring process from the basement membrane. The frequent presence of PMN cells in capillary lumina where the endothelium is disturbed may follow, rather than cause, endothelial injury. Partial occlusion of many capillaries, due to the combined effects of endothelial cell swelling, platelet aggregation in areas of stripped endothelium, and arterial spasm, occurs within a few hours of revascularization. The platelet aggregates at this stage are not associated with fibrin and are reversible.

Blood flow in nonimmunosuppressed allografts changes dramatically between the second and fifth days. Progressive afferent vascular spasm ensues, decreasing perfusion to 10 percent or less by the fifth day. Edema, patchy areas of infarction, and ultimately complete cessation of blood flow follow. Since interstitial edema and mononuclear cell infiltration occur before the final event of infarction, it was thought that extrinsic interstitial pressure occluded the vessels. However, the autoradiographic demonstration that ischemia originates from the cortex and is random and limited rather than concentric emphasizes the

role of vascular spasm. The reduction in capillary flow was then attributed to partial occlusion by large, specifically sensitized lymphocytes adhering to the capillary endothelium. Yet the functional abnormalities of increased vascular permeability, vascular spasm, and decreased cortical perfusion occur before anatomical abnormalities can be detected. In this way they resemble immediate hypersensitivity reactions rather than delayed cellular reactions [52].

Mononuclear cells of the lymphocytic series infiltrate the interstitium only after 24 to 72 hours. Recent work suggests that the mononuclear cells, long diagnostic of the rejection process, do not directly damage renal tubular cells [87]. Hattler et al. have shown that MLC-reactive cells disappear from the canine recipient's blood within 24 to 48 hours after grafting and reappear only when blood flow to the graft ceases [59, 103]. The MLC-reactive cells can be recovered from the kidney. Nearly simultaneous with this process is the occurrence of serum factors which block both MLC reactivity and lymphoid cell cytotoxicity. Lymphoid cells removed from a kidney graft undergoing rejection display in vitro MLC reactivity and cell-mediated cytotoxicity (CMC) only after such factors are removed.

The kinetics of two parameters of the immune response to an experimental allografted kidney is illustrated in the top half of Figure 17-10. Specific cytotoxic cells (A) appear in lymph nodes on the third day after grafting and persist for about 10 days. Cytotoxic antibody (B) is not detected until the sixth day. Renal function, as measured by serum creatinine (C), begins to increase on the sixth day, and the kidney becomes functionless on the eleventh or twelfth day [93, 107]. The disappearance of the cytotoxic effector cells and the persistence of the antibody are of major importance.

The in vivo cytotoxicity of T-lymphocyte effector cells in the renal interstitium remains undemonstrated. In fact, the extent of mononuclear cell infiltration is not correlated

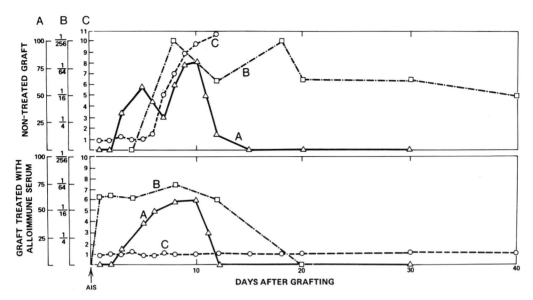

FIGURE 17-10. *Renal function and immunological response to allogeneic renal graft (in rats, Lx BN F₁ kidney to Lewis). Ordinate axis: A. Percent cytotoxicity mediated against donor fibroblasts by spleen cells from the recipient. B. Titer of cytotoxic antibody against donor lymphocytes in serum from the recipient. C. Serum creatinine, mg per 100 ml plasma, from recipients (with bilateral nephrectomy of own kidneys). Upper and lower figures represent animals given nonimmune or alloimmune serum. (Unpublished data of Z. J. Lucas and K. Enomoto.)*

with the ultimate function of the graft. Fibrin deposition in blood vessels and medial necrosis of medium-sized arteries are the only histological features of irreversible rejection.

These observations suggest that allograft destruction results from injury to the vasculature with resultant parenchymal ischemia. Additional evidence indicates that both the clotting and the fibrinolytic sequence of blood reactions accompany acute rejection. Fibrin split products appear in high concentration in the urine from the fourth day on; radio-labeled antifibrin globulins are concentrated in the rejecting kidney of experimental animals but not by the normal kidney [18, 22].

Hyperacute Rejection

Placing an organ in a sensitized recipient almost invariably results in rapid graft destruction. This may be catastrophically rapid—within minutes of grafting (xenograft rejection or hyperacute rejection in allo-

grafts) [130]—or it may evolve over one to two days (accelerated rejection) [91]. In contrast to the success of immunosuppression in the prevention, amelioration, or reversal of acute rejection, no successful method of avoiding rejection in a sensitized recipient has been devised.

Most presensitized recipients have cytotoxic antibody to donor antigens. Its demonstration is the basis for preoperatively identifying presensitized recipient-donor combinations (antibody crossmatch). Transplantation to presensitized recipients is avoided whenever possible. There is a correlation between the level of antibodies against histocompatibility antigens and the rate of second set rejection [91]. Sensitization is presumed to result from multiple transfusions, multiple pregnancies, or a prior rejected allograft. Sensitization is thought to be constitutive in xenogeneic combinations. The initial, and apparently the only necessary, event for beginning accelerated forms of rejection is the reaction of antibody with the vascular endothelium.

Platelet aggregates in capillaries are a prominent feature of rejected xenografts. Marked platelet sequestration also occurs in hyperacutely rejecting allografts in the absence of significant fibrin deposition. Aspirin or heparin in concentrations preventing both platelet aggregation and thrombosis has not prevented such reactions. However, complement depletion or antibody adsorption does result in xenograft prolongation.

The current concept is that antibodies react with transplantation antigens present on endothelial cell membranes, bind complement, and set off a chain of secondary thrombotic and nonspecific inflammatory reactions which involve PMN leukocytes, kinins, platelet factors, leukocytic proteolytic enzymes, and anaphylatoxin components of complement. This rapidly leads to massive thrombosis. If thrombosis is prevented by anticoagulation, tissue perfusion remains at a standstill because of the marked disintegration of endothelium and basement membrane.

"Chronic" Rejection

Sustained low-grade injury to all transplanted organs, regardless of the excellence of clinical function, occurs. Biopsies show varying degrees of interstitial fibrosis and ob-

TABLE 17-8. *Rejection Syndromes in Renal Transplantation*

	Hyperacute	Accelerated	Acute	Chronic
Synonym in skin grafts	"White graft" reaction	Second set	First set	
Onset	1–2 hours	1–4 days	5–8 days	Many months
Predominant cell type	Granulocytes	Granulocytes	Mononuclear cells	Mononuclear cells or very little infiltrate
Pathological feature	Cortical thrombosis	Glomerulonecrosis; vasculitis	Lymphocytic infiltration	Scarred glomeruli; onion peeling of vessels (vasculitis); parenchymal atrophy and scarring
Differential clinical diagnosis	Renal vein thrombosis	Acute tubular necrosis (ATN); acute renal failure (low perfusion); renal artery obstruction	Prolonged ATN; prolonged acute ischemic renal failure	Recurrence of original immune disease
Antibody detected on homograft	Rarely demonstrable	Usually prominent	Rarely	Almost invariably
Antibodies in serum	Positive by cytotoxicity testing	Requires more sensitive assay than cytotoxicity assay	No	MLC-blocking antibodies; lymphocyte-dependent antibody lysis sporadically present

Table 17-8 (continued).

	Hyperacute	Accelerated	Acute	Chronic
Antigen to which immune response is directed	Transplantation; ABO incompatibility	Transplantation	Transplantation	a. Transplantation b. Glomerular basement membrane (original GBM disease) c. Original soluble complex (causing original glomerulonephritis) d. Renal antigen (secondary to release of autoantigens during acute rejection)—an autoimmune disease of the graft e. Newly acquired viral or other antigenemia (new glomerulonephritis) f. Iatrogenic antigen-antibody complex disease, as from horse antilymphocyte serum

literative arteritis [116]. Intimal thickening has been attributed to the chronic organization of microplatelet thrombi adjacent to the areas of endothelial damage. It has been suggested that the hyperacute, accelerated, acute, and even chronic forms of rejection may be various manifestations of a similar injurious process which differs in intensity depending on the amount of alloantibody present to bind to the vascularized graft [91]. Characteristic features of the rejection types described thus far are summarized in Table 17-8.

Delayed Vascularized Grafts

First Set Graft Rejection

Studies on the fate of human skin grafts confirm the observations made in animals. There is no detectable difference in the gross or stereomicroscopical appearance of the microvasculature of autografts or allografts for several days. Each remains blanched for 24 hours, becoming pink by the third or fourth day. Initially, superficial capillaries are dilated and filled with blood. Flow begins on the third to fourth day, becoming generalized in two more days. Autografts have desquamation of the superficial epithelium, with simultaneous regeneration; by the sixth or seventh day the graft and host epidermis merge.

With allografts a halo of erythema and edema becomes increasingly prominent on day 6 to day 7. The color becomes cherry red, then cyanotic. Allografts become progressively more edematous. Cyanosis is followed by hemorrhage, desiccation, and ultimately eschar formation. These changes relate to alterations in the new blood supply; the superficial capillaries progressively dilate, blood flow stops by the eighth or ninth day, and the vessels thrombose shortly thereafter.

Histological changes similar to those in acutely rejecting kidneys occur, with one exception. Mononuclear cell infiltration is distributed in two layers: in the graft, somewhat localized in the subdermal area; and in the top of the host bed, the true interface between donor and host.

Second Set Rejection

The interval between the first and second grafts has a profound effect on the survival of second set grafts. If it is less than seven days following removal of the rejected first graft, a second graft from the same donor induces a *white graft* reaction. The graft never becomes vascularized. Twenty-four hours after placement a prominent band of edema fluid filled with PMN leukocytes separates the graft from the underlying host tissues. Twenty-four hours later, necrosis of the graft with dense infiltration of PMN cells takes place. This corresponds to the hyperacute rejection syndrome in organ grafts.

Extending the interval between grafts beyond 12 days causes an accelerated type of response. The grafts show the usual characteristics of an early take, but the rejection process is telescoped into five to seven days, about four days faster than first set grafts. The histological features, similar to those of acute rejection, occur more rapidly in *accelerated rejection*.

Lastly, if the interval between the two grafts is extended to 80 days, the second set graft rejects the same way a first set graft does.

Differences in Rates of Rejection and in Response to Modification of the Immune Response Between Delayed and Immediately Vascularized Grafts

Allografted skin is more rapidly rejected than other organs, such as kidney and heart, and its survival is less easily prolonged by modifying the immune response. There are many explanations for this phenomenon:

1. The rate of vascularization, slow in skin, may result in ischemic damage with greater vulnerability to immunological attack.

2. Skin has a relatively rich lymphatic drainage system which is rapidly established after grafting. Indeed, Barker and Billingham have demonstrated that the lymphatics are a prime source of sensitization in skin [4]. If skin grafting is performed so as to prevent reestablishment of the lymphatic drainage, survival is prolonged 20 to 50 days. Similar isolations of kidney grafts do not alter rejection rates.

3. Evidence is accumulating that there are quantitative and/or qualitative differences in the antigenicity of skin and other organs [83].

4. Organs with immediate vascularization may evoke more of a humoral than a cellular reaction and thus may autoregulate the immune response.

One approach to this problem was attempted by Gruber and Lucas, who performed four types of skin grafts differing in the rate of reestablishing vascular or lymphatic connections [56]. Schematic summary of the types of grafts is shown in Figure 17-11. The conventional skin graft has

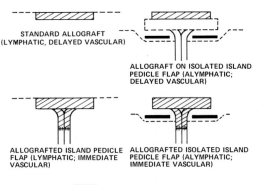

STANDARD ALLOGRAFT (LYMPHATIC, DELAYED VASCULAR)

ALLOGRAFT ON ISOLATED ISLAND PEDICLE FLAP (ALYMPHATIC; DELAYED VASCULAR)

ALLOGRAFTED ISLAND PEDICLE FLAP (LYMPHATIC; IMMEDIATE VASCULAR)

ALLOGRAFTED ISOLATED ISLAND PEDICLE FLAP (ALYMPHATIC; IMMEDIATE VASCULAR)

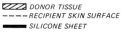

DONOR TISSUE
RECIPIENT SKIN SURFACE
SILICONE SHEET

FIGURE 17-11. *Four possible models of allogeneic skin grafting, employing different combinations of vascular and lymphatic reconstitution. (From R. P. Gruber and Z. J. Lucas. In B. D. Jankovic and K. Isakovic [Eds.],* Microenvironmental Aspects of Immunity. *New York: Plenum Press, 1973. P. 545.)*

TABLE 17-9. *Survival Times of Skin Grafts from LxBN to Lewis Rats Differing in Vascular and Lymphatic Reconstitution*[a]

Treatment	Lymphatic: Vascular:	Conventional Immediate Delayed	Isolated Pedicle Delayed Delayed	Micro-vascular Anas-tomosis Immediate Immediate	Isolated Anas-tomosis Delayed Immediate
No treatment		6, 7, 8, 8, 8, 8, 8, 8	12, 12, 16, 16, 17, 22	6, 7, 7, 7, 7, 8, 9, 9, 9, 9, 9, 9	8, 8, 8, 8, 8, 9
		7.4	15.8[b]	8.0	8.2
Enhancing serum		7, 8, 8, 11	—	9, 9, 9, 10, 10	11, 11, 12, 14, 14
		8.5		9.4	12.4[b]
Cyclophosphamide		10, 11, 11, 12	10, 12	9, 11, 16, 17	6, 6, 7, 7, 7
		11	11	13.3[b]	6.6
Enhancing serum and cyclophosphamide		9, 9, 10, 10, 12, 12	—	10, 13, 13, 13	16, 17, 21, 22
		10.3		12.3[b]	16.5[b]

[a]Individual survival times in days. Mean survival time is underlined.
[b]Statistically different from conventional grafts or from untreated grafts of the same type by the Mann Whitney U test; $p \leq .01$.
Source: From unpublished results of K. Wustrack and Z. J. Lucas.

immediate reestablishment of lymphatic drainage, but vascularization occurs on the fourth to fifth day. An allograft placed on an isolated island pedicle flap, with lymphatics stripped from the sole artery and vein and prevented from reestablishing connections by a silicone sheet placed between the flap and its bed, has both delayed lymphatic and delayed vascular connections (Barker-Billingham technique). A skin graft pedicle with its central blood vessels anastomosed to the femoral vessels of the recipient creates both immediate lymphatic and vascular connections. Lastly, an allogeneic pedicle may be directly anastomosed to recipient vessels but have other contact prevented by a silicone sheet interposed between graft and host. In this case there is immediate vascularization with delayed lymphatic connection. Table 17-9 presents the MST of such grafts from

Lewis x Brown Norway F_1 hybrids (LBN) to parental (Lewis) rats. Without therapy, only delay in reconstitution of *both* lymphatic and vascular connections affects survival, the implication being that the lymphatic and vascular routes are both equally effective in inducing sensitization. The relative importance of vascular or lymphatic connections with respect to the effects of immunosuppression and enhancement will be discussed in subsequent sections.

REGULATION OF THE IMMUNE RESPONSE

Autoregulation of the Immune Response

A central feature of the immune response is that under ordinary conditions an animal does not develop effector cells or antibodies reacting against its own antigens. In the last 20 years the concept has emerged that, although the host has the capacity to react against itself, it doesn't do so because a state of "natural tolerance to self-antigens" exists. Its termination results in *autoimmunity*. Autoimmunity is most readily initiated when the host contacts an antigen related to, or cross-reacting with, a tissue constituent. Clinically, this occurs occasionally by infection with streptococci (which share determinants with HL-A and myocardial antigens) or trauma. An example of the latter is *sympathetic ophthalmia*, a severe inflammation of the uveal tract of the uninjured eye occurring four to seven days after an injury involving the uveal tract of the other eye.

An operational basis for the study of autoregulation of the immune response was provided by Burnet and Fenner, who postulated that exposure of primitive antigen-sensitive cells to antigen in early fetal life would render those cells incapable of clonal multiplication [24]. The continuous presence of self-antigens would then forever prevent the emergence of such "forbidden clones" of cells responding to self-antigens. This prediction was proved correct when Billingham, Brent, and Medawar induced *tolerance* or *immunological unresponsiveness* in mice to histocompatibility antigens by neonatal injection of viable lymphocytes [15]. Since then, immunological unresponsiveness has been induced to a variety of antigens in neonatal animals and, under certain conditions, in adult animals. Its initiation is dependent on the nature of the antigen, its dose, and the immunocompetence of the animal.

Another state of unresponsiveness, *immunological enhancement*, is mediated by antibody reacting with the specific antigen. This was first noted in 1903 when Flexner and Jobling observed that tumor injected into animals simultaneously with immune serum from other animals dying of the same tumor grew much faster than in animals injected with nonimmune serum or sera from animals injected with other types of tumors [43]. En-

hanced tumor growth was subsequently found to result from further inhibition of an already ineffectual immune response, leading to earlier death of the animal.

Antibody suppression of antibody synthesis is seen in other situations, as part of the natural temporal sequence of the immune response and as a result of experimental manipulation. Thus, early IgM synthesis is shut off by later IgG synthesis; also, IgG antibody of high avidity for antigen shuts off production of IgG of lower avidity. Similarly, mice given antisheep RBC simultaneously with immunization with sheep RBC do not develop hemolysins or hemagglutinins to sheep RBC. This section will discuss basic concepts concerned with four aspects of immunological unresponsiveness to specific antigens: tolerance, the maintenance of unresponsiveness to self-antigens (autoimmunity), immunological enhancement, and antibody suppression of antibody synthesis.

Tolerance

THE ABSENCE OF REACTIVE CELLS. The first systematic explanation of immunological tolerance to self-antigens was incorporated into Burnet's clonal selection theory [24]. Burnet suggested that during early life, before maturation of the immune process, animals develop a specific unresponsiveness to their own body components. The mechanism of how they do so is unknown. Presumably, antigen combines with the receptors of primitive antigen-sensitive cells (ASCs) and eliminates them before lymphocytes become immunocompetent. These ASC were "forbidden clones." In 1953 Medawar's group realized Burnet's prediction that exposure of immunologically immature animals (fetuses or neonates) to foreign antigens would render them subsequently unresponsive to that antigen in adult life [14].

CONDITIONS AFFECTING INDUCTION, MAINTENANCE, AND REVERSAL OF IMMUNOLOGICAL TOLERANCE. In the last two decades a great deal of work has been expended in defining the tolerant state induced not only by neonatal exposure to antigen but also by manipulations of the immune system in adult animals. The induction of tolerance depends on (1) the immunocompetence of the host, (2) species and strain of animal, and (3) nature, dose, and route of administration of the antigen. The following general facts have emerged:

1. It is easier to induce tolerance in immunologically incompetent animals than in normal adults. Methods utilized to abolish or to interfere with the immunocompetence of the host just prior to the administration of antigens are irradiation [35], immunosuppressive drugs [121], thoracic duct drainage [123], and treatment with antilymphocyte globulin (ALG) [148]. Thus, all rabbits given 500 rads of whole-body irradiation and injected two to seven days later with bovine serum albumin (BSA) did not form antibody to a subsequent injection of BSA given in Freund's adjuvant two months later [88, 141].

Only six drugs (or classes of drugs) have been demonstrated capable of inducing specific unresponsiveness to soluble antigens: 6-mercaptopurine (and presumably azathioprine) [121], amethopterin [5], cyclophosphamide [98], cytosine arabinoside [53], and acriflavine [39].

2. The ease of immunological tolerance depends upon the species and strain of animal. Completely unresponsive states of long duration can be induced in rabbits and mice, similar shorter states in guinea pigs, and only hyporesponsive states in chickens [141]. Even greater variation occurs among various strains within a species. Cross-mating these strains suggests that unresponsiveness is inherited.

3. The nature, dose, and route of administration of antigen are major factors in the degree and the duration of tolerance. Many protein antigens can aggregate in concentrated solution to form polymers. In general, the aggregated or polymeric forms are excellent *immunogens* (a form of a substance that induces immunity); deaggregated or monomeric forms of the same antigen are more likely to induce unresponsiveness to a subsequent injection of the immunogenic form. These are called *tolerogens* (a form of antigen that induces tolerance). Examples of immunogens and tolerogens are aggregated and deaggregated gamma globulins and serum albumins.

Antigen rapidly equilibrating between vascular and extravascular spaces is likely to induce tolerance, presumably because the antigen comes in contact with all antigen-reactive cells. Heterologous serum proteins, contrasting with bacterial and viral antigens or heterologous erythrocytes, are examples of substances to which tolerance is readily induced. Erythrocytes are rapidly removed from blood, do not equilibrate between the vascular and extravascular compartments, and usually induce only hyporesponsive states.

A substance has to be metabolizable in order to be immunogenic. Various bacterial polysaccharides (pneumococcal polysaccharide, detoxified *Escherichia coli* endotoxin) or synthetic polypeptides composed of D-amino acids are not degraded by mammalian enzymes; they persist in tissues for extremely long times. Very small doses of these materials induce unresponsiveness of long duration.

In general, the larger the dose of tolerogen injected, the more complete and the longer the duration of unresponsiveness. With certain antigens there appear to be two dosage ranges, one high and one low, that induce tolerance, and an intermediate dose of antigen that induces immunity. This is not the case when a completely deaggregated antigen is used and may reflect a competition between antigen-sensitive cells and the tolerogenic and immunogenic forms of the antigen [141].

Intravenous administration of antigen is required for tolerance induction because of the rapid distribution of antigen to all antigen-reactive cells.

Although induced tolerance is often maintained for long periods, immunity returns without further administration of tolerogen. Spontaneous termination of tolerance coincides with the disappearance of antigen from tissue fluids. Injection with a chemically altered tolerogen or antigens cross-reacting with the tolerogen may immunologically terminate tolerance at any time. The techniques for terminating tolerance are the same methods that induce autoimmunity, or the loss of tolerance to self-antigens. This is a fact of major interest.

THE PRESENCE OF NONREACTIVE CELLS. The finding that antibody response is most readily explained by the mode in which the antigen was presented, either on the surface of helper T cells or macrophages or in an aggregated state, requires modification of the "forbidden clone" theory. Thus, an antigen-sensitive lymphocyte, upon contact with an antigen, has essentially two courses of action: to become unresponsive (or tolerant) or to become responsive (or activated). The course taken is a property of the antigen rather than the ASC [105, 141]. It must be realized that, experimentally, to distinguish between the absence of reactive cells and the presence of nonreactive cells is very difficult.

THE PRESENCE OF IMMUNOLOGICALLY ACTIVE LYMPHOCYTES BLOCKED BY SERUM FACTORS. The Hellstroms detected cytotoxic lymphocytes in mice rendered tolerant by neonatal injection of allogeneic lymphoid cells [61]. Furthermore, sera from such "tolerant" animals prevented the cytotoxic cells from destroying the targets. These experiments suggested that tolerance was a variant of immunological enhancement and mediated by antibody.

Medawar's group reexamined the murine system used by the Hellstroms and found that their animals were only *partially* tolerant [12]. By varying the numbers of injected cells into the newborn mice, they induced different degrees of partial or complete tolerance as assessed by duration of skin graft survival. Cytotoxic cells were detected only where tolerance was partial; blocking factors were seen only with very minimal states of unresponsiveness, and then as a transient phenomenon. Characteristics of various immunological unresponsive states are summarized in Table 17-10. Complete or true tolerance is still best characterized as an *unresponsive* state, an inhibition of the central phase of immune reactivity.

SUPPRESSIVE OR REGULATORY EVENTS ON IMMUNE REACTIONS MEDIATED BY LYMPHOCYTES. Various findings suggest the possibility of a lymphocyte population involved in actively promoting tolerance or in suppressing the normal immune response. Thus, if an animal made tolerant to an antigen is irradiated before being challenged with the antigen, tolerance can be terminated [40]. Perhaps an x-ray–sensitive cell maintains the tolerant state. Similarly, Cohen and Wekerle's sensitization in vitro against both syngeneic and isogeneic cells (e.g., self-antigens) demonstrates that tolerance can be overcome without a new generation of bone marrow–derived primeval lymphocytes [29].

There is direct evidence for a population of regulatory lymphocytes functioning as a control system for tolerance. "Suppressor" cell activity has been found in antigen competition systems, tolerance to soluble and cellular antigens [48, 49], allotype suppression [71], nonreactivity to autoantigens [97], and the "immunosuppression" accompanying graft-vs.-host (GVH) reactions [57]. Unresponsiveness cannot be broken by transfer of normal or even immune syngeneic cells. Thus, one subpopulation of T cells is required for helper function and another to suppress antibody formation. Nonreactivity is dominant over reactivity.

Autoimmunity

During early life, before maturation of the immune mechanism, animals develop specific unresponsiveness to most of their self-

TABLE 17-10. *Summary of Characteristics of Immunologically Unreactive States*

State	Method of Induction	Immunological Reactivity to									
		Histocompatibility Antigens						Other Antigens	Lymphocyte Chimera	Serum Blocking Factors	Suppressor Cells
						Graft Survival					
		MLC	CMC	GVH	Antibody	Kidney	Skin	Antibody			
Normal	—	+	+	+	+	No	No	+	No	No	No
Natural tolerance to self-antigens	—									No	Yes
Experimentally induced tolerance											
a. Partial	Low-dose antigen (as, 10–25 × 10⁶ cells); neonate	+	+ (some animals)	n.t.a	n.t.	n.t.	Slight increase	n.t.	Slight	Transient, in animals without CMC	n.t.
b. Complete	High-dose antigen; neonate or immunosuppressed adult	−	−	−	−	Long survival	Long survival	No	Yes	No	Yes
Enhancement	Immune serum	+	+	+	+	Long survival	Little or no increase	No	No	Yes	No

a n.t. = not tested.

315

antigens. Available data suggest that this results from direct contact between the self-antigen and the receptors on the antigen-sensitive cells. The unresponsive state is maintained by persistent levels of the self-antigen in tissue fluids, present in a *tolerogenic* form.

As discussed in the section on Tolerance, the same manipulations leading to terminating induced tolerance result in the induction of autoimmunity. From such studies, Chiller et al. postulated that natural tolerance to self-antigens is due to the inability of T cells to function because they have been made unresponsive [27]. Numerous experiments demonstrate that B cells properly stimulated with adjuvant can respond to self-antigens.

Any manipulation bypassing T-helper function should elicit autoantibody formation. Three major methods are recognized: virus infection, modification of a self-antigen by a hapten or drug, and effects of allogeneic cells and adjuvants. Also, it is well recognized clinically that many human virus infections are sometimes followed by autoimmune phenomena (antibody-mediated thrombocytopenia; Coombs' positive hemolytic anemia).

Induced immune thyroiditis best illustrates hapten-induced autoimmunity. Rabbits sensitized to a hapten on one carrier will develop antithyroglobulin and thyroiditis when injected with the same hapten covalently linked to rabbit thyroglobulin [140]. Human examples are the hemolytic anemia observed in some patients treated with α-methyldopa and the lupus-like syndrome associated with hydralazine or isoniazid.

Lastly, injections of allogeneic cells may eliminate the requirement for helper T cells. The ongoing, immunologically irrelevant T-cell activation nonspecifically stimulates B cells to synthesize antihapten antibody. Immunological adjuvants stimulate T cells nonspecifically, causing lymphoblastic transformation and proliferation. Adjuvants capable of bypassing specific T-cell requirements for antibody synthesis are complete Freund's adjuvant (heat-killed mycobacteria, light mineral oil, and emulsifier), pertussis vaccine, and *Corynebacterium parvum* vaccine.

Immunological Enhancement

The concept that passive immunity can block active immunization was established over 60 years ago [127]. The term *immunological enhancement* is restricted to the indefinitely prolonged survival or the delayed rejection of allografts resulting from the presence of specific antigraft antibody in the host [74]. The mechanism is unknown except that it is mediated by antibody. This is a sine qua non, separating enhancement from immunological unresponsiveness (tolerance).

Several centers began clinical application of this principle in the 1960s by using Rh immunoglobulin to prevent Rh sensitization in nonimmunized Rh-negative mothers [46]. Marked clinical success resulted; of a total of 582 Rh immunoglobulin–protected, Rh-negative mothers (with Rh+ fetuses), none was actively immunized; 65 of 537 control mothers became actively immunized to Rh antigen [45].

GENERAL FEATURES OF GRAFT SURVIVAL. Enhancement was first observed with tumor grafts, where much of the initial work was done. Accelerated growth of strain-specific tumors occurs in allogeneic recipients that have been pretreated with an antiserum directed against the tumor (passive enhancement) or with injection of antigenic material derived from the tumor genotype (active enhancement). Accelerated tumor growth represents a more successful "take" of the tumor graft. Different tumor cell types show a large variability in their response to enhancing antibodies in vivo. In general, the more sensitive the cell is to lysis by cytotoxic antibodies in vitro, the more difficult the attainment of enhancement in vivo.

Until recently, the application of passive immunity to tissue grafts other than tumor cells has been only partially successful. Brent and Medawar prolonged skin graft survival by pretreating incompatible hosts with either passively administered antibodies or lyophilized tissue, but the effect was of short duration [21].

OPTIMAL PRETREATMENT WITH ANTIGEN FOR ACTIVE ENHANCEMENT OR PREPARATION OF SERUM FOR PASSIVE ENHANCEMENT. Enhancement is an interplay between the antigen, the antibody it elicits, and the host cellular immune response. The type of antigen and the route by which it is administered largely determine the optimal timing for grafting. Sensitization by allogeneic lymphocytes or solubilized antigen given intravenously does not elicit a cytotoxic cellular response. Kidneys will have prolonged survival if placed three to six days after one intravenous injection or seven days after two intravenous injections 14 days apart. Sera

obtained at those times from the sensitized animals will passively confer indefinite enhancement [36]. These results are illustrated in Figure 17-12. In this system transferable enhancing activity is detected before cytotoxic antibody.

Other methods of inducing sensitization (e.g., repeated intradermal inoculations of lymphocytes with or without Freund's adjuvant, primary skin or kidney graft) do generate cytotoxic lymphocytes and a hyperimmune humoral response with high titers of hemolytic, cytolytic, and agglutinating antibodies. A test graft placed too soon after such stimulation experiences accelerated rejection, but as the time interval between sensitization and grafting increases, enhancement occurs.

Skin grafts are much more difficult to enhance than either kidney or heart grafts in the same experimental model. Comparison

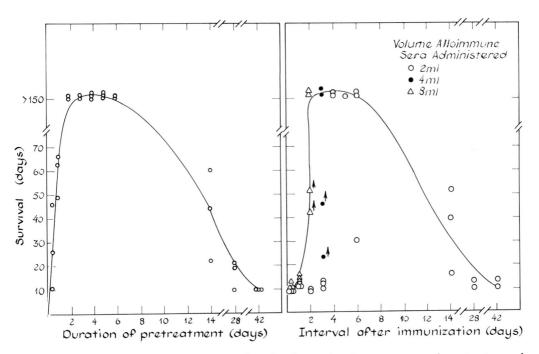

FIGURE 17-12. *Survival of allogeneic renal grafts after antigenic pretreatment of varying intervals between pretreatment and grafting (left) or administration of alloimmune sera obtained at varying intervals after single intravenous immunization with BN spleen cells (right). ↑ indicates animals still surviving (but less than 150 days when the graph was charted). All grafts were LxBN F$_1$ hybrid to Lewis. (From K. Enomoto and Z. J. Lucas,* Transplantation *15:8, 1973.)*

of survival times of grafts surgically anastomosed so that rates of reestablishment of lymphatic and vascular supply differ shows that *only* simultaneous delay in establishing *both* circulations increases survival (Table 17-9). Sensitization by either vascular or lymphatic routes seems equally efficient. Enhancing serum prolongs graft survival in grafts having immediate vascular continuity, but significantly more so in grafts with delayed lymphatic connections. This last group most closely resembles the renal graft. The results suggest that in vascularized grafts the reaction occurring between endothelial cells and antigen-sensitive lymphocytes is most important in effecting enhancement.

CHARACTERIZATION OF THE ANTIBODY(IES) MEDIATING ENHANCEMENT. Transferable enhancing activity has many serological characteristics of immunoglobulin: stability for prolonged times in the frozen state, activity in small amounts, timing of appearance after immunization, and exquisite specificity for the mismatched antigens. Kaliss presented the first evidence that antibodies mediate enhancement [73]. However, investigations of over a decade have not further characterized enhancing antibody.

Suppression of Antibody Synthesis

The regulation of antibody synthesis remains incompletely understood. Since an antigen elicits antibody production, it is plausible to suppose that the removal of antigen inhibits antibody synthesis. Uhr and Moller conclude that newly synthesized antibody binds the immunizing antigen, resulting in less and less available to stimulate antibody production [136]. This regulation of antibody synthesis by the antibody itself is termed *feedback inhibition*.

A study by Wigzell is a prototype of many in vivo experiments on antibody's regulatory role on its own synthesis [143]. Mice given sheep RBC (SRBC) begin a 19S antibody response after two days with the characteristic rise and subsequent fall at four weeks, at

which time the 7S response begins. If anti-SRBC serum is given at four weeks, the 7S response fails to appear. The 19S response can also be suppressed, but only after a 48-hour lag. If antibody is added after the 7S antibody appears, a 48-hour lag also elapses before shutdown. Several months after antigen stimulation, no dose of antibody will eliminate 7S antibody. Since the majority of rodent plasma cells have life spans of about 48 hours, it appears that an antibody-producing cell cannot be stopped while making its product. Antibody could interfere with cells not yet stimulated by the antigen by removal of that antigen.

Late 7S antibody to SRBC was more effective than early 7S or 19S antibody in inhibiting the immune response. Since late antibody is known to be of higher affinity than early antibody, its efficiency presumably results from better antigen removal. Memory lymphocytes apparently have surface antibody molecules which, upon interaction with the specific antigen, lead to synthesis of antibody with affinity similar to that of the receptor. The most efficient antibody to compete with the lymphocyte receptor for antigen would be late, high-affinity 7S antibody.

IDIOTYPIC ANTIBODIES. Idiotypic antibodies are a homogeneous population of immunoglobulins that induce antisera in another animal of the same immunoglobulin allotype. Other homogeneous antibodies such as myeloma protein, Bence Jones protein, and pathological macroglobulins also induce antisera, as has been shown in heterologous species, which cannot be adsorbed out with normal, pooled immunoglobulin. Antibody to which antisera are raised in heterologous species is said to possess *individual antigenic determinants*, while antibody to which antisera are raised in homologous species is said to possess *idiotypic determinants*. Regardless of the species raising the antisera, the antigenic determinants are probably the same or very similar [67].

Since the discovery of immunoglobulins, homogeneous antibodies have been sought to determine amino acid composition and molecular structure. Human myeloma proteins and artificially induced mouse myelomas have led to homogeneous antibody populations for sequencing studies. These pathological antibodies are postulated to be the product of a single clone of antibody-producing cells.

The area of the idiotypic antibody which is most likely to be responsible for its antigenicity is the variable N-terminal region because antisera may be raised in animals of the same allotype as the donor. Rabbits of the same allotype have the same constant regions for H and for L chains. Brent and Nisonoff showed that the combining site is part of or near the idiotypic determinant [20]. Rabbit donor antibody against *p*-amino benzoic acid (PABA) conjugated to bovine gamma globulin was injected as a complex polymerized with glutaraldehyde into rabbits of the same allotype as the donor. Between four and six weeks antibody to anti-PABA was detected. However, if PABA were added, the hapten strongly inhibited precipitation of the antibody and antiantibody. The combining site was thus concluded to be the idiotypic site.

SUGGESTED MECHANISMS FOR ANTIBODY REGULATION OF THE IMMUNE RESPONSE. The previous two sections stress that the immune response is biphasic (initially cellular, then humoral) and cyclic. Enhancement of organ grafts depends on a diminished cellular immunity, increased humoral antibody, probably high avidity, and low cytotoxic efficiency.

Historically, enhancing sera has been thought to act at any of the three sequential phases of the immune response: afferent, central, or efferent. Current views suggest that all phases are affected. It is now clearly established that, upon injection into a recently grafted animal, enhancing antibody (radio-labeled alloimmune globulin) rapidly binds to the exposed antigens of renal grafts [107]. Decreased cytotoxicity of administered enhancing serum [47] indirectly demonstrates binding of alloantibodies to the graft. Similar results occur with skin grafts, although manifestation of binding to the graft is delayed for four days, coinciding in time with establishment of vascular continuity between graft and host [72]. Data are contradictory for what appears thereafter. Decreased antigenicity of the "enhanced" kidney was observed by one group [107] but not by another group [42]. However, decreased antigenicity is possible since antibody combining with alloantigen on the cell surface in vitro is released into the supernatant culture medium as an altered antigen-antibody complex [42]. This left a viable cell insusceptible to lysis by cytotoxic antibodies (and presumably devoid of histocompatiblity antigens) for four to eight hours, the time necessary to resynthesize such antigens.

Enomoto and Lucas confirmed what had long been suspected [36]. Passively administered enhancing sera cannot prolong renal graft survival in the absence of a host immune response; enhancement does not occur in splenectomized recipients given 10 times as much enhancing serum as nonsplenectomized recipients. It appears as if the spleen responds differently to a stimulus by antigen complexed to alloantibody from the way it does to antigen alone, elaborating a specific immunological factor causing persistent immunological blockade. This sequence suggests that the factor differs from the antibody directed to the mismatched transplantation antigen.

Ramseier and Lindenmann recently observed that F_1 hybrid animals injected with parental strain lymphoid cells develop antibodies specifically reacting with parental receptors or "recognition structures" (RS) for histocompatibility antigens [119]. These RS are analogous to idiotypic antibodies. Anti-RS of the appropriate specificity inhibits GVH reactions in mice and enhances renal graft survival in rats [92]. Because antibodies made to alloantibody can also inhibit these cellular immune reactions [92, 99, 132], immunoglobulin may be the elusive T-cell receptor. It appears that optimal anti-idiotypic antibody response is obtained only when the antibody is aggregated, as on the surface of cellular antigens [67, 92], or polymerized with glutaraldehyde [20, 99].

Thus, a current operational view of immunological enhancement is that passively administered alloantibody rapidly binds to alloantigen on the graft and is released into the circulation as antigen-antibody complexes, eliciting the formation, initially in the spleen, of a second type of antibody, directed against the idiotypic combining sites of the alloantibody or T-cell receptor sites.

Alternative hypotheses suggest that the active inhibitor is the antigen-antibody complex itself [125], acting on cells possessing antigen receptors, which renders the effector cell ineffective. Removal of the complex (as by transfer of washed lymphocyte to in vitro assay tubes) restores activity. These models are presented in Figure 17-13.

In summary, the immune response, like

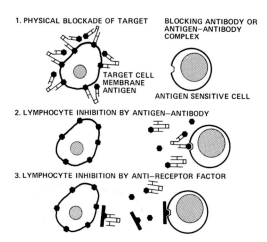

FIGURE 17-13. *Hypothetical models for the mechanism of immunological enhancement.* Physical blockade of target *implies a normally competent sensitized lymphocyte that is prevented from coming into contact with the target cell.* Lymphocyte inhibition by antigen-antibody *or by* antireceptor factor *implies an inactivation of the sensitized lymphocyte.*

blood clotting, hormone release, and other body functions, is physiologically regulated by a complex pattern of positive and negative checks and counterchecks. Antigen and antigen-sensitive T effector, T helper, and B cells furnish positive control. Antibodies of increasing avidity for the antigen (by antigen sequestration), suppressor T cells, and the postulated anti-idiotypic antibodies to antigen-reactive receptors or antibodies provide negative control. Understanding of these mechanisms is far from complete. Such intelligence will provide the future successful use of immunotherapy in organ grafts and cancer treatment.

Extrinsic Regulation

The objective of extrinsic regulation of the immune response in transplantation is to effect graft survival without producing toxicity or crippling body defenses against microbes. Immunosuppressive therapy includes the use of drugs or chemicals, serological agents such as heterologous antilymphocyte globulin, and physical agents such as irradiation. Many different drugs and combined regimens, measuring parameters of skin graft survival, delayed skin reactions, or antibody levels, have been tried experimentally in animals, only to be discarded because any immune suppression coincided with severe leukopenia or thrombocytopenia. This section concludes with a summary of clinically effective immunosuppressive regimens.

Immunosuppression by Drugs

Immunosuppressive drugs cause enzyme inhibition, DNA or RNA template damage leading to reduced or misdirected nucleic acid and protein synthesis, intracellular structural disorganization leading to cell death, or mitotic inhibition.

ANTIMETABOLIC DRUGS. An *antimetabolite* is a substance that can take the place of a natural metabolite in its reaction with an enzyme. This event is possible because the antimetabolite and the natural substrate are structurally similar in the portion of the molecule combining with the active site of the enzyme. Inhibition of a biosynthetic process happens either because the antimetabolite competes with the natural substrate or because it is utilized and a fraudulent (nonfunctional) product accumulates. The fraudulent metabolite may inhibit because it cannot be utilized in subsequent reactions or because it acts as a feedback inhibitor of an earlier step in the reaction sequence.

1. Purine analogues are the most effective immunosuppressant agents available. The synthesis of nucleic acids requires the formation of purine and pyrimidine ribonucleotides from simple precursors, their phosphorylation to triphosphates, and their polymerization to form RNA or DNA. 6-Mercaptopurine (6-MP) is converted to 6-mercaptopurine ribotide, which accumulates because it is not utilized as a substrate for incorporation into nucleic acid chains. High levels of 6-MP ribotide exert an end product feedback inhibition on the first enzymatic step in the synthesis of the purine bases adenine and guanine. Azathioprine, a drug specifically synthesized to decrease the toxicity of 6-MP, is enzymatically converted to 6-MP in vivo. Skin allograft survival has been markedly prolonged in many animal systems with azathioprine; it is the most widely used immunosuppressive drug in clinical organ transplantation. Its end effect inhibits both lymphocyte differentiation into blast or effector cells and lymphocyte replication and clonal expansion.

2. Pyrimidine analogues, 5-fluorouracil, 5-fluorodeoxyuridine, and cytosine arabinoside, have been effective in cancer chemotherapy. They function both as end stage feedback inhibitors of the synthesis of pyrimidine nucleotides and in the substitution as fraudulent bases into nucleic acid templates. These drugs suppress antibody formation in animals but have little effect on prolonging renal grafts in animals.

3. Folic acid antagonists are useful antimetabolic drugs. Methotrexate competitively inhibits the enzyme folic acid reductase, which normally converts folic acid to a cofactor involved in the methylation of nucleic acid bases. It has been used extensively in the treatment of gestational choriocarcinoma. It and other folic acid antagonists (e.g., aminopterin) are potent immunosuppressants in man (as established by antibody formation to tetanus toxoid).

ALKYLATING AGENTS. Alkylating drugs (mechlorethamine, triethylenemelamine, chlorambucil, thiotepa, nitrogen mustard, L-phenylalanine mustard, methylhydrazine, and cyclophosphamide) cross-link the two strands of double-stranded DNA, destroying its template function. The most widely used alkylating agent in both laboratory and clinical transplantation is cyclophosphamide. It effectively suppresses antibody formation in man and has been used extensively as the primary immunosuppressant in human liver transplants. It is superior to azathioprine in hepatic transplants because the latter drug occasionally causes severe hepatic necrosis. In rodent systems cyclophosphamide suppresses the humoral response better than the cellular, whereas azathioprine has the opposite effect. However, combined therapy with both drugs yielded a high incidence of infectious complications in human kidney transplants and has been abandoned [131].

ANTIBIOTICS. Actinomycin D binds to deoxyguanosine residues of DNA, prevents transcription by RNA polymerase, and inhibits both differentiation and replication. In man effective immunosuppressive doses are accompanied by severe bone marrow depression.

STEROIDS. Corticosteroids have long been used in treating "immunological" diseases—asthma, anaphylaxis, severe allergy. When combined with metabolic inhibitors, they are effective agents in prolonging graft survival. The mechanisms by which steroids bring about immunosuppression are unknown. Cortisone destroys a large fraction of both T and B cells, but resistant cells survive to re-populate the lymphocyte pools with undiminished functional capacity.

Prednisone is commonly used as an adjunct to azathioprine in sustained immunosuppression, usually at doses of 0.1 to 0.5 mg per kilogram per day. Acute rejection in patients is treated in one of two ways: Oral prednisone is increased to 1.5 to 6.0 mg per kilogram per day, with stepwise decreases of 0.5 to 1.0 mg per kilogram per day every three to five days until usual maintenance levels are reached. Alternatively, methylprednisolone is given intravenously (1 to 3 gm in 100 ml 5% G/W for 30 minutes) [94, 135]. Large bolus treatment is repeated daily or every other day until rejection is reversed. It is thought that because the half-life of methylprednisolone is short (30 to 90 minutes) the pharmacological side-effects will be minimized while obtaining a maximum lympholytic response. During acute rejection, treatment with daily azathioprine is maintained.

Serological Agents

Heterologous antilymphocyte serum (ALS) has become very important in experimental manipulation of the immune response in animals, although its role in clinical transplantation remains undefined. The long-known fact that specific antibody plus complement could lyse lymphoid cells both in vivo and in vitro provided the rationale for developing ALS. However, following ALS manufacture and application, investigators noted that the immunosuppressive properties of ALS did not correlate with its titer of cytotoxic antibodies (or of any other in vitro measure of antilymphocyte activity) [8]. Currently, immunosuppressive properties of an ALS prepared for clinical use must be tested on skin grafts exchanged between monkeys or directly in man.

Antisera have been made against human splenic lymphocytes [75], lymphoblastoid cells in continuous culture [124], and thymus cells [124] in horses, goats, and rabbits. Globulin fractions containing antibody are purified from the sera for clinical use (antilymphocyte globulin [ALG]).

Two problems emerge for assessing the role of ALG in human immunosuppression. First, ALG is a foreign protein, and, despite concurrent immunosuppression with other drugs as well as the ALG, an immune response, both humoral and cellular, to the heterologous globulin is made. A humoral response rapidly inactivates ALG, leading to its increasing ineffectiveness as an immunosuppressant. Antigen-antibody complexes will also induce serum sickness–like syndromes. Anaphylaxis due to cellular immune reactions may necessitate its discontinuance. Incorporating ultrafilters into the intravenous infusion to remove aggregates has made ALG less immunogenic. Groups attempting to induce tolerance to heterologous ALG by high-dose sustained administration have neither induced tolerance nor achieved longer survivals [50] than centers using it for only the first two weeks after transplantation [95]. Second, because ALG is not suited for long-term treatment, long-term survival may not accurately reflect its short-term immunosuppressive properties. Thus, experienced transplant surgeons note that adding ALG to the regimen of azathioprine and prednisone simplifies the difficulties of shepherding a patient through the high-risk period after transplantation (the first three months). Survival figures at one and two years following transplant reflect only a slight, if any, advantage over azathioprine and prednisone alone [80].

X-Irradiation

Whole-body irradiation provided immunosuppression for the first 34 renal grafts in the 1950s [11, 109]. Because of irreversible bone marrow suppression only 10 percent of the patients survived beyond a few weeks. Death ensued from infection or uncontrolled bleeding. Current application is limited to marrow transplantation (where one wants to destroy *all* leukemic cells in the marrow) and to radiation of the transplanted kidney. Rationale for the latter usage rests on two premises: Effector cytotoxic cells are radiosensitive; and sensitization may be reduced or delayed by eliminating passenger leukocytes in the renal graft. Clinical results have been ineffective, and most centers have abandoned its usage.

Useful Clinical Immunosuppressive Regimens

Transplant recipients require sustained immunosuppression to maintain graft function. The most useful drugs (summarized in Table 17-11) are azathioprine plus prednisone. Cyclophosphamide or methotrexate, at about equal weight doses, can be substituted for azathioprine. Acute rejection occurs 5 to 10 days after grafting in about 85 percent of non-HL-A identical combinations. Treatment by increasing the dosage of azathioprine carries a great risk of severe bone marrow depression. Most centers, therefore, leave the azathioprine dosage unchanged and either increase oral prednisone or give high doses of methylprednisolone intravenously. If renal function continues to deteriorate, ALG may be given alone or in addition to methylprednisolone for the first two weeks to three months after grafting, or until sensitization to heterologous serum protein occurs. With this regimen there are fewer acute rejections. Long-term maintenance rests on "low-dose" Imuran and prednisone. The prednisone dose in many patients with chronically surviving renal grafts is very low (0 to 5 mg per day). However, optimal long-term dosage has not been critically studied; because of the late appearance of "chronic rejection" syndromes that histologically resemble soluble antigen-antibody complex glomerulonephritis, a safer compromise between renal survival and toxic drug effects is 10 to 15 mg per day.

"Graft adaptation," which occurs around the second to third month, is extremely beneficial to the patient and is probably the most important process in renal transplants. After that interval, acute rejection crises are less likely to occur, and high-dose immunosuppression can be reduced to levels compatible with adequate host defenses against opportunistic infections. *Graft adaptation* is a poor term, grouping together aspects of tolerance and enhancement, processes that regulate the recipient's response to the graft.

PARADOXICAL RESULTS OF THE IMMUNE RESPONSE TO TUMOR AND ORGAN GRAFTS

Demonstration of Tumor Immunity

Tumor-specific immunogenicity of most transplantable neoplasms is well established [77]. Although this area had been investigated for over 50 years, it was only 15 years ago that, with the aid of inbred strains of animals, immunity due to tumor-specific transplantation antigens (TSTA) was differentiated from immunity brought about by histocompatibility antigens. The current view is that most, and perhaps all, neoplasms are antigenic in the animal of origin. Only critical detection methods [78] can demonstrate the antigenicity.

Investigation in tumor immunology, which has proliferated markedly in the last five years, is reviewed in detail by Smith [126]. Several general principles emerge from this mass of data: (1) Almost all animal and human tumors are immunogenic to the bearer. (2) Immunosurveillance seems to be an important mechanism in preventing the establishment of potential or nascent tumors. (3) Tumor bearing is associated with apparent nonspecific depression of cell-mediated immunocompetence in the host. This may be due to immunodepressant factors elaborated by tumor cells. (4) Tumors present the host with a heavy and continuously shed burden of tumor cells, cell membranes, cell components, and other products distributed through the blood and lymphatics. (5) Every component of the immune response evoked

TABLE 17-11. *Useful Clinical Immunosuppressive Regimens*

Time	Azathio-prine[a]	Cyclophos-phamide	Prednisone	ALG	Systemic Methyl-prednisolone
Pretransplant	2–4 mg/kg per day for 3 days before				
At time of transplant					1–3 gm IV in 100 ml 5% G/W
Early post-operative maintenance (1–3 months) (daily)	2–4 mg/kg per day (lower limit if ALS is used)	2–3 mg/kg per day (a substitute for azathioprine)	0.5–2.0 mg/kg per day[b] (lower limit if ALS is used)	2–20 mg/kg per day (depends on potency— empirically determined) (2 weeks to 3 months)	
Used in reversal of acute rejection episodes	4–6 mg/kg per day, rapidly decreasing to 2 mg/kg per day				
	2–4 mg/kg per day		2–6 mg/kg per day, tapering by 0.5 mg/kg per day every 3–5 days		
	2–4 mg/kg per day		0.5–2.0 mg/kg per day	2–20 mg/kg per day IV if not included in daily regimen	
	2–4 mg/kg per day		0.5–2.0 mg/kg per day		1–3 gm IV in 100 ml 5% G/W over 30-minute period; daily or every other day until rejection reversed
Late maintenance	2 mg/kg per day[c]		0–0.1 mg/kg per day	None	None

[a]Must be monitored by creatinine clearance, urine output, and WBC. Decrease dosage or use cyclophosphamide if hepatic dysfunction is present.
[b]All patients develop Cushingoid features within 3 months on this dosage; may either lower dosage or use alternate-day therapy (double the dosage but take only on alternate days).
[c]Leukopenia at this dose occurs only if renal or hepatic function is impaired.

by foreign tissue antigens, both cell and antibody mediated, is stimulated by tumors.

The conclusion is that, once established, the tumor and the host act synergistically in favoring growth of the tumor—the tumor contributing through its antigen and special factor-producing capabilities, and the host, paradoxically, through its own highly active immunological machinery.

Given the appropriate immunization procedures, one may demonstrate both inhibition and acceleration of tumor growth. In animals, adoptively transferred lymphoid cells or passively transferred serum from immunized or tumor-bearing animals will inhibit or accelerate tumor growth, respectively. Heppner demonstrated both specific cytotoxicity of autochthonous* lymph node cells of animals with progressively growing mammary tumor virus (MTV)–induced mammary tumors and the blocking of those cytotoxic cells by serum factors from the same animals [62]. The serum factors from MTV-infected mice were uniquely tumor specific. This protective action of serum, also shown in a number of other tumor systems [60], represents an in vitro demonstration of an in vivo mechanism permitting the progressive growth of the tumor in an animal with lymphocytes reactive against the tumor cells.

Examination of a Paradox: Why Tumors to Which Immunity Is Demonstrated Go On to Kill the Host

Solid tumor grafts differ from organ tissue grafts in two major ways: (1) Tumors are comprised of cells with a marked mutational potential and capacity to physiologically adapt to or modify the host environment. (2) The tumor develops its vascular supply from ingrowths of host endothelium. Its blood vessels contain isogeneic rather than foreign histocompatibility antigens.

The growth of a typical solid tumor is conceptualized in Figure 17-14. Exponential rate of growth occurs soon after the initial cell

Autochthonous refers to lymphocytes from the *same* animal from which the tumor was obtained.

undergoes oncogenic transformation. At a mass of about 10^4 cells, growth essentially stops, presumably because a size optimal for diffusion of nutrients into the mass of tumor cells and diffusion of metabolites out of the tumor has been reached. Growth recurs only after host capillaries begin to grow into the tumor. In certain experimental tumors this event coincides with the elaboration by the tumor of a substance that promotes capillary growth (tumor angiogenesis factor [TAF]) [44]. Tumor growth is again exponential until the preterminal state (total body burden of tumor cells about 10^{11}), when the tumor causes general inanition. Clinical detection of most tumor masses occurs with a diameter of 1 cm— about 10^9 cells. Before generalized inanition, tumor-bearing hosts develop a nonspecific depression of cellular immunity which may be due to the release of a specific factor elaborated by tumors (inhibitor of cellular immunity [ICI]). Tests of immune reactivity to tumors or their products have not been correlated with body burdens of tumor cells less than 10^8 to 10^9.

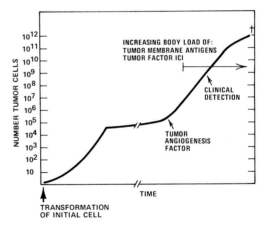

FIGURE 17-14. *Conceptualized growth curve of a solid malignant tumor. Particularly, note tumor growth lags occurring around 10^4 cells, probably related to development of vascular supply, and around 10^{11} cells, where nutrients in the tumor-bearing animal probably become rate limiting. Tumor factor ICI refers to* inhibitor of cellular immunity.

Explanations for the paradoxical ineffectiveness of tumor immunity include the following:

1. General nonspecific depression of the immune response by a tumor product has been detected only in advanced stages of human malignant disease. Lethal tumors can be produced by transplantation of a very few tumor cells so that this cannot be an essential feature of oncogenesis unless local concentrations of such inhibitors are greater than systemic concentrations.

2. The host is unable to recognize the tumor antigen as foreign. Specific tolerance is now considered unlikely as better assays are demonstrating at least qualitatively intact cellular and humoral responses in virtually all systems tested.

3. Antigenicity or modulation of tumor cells is lost [112].

4. The animal is unable to continue producing an immune response to the tumor. The last two possibilities are largely refuted by recent work in which patients with disseminated malignant melanoma responded to autoimmunization with their own tumor cells by producing cytotoxic sera.

5. The tumor acts as an antigen "sponge," soaking up all available antibody, or as an overwhelming antigen source, shedding cells or membranes into the circulation. This action neutralizes specific immunoglobulin receptors on sensitized cells. Tumor cells have been assayed for antibodies contained on their membranes with conflicting results; Fairley et al. found no membrane antibodies by indirect or direct immunofluorescence on malignant melanoma cells [38] whereas Witz et al. found immunoglobulins by extracting benzapyrene-induced primary tumors and spontaneous mammary carcinoma in C3H mice [147].

6. "Enhancing" antibodies are readily formed to tumor cells [106]. As discussed under Immunological Enhancement, above, serum from tumor-bearing animals enhances the growth of their specific tumors in vivo and blocks cellular cytotoxic reactions against the tumor cells in vitro. In addition, Lewis et al. has demonstrated that many patients with localized malignant melanoma have antibodies cytotoxic to their own melanoma cells but lose this antibody when the tumor becomes disseminated [86]. The loss is associated with a new immunoglobulin which precipitates with the cytotoxic antibody in diffusion gels and neutralizes it on cytotoxic assay. This may be an anti-idiotypic antibody.

FUTURE EXPECTATIONS

"We expect too much from the student, and we try to teach him too much. Give him good methods and a proper point of view, and all other things will be added as his experience grows" [113].

Part VI has endeavored to provide a proper immunological point of view. It has presented current views on the cellular and molecular mechanisms constituting the immune response. Considerable insight has been gained in defining the genetic basis of histocompatibility, the requirements for triggering activation of antigen-sensitive lymphocytes, and the functional separation of lymphocytes into T and B cells, and in developing methods for detecting cellular immunity in vitro. Immune response to tumors has been demonstrated. Clinically, transplant surgeons have unknowingly taken advantage of physiological controls on the immune response to judiciously employ poisonous immunosuppressant drugs to effect long-term renal survival. Our knowledge of the intrinsic feedback controls on the immune response should expand in the near future to permit the clinical induction of tolerance or enhancement and to achieve specific, rather than nonspecific, control of the response to a graft. Understanding immune regulatory mechanisms will make it clear why malignancy can circumvent a normally protective immune response. This knowledge will lead to effective combinations of immunotherapy with surgery, radiation, or chemotherapy for the treatment of malignancy.

REFERENCES

1. Alexander, P., and Evans, R. Endotoxin and double stranded RNA render macrophages cytotoxic. *Nature [New Biol.]* 232:76, 1971.

2. Amos, D. B., Seigler, H. F., Southworth, J. G., and Ward, F. E. Skin graft rejection between subjects genotyped for HL-A. *Transplant. Proc.* 1:342, 1969.

3. Bailey, D. W., and Mobraaten, L. H. Estimates of the number of histocompatibility loci at which the Balb/C and C57BL/G strains of mice differ. *Genetics* 50:233, 1964.

4. Barker, C. E., and Billingham, R. E. The role of afferent lymphatics in the rejection of skin homografts. *J. Exp. Med.* 128:197, 1968.

5. Barlow, J., and Hutchin, J. Induction of persistent tolerant infection with lymphocytic choromeningitis virus in adult mice by amethopterin treatment. *Annu. Rep. N.Y. Dept. Health,* 1962. P. 39.

6. Barnett, K., and Hansen, W. H. Undulations in the time-response curve for tumor immunity after primary immunization with washed erythrocytes. *J. Natl. Cancer Inst.* 18:57, 1957.

7. Baronio, G. *Degli Innesti Animati.* Milan, 1804.

8. Barth, R. F., and Corroll, G. F. Immunosuppressive effects of antilymphocyte serum in complement-deficient mice: Evidence that immune cytolysis is not essential for ALS activity. *J. Immunol.* 104:522, 1970.

9. Benacerraf, B., Green, I., and Paul, W. E. The immune response of guinea pigs to hapten-poly-L-lysine conjugates as an example of the genetic control in the recognition of antigenicity. *Cold Spring Harbor Symp. Quant. Biol.* 32:569, 1967.

10. Benacerraf, B., and McDevitt, H. O. Histocompatibility-linked immune response genes. *Science* 175:273, 1972.

11. Berenbaum, M. C. Immunosuppressive agents and allogeneic transplantation. *Symp. Tissue Org. Transplant.* (Suppl. *J. Clin. Pathol.* 20:471) 1967.

12. Beverley, P. C. L., Brent, L., Brooks, C., Medawar, P. B., and Simpson, E. *In vitro* reactivity of lymphoid cells from tolerant mice. *Transplant. Proc.* 5:679, 1973.

13. Billing, R. J., Mittal, K. K., and Terasaki, P. I. Isolation of soluble HL-A antigens from normal human sera by ion exchange chromatography. *Tissue Antigens* 3:251, 1973.

14. Billingham, R. E., Brent, L., and Medawar, P. B. Actively acquired tolerance to foreign cells. *Nature* (Lond.) 172:603, 1953.

15. Billingham, R. E., Brent, L., and Medawar, P. B. Quantitative studies on tissue transplantation immunity: III. Actively acquired tolerance. *Philos. Trans. R. Soc. Lond.* [*Biol.*] 239:357, 1956.

16. Billingham, R. E., Brent, L., Medawar, P. B., and Sparrow, E. M. Quantitative studies on tissue transplantation immunity: I. The survival times of skin homografts exchanged between members of different inbred strains of mice. *Proc. R. Soc. Lond.* [*Biol.*] 143:43, 1954.

17. Billingham, R. E., Krohn, P. L., and Medawar, P. B. Effects of cortisone on survival of skin homografts in rabbits. *Br. Med. J.* 1:1157, 1951.

18. Blaney, R. W., Renney, J. T. G., Baxter, T. J., and Deans, B. J. The use of ^{125}I-fibrinogen in the detection of renal allograft rejection. *Transplantation* 16:5, 1973.

19. Bloom, B. R., and Glade, P. R. (Eds.). *In Vitro Methods in Cell-Mediated Immunity.* New York: Academic, 1971.

20. Brent, B. W., and Nisonoff, A. Quantitative investigations of idiotypic antibodies: IV. Inhibition by specific haptens of the reaction of antihapten antibody with its anti-idiotypic antibody. *J. Exp. Med.* 132:951, 1970.

21. Brent, L., and Medawar, P. B. Quantitative studies on tissue transplant immunity: V. The role of antiserum in enhancement and desensitization. *Proc. R. Soc. Lond.* [*Biol.*] 155:392, 1962.

22. Brown, W. E., and Merrill, J. P. Urine fibrinogen fragments in human renal allografts: A possible mechanism of renal

injury. *New Engl. J. Med.* 278:1366, 1968.

23. Burnet, F. M. *The Clonal Selection Theory of Acquired Immunity.* Nashville, Tenn.: Vanderbilt University Press, 1959.

24. Burnet, F. M., and Fenner, T. *The Production of Antibodies.* Melbourne, Australia: Macmillan, 1949.

25. Carrel, A. La technique opératoire des anastomoses vasculaires et la transplantation des viscères. *Lyon Med.* 98:859, 1902.

26. Ceppellini, R., Mattiuz, P. L., Scudellei, G., and Visetti, M. Experimental allotransplantation in man: I. The role of HL-A system in different genetic combinations. *Transplant. Proc.* 1:385, 1969.

27. Chiller, J. M., Habecht, G. S., and Weigle, W. O. Kinetic differences in unresponsiveness of thymus and bone marrow cells. *Science* 171:813, 1971.

28. Chused, T. M., Steinberg, A. D., and Parker, L. M. Enhanced antibody response of mice to polyinosinic-polycytidylic acid by antithymocyte serum and its age dependent loss in NZB/W mice. *J. Immunol.* 111:52, 1973.

29. Cohen, I. R., and Wekerle, H. Regulation of autosensitization. The immune activation and specific inhibition of self-recognizing thymus derived lymphocytes. *J. Exp. Med.* 137:224, 1973.

30. Converse, J. M., and Carson, P. R. The Historical Background of Transplantation. In Rappaport, F. T., and Dausset, J. (Eds.), *Human Transplantation.* New York: Grune & Stratton, 1968. P. 3.

31. Cooper, H. L. Studies on RNA metabolism during lymphocyte activation. *Transplant. Rev.* 11:3, 1972.

32. Dausset, J., and Colombani, J. Isoanticorps anti-leucocytaires et anti-plaquettaires serologie et importance practique en particulier pour les greefes. Proceedings, 8th Congress, International Society for Blood Transfusion, 1960. *Bibl. Haematol.* 13:324, 1962.

33. David, J. R. Macrophage migration. *Fed. Proc.* 27:6, 1968.

34. Dempster, W. J., Lennox, B., and Boag, J. W. Prolongation of survival of skin homografts in the rabbit by irradiation of the host. *Br. J. Exp. Pathol.* 31:670, 1950.

35. Dixon, F. J., and Maurer, P. H. Immunologic unresponsiveness induced by protein antigens. *J. Exp. Med.* 101:245, 1955.

36. Enomoto, K., and Lucas, Z. J. Immunologic enhancement of renal allografts in the rat: III. Role of the spleen. *Transplantation* 15:8, 1973.

37. Evans, R., and Alexander, P. Role of macrophages in tumor immunity: II. Involvement of a macrophage cytophilic factor during syngeneic tumor growth inhibition. *Immunology* 22:627, 1972.

38. Fairley, G. H., Lewis, M. G., Ikonopisov, R. L., Nairn, R. C., and Alexander, P. Detection of tumor specific immune reactions in human melanoma. *Ann. N.Y. Acad. Sci.* 177:286, 1971.

39. Farr, R. S., Samuelson, J. S., and Stewart, P. B. The suppression of antibovine serum albumin production in rabbits by acriflavine hydrochloride, N.F. *J. Immunol.* 94:682, 1965.

40. Fefer, A., and Nossal, G. J. V. Abolition of neonatally-induced homograft tolerance in mice by sublethal irradiation. *Transplant. Bull.* 29:73, 1962.

41. Feldmann, M., and Basten, A. Cell interactions in the immune response *in vitro:* IV. Comparison of the effects of antigen-specific and allogeneic thymus-derived cell factors. *J. Exp. Med.* 136:722, 1972.

42. Fine, R. N., Batchelor, J. R., French, M. E., and Shumak, K. H. The uptake of ^{125}I-labeled rat alloantibody and its loss after combination with antigen. *Transplantation* 16:641, 1973.

43. Flexner, S., and Jobling, J. W. On the promoting influence of heated tumor emulsions on tumor growth. *Proc. Soc. Exp. Biol. Med.* 4:156, 1907.

44. Folkman, J. E., Merler, E., Abernathy, C., and Williams, G. Isolation of a tumor factor responsible for angiogenesis. *J. Exp. Med.* 133:275, 1971.

45. Freda, V. J., Gorman, J. G., and Pollock, W. Suppression of the primary Rh immune response with passive Rh IgG

immunoglobulin. *N. Engl. J. Med.* 277:1022, 1967.

46. Freda, V. J., Robertson, J. G., and Gorman, J. J. Antepartum management and preventions of Rh isoimmunization. *Ann. N.Y. Acad. Sci.* 127:909, 1965.

47. French, M. E. Antibody turnover in enhanced rat kidneys. *Transplant. Proc.* 5:621, 1973.

48. Gershon, R. K., Lance, E. M., and Kondo, K. Immuno-regulatory role of spleen localizing thymocytes. *J. Immunol.* 112:546, 1974.

49. Gershon, R. K., and Kondo, K. Cell interactions in the induction of tolerance: The role of thymic lymphocytes. *Immunology* 18:723, 1970.

50. Gewurz, H., Moberg, A. W., Johnson, D., Simmons, R. L., and Najarian, J. S. Induction of tolerance to horse gamma globulin (HoGG) and antilymphocyte globulin (HoALG) in humans and experimental animals. *Transplant. Proc.* 3:737, 1971.

51. Gibson, T., and Medawar, P. B. The fate of skin homografts in man. *J. Anat.* 77:299, 1943.

52. Glassock, R. J., Feldman, D., Reynolds, E. S., Dammin, G. J., and Merrill, J. P. Human renal isografts: A clinical and pathologic analysis. *Medicine* 47:411, 1968.

53. Gordon, R. O., Wade, M. E., and Mitchell, M. S. The production of tolerance to human erythrocytes in the rat with cytosine arabinoside or cyclophosphamide. *J. Immunol.* 103:233, 1969.

54. Graff, R. J., Silber, W. K., Billingham, R. E., Hildemann, W. H., and Snell, G. D. The cumulative effect of histocompatibility antigens. *Transplantation* 4:605, 1966.

55. Green, J. A., Cooperband, S. R., Rutstein, J. A., and Kibrick, S. Inhibition of target cell proliferation by supernatants from cultures of human peripheral lymphocytes. *J. Immunol.* 105:48, 1970.

56. Gruber, R. P., and Lucas, Z. J. The Effect of Lymphatic Interruption and Immediate Vascularization on the Afferent Arc of Skin Graft Rejection. In Jankovic, B. D., and Isakovic, K. (Eds.),

Microenvironmental Aspects of Immunity. New York: Plenum, 1973. P. 545.

57. Hardin, J. A., Chused, T. M., and Steinberg, A. D. Suppressor cells in the graft vs host reaction. *J. Immunol.* 111:650, 1973.

58. Hart, D. A., Jones, J. M., and Nisonoff, A. Mitogenic factor from inbred guinea pigs: 1. Isolation of the factor. *Cell. Immunol.* 9:173, 1973.

59. Hattler, B. G., Miller, J., and Johnson, M. C. Cellular and humoral factors governing canine mixed lymphocyte cultures after renal transplantation: II. Cells. *Transplantation* 14:47, 1972.

60. Hellstrom, I., Hellstrom, K. E., Evans, C. A., Heppner, G. H., Pierce, G. E., and Yang, J. P. S. Serum mediated protection of neoplastic cells from inhibition by lymphocytes immune to their tumor-specific antigens. *Proc. Natl. Acad. Sci. U.S.A.* 62:362, 1969.

61. Hellstrom, K. E., Hellstrom, I., and Allison, A. C. Neonatally induced allograft tolerance may be mediated by serum-borne factors. *Nature* (Lond.) 230:49, 1971.

62. Heppner, G. H. Studies on serum-mediated inhibition of cellular immunity to spontaneous mouse mammary tumors. *Int. J. Cancer* 4:608, 1969.

63. Hildemann, W. H. Components and concepts of antigenic strength. *Transplant. Rev.* 3:5, 1970.

64. Hirschhorn, K., Bach, F., and Kolodny, R. L. Immune response and mitosis of human peripheral blood lymphocytes *in vitro. Science* 142:1185, 1963.

65. Hodgers, C. V., Pickering, D. E., Murray, J. E., and Goodwin, W. E. Kidney transplant between identical twins. *J. Urol.* 89:115, 1963.

66. Holman, E. Protein sensitization in iso skin grafting. Is the latter of practical value? *Surg. Gynecol. Obstet.* 38:100, 1924.

67. Hopper, J. E., and Nisonoff, A. Individual antigenic specificity of immunoglobulins. *Adv. Immunol.* 13:57, 1971.

68. Horton, J. E., Raisz, L. G., and Simmons, H. A. Bone resorbing activity in supernatant fluid from cultured human

peripheral blood leucocytes. *Science* 177:493, 1972.

69. Houck, J. C., Irausquin, H., and Leikin, S.   Lymphocyte DNA synthesis inhibition. *Science* 173:1139, 1971.

70. Hume, D. M., and Egdahl, R. H.   Progressive destruction of renal homografts isolated from the regional lymphatics of the host. *Surgery* 38:194, 1955.

71. Jacobson, E. B., and Herzenberg, L. A.   Active suppression of immunoglobulin allotype synthesis: I. Chronic suppression after perinatal exposure to maternal antibody to paternal allotype in (SJL × BALB/c) F_1 mice. *J. Exp. Med.* 135:1151, 1972.

72. Jones, J. M., Peter, H. H., and Feldman, J. D.   Binding *in vivo* of enhancing antibodies to skin allografts and specific allogeneic tissues. *J. Immunol.* 108:301, 1972.

73. Kaliss, N.   Regression or survival of tumor homografts in mice pretreated with injections of lyophilized tissue. *Cancer Res.* 12:110, 1952.

74. Kaliss, N.   The elements of immunologic enhancement: A consideration of mechanisms. *Ann. N.Y. Acad. Sci.* 101:64, 1962.

75. Kashrivagi, N., Brantigan, C. O., Brettschneider, L., Groth, C. G., and Starzl, T. E.   Clinical reactions and serologic changes after the administration of heterologous antilymphocyte globulin to human recipients of renal homografts. *Ann. Intern. Med.* 68:275, 1968.

76. Katz, D. H., and Benacerraf, B.   The regulatory influence of activated T cells on B cell responses to antigen. *Adv. Immunol.* 15:2, 1972.

77. Klein, G.   Tumor antigens. *Annu. Rev. Microbiol.* 20:223, 1966.

78. Klein, G.   Experimental studies in tumor immunology. *Fed. Proc.* 28:1739, 1969.

79. Koch, C. T., Eysvoogel, V. P., Fredericks, E., and van Rood, J. J.   Mixed-lymphocyte culture and skin graft data in unrelated HL-A identical individuals. *Lancet* 2:1334, 1971.

80. Kountz, S. L.   Clinical transplantation —an overview. *Transplant. Proc.* 5:59, 1973.

81. Krahenbuhl, J. L., Rosenberg, L. T., and Remington, J. S.   The role of thymus-derived lymphocytes in the *in vitro* activation of macrophages to kill *Listeria monocytogenes*. *J. Immunol.* 111:992, 1973.

82. Kyger, E. R., and Salyer, K. E.   The role of donor passenger leucocytes in rat skin allograft rejection. *Transplantation* 16:537, 1973.

83. Lance, E. M., Boyse, E. A., Cooper, S., and Carswell, E. A.   Rejection of skin allografts by irradiation chimeras: Evidence for skin-specific transplantation barrier. *Transplant. Proc.* 3:864, 1971.

84. Landsteiner, K.   *The Specificity of Serological Reactions* (rev. ed.).   New York: Dover, 1962.

85. Lawrence, H. S.   Transfer Factor. In Lawrence, H. A., and Landy, M. (Eds.), *Mediators of Cellular Immunity.* New York: Academic, 1969. P. 145.

86. Lewis, M. G., Phillips, T. M., Cook, K. B., and Blake, J.   Possible explanation for loss of detectable antibody in patients with disseminated malignant melanoma. *Nature* (Lond.) 232:52, 1971.

87. Lindquist, R. R., Guttmann, R. D., and Merrill, J. P.   Electron microscope studies of the mononuclear cells accumulating in rejecting renal allografts. *Transplantation* 12:1, 1971.

88. Linscott, W. D., and Weigle, W. O.   Induction of tolerance to bovine serum albumin by means of whole body irradiation. *J. Immunol.* 94:430, 1965.

89. Lischner, H. W., and DiGeorge, A. M.   Role of the thymus in humoral immunity. *Lancet* 2:1044, 1969.

90. Lucas, Z. J.   Regulatory Control of Nucleic Acid Synthesis During Blastogenesis of Lymphocytes in Culture. In Mihich, E. (Ed.), *Drugs and Cell Regulation.* New York: Academic, 1971. P. 159.

91. Lucas, Z. J., Coplon, N., Kempson, R., and Cohn, R.   Early renal transplant

failure associated with subliminal sensitization. *Transplantation* 10:522, 1970.

92. Lucas, Z. J., and Enomoto, K. Enhancement of renal grafts by anti-"receptor-site" serum. *Fed. Proc.* 32:971, 1973. (Abstract.)

93. Lucas, Z. J., Markley, J., and Travis, M. Immunologic enhancement of renal allografts in the rat: I. Dissociation of graft survival and antibody. *Fed. Proc.* 29:2041, 1970.

94. Lucas, Z. J., Palmer, J. M., Payne, R., Kountz, S. L., and Cohn, R. Human renal transplantation: I. Systemic immunosuppressive treatment. *Arch. Surg.* 100:113, 1970.

95. Mannick, J. A., Davis, R. C., Cooperband, S. R., Glasgow, A. H., Williams, L. F., Harrington, J. T., Cavallo, T., Schmitt, G. W., Idelson, B. A., Olsson, C. A., and Nasbeth, D. C. Clinical use of rabbit antihuman lymphocyte globulin in cadaver-kidney transplantation. *N. Engl. J. Med.* 284:1109, 1971.

96. McCluskey, R. T., Benacerraf, B., and McCluskey, J. W. Studies on the specificity of the cellular infiltrates in delayed hypersensitivity reactions. *J. Immunol.* 90:466, 1963.

97. McDevitt, H. O. Genetic control of the antibody response. *Hosp. Pract.* 8:61, 1973.

98. McGuire, H. C., and Maibach, H. I. Specific immune tolerance to anaphylactic sensitization (egg albumin) induced in the guinea pig by cyclophosphamide (Cytoxan). *J. Allergy* 32:406, 1961.

99. McKearn, T. J. Antireceptor antiserum causes specific inhibition of reactivity to rat histocompatibility antigens. *Science* 183:94, 1974.

100. Medawar, P. B. The behavior and fate of skin autografts and skin homografts in rabbits. *J. Anat.* 78:176, 1944.

101. Medawar, P. B. Second study of behavior and fate of skin homografts in rabbits. *J. Anat.* 79:157, 1945.

102. Mickey, M. R., Kreisler, M., Sebert, E. D., Tanaka, N., and Terasaki, P. I. Analyses of HL-A incompatibility in human renal transplants. *Tissue Antigens* 1:57, 1971.

103. Miller, J., Hattler, B. G., and Johnson, M. C. Cellular and humoral factors governing canine mixed lymphocyte cultures after renal transplantation: III. Further studies with antibody. *Transplantation* 14:57, 1972.

104. Mischell, R. I., and Dutton, R. W. Immunization of dissociated spleen cell cultures from normal mice. *J. Exp. Med.* 126:423, 1967.

105. Mitchison, N. A. Cell Cooperation in the Immune Response: The Hypothesis of an Antigen Presentation Mechanism. In Miescher, P. A. (Ed.), *Immunopathology, VIth Symposium, 1970.* Basel: Schwabe, 1971.

106. Moller, G. Studies on the mechanisms of immunological enhancement of human homografts: II. Effect of isoantibodies on various tumor cells. *J. Natl. Cancer Inst.* 30:1177, 1963.

107. Morris, R., and Lucas, Z. J. Immunologic enhancement of rat kidney grafts: Evidence for peripheral action of homologous antiserum. *Transplant. Proc.* 3:697, 1971.

108. Murray, J. E., Barnes, B. A., and Atkinson, J. Fifth report of the human kidney transplant registry. *Transplantation* 5:752, 1967.

109. Murray, J. E., Merrill, J. P., Dammin, G. J., Dealy, J. B., Alexander, G. W., and Harrison, J. H. Kidney transplantation in modified recipients. *Ann. Surg.* 156:337, 1962.

110. Nakamuro, K., Tanigaki, N., and Pressman, D. Multiple common properties of human β_2-microglobulin and the common portion fragment derived from HL-A antigen molecules. *Proc. Natl. Acad. Sci. U.S.A.* 70:2863, 1973.

111. Nowell, P. C. Phytohemagglutinin: An initiator of mitosis in cultures of normal human lymphocytes. *Cancer Res.* 20:462, 1960.

112. Old, L. J., Stockert, E., Boyse, E. A., and Kim, J. H. Antigenic modulation.

Loss of TL antigen from cells exposed to TL antibody. Study of the phenomenon *in vitro. J. Exp. Med.* 127:523, 1968.

113. Osler, W. *Aequanimitas, and Other Addresses to Medical Students, Nurses, and Practitioners of Medicine* (3rd ed.). New York: Blakiston Div., McGraw-Hill, 1932. P. 201.

114. Pick, E., Kreja, J., Cech, K., and Turk, K. L. Interaction between "sensitized lymphocytes" and antigen *in vitro:* I. The release of a skin reactive factor. *Immunology* 17:741, 1969.

115. Polley, M. J. Ultrastructural Studies of C1a and of Complement-Membrane Interactions. In Amos, B. (Ed.), *Progress in Immunology.* New York: Academic, 1971. P. 597.

116. Porter, K. A. Morphological aspects of renal homograft rejection. *Br. Med. Bull.* 21:171, 1965.

117. Raff, M. C. Role of thymus-derived lymphocytes in the secondary humoral immune response in mice. *Nature* (Lond.) 226:1257, 1970.

118. Raju, S., and Grogan, J. B. Immunology of anterior chamber of the eye. *Transplant. Proc.* 3:605, 1971.

119. Ramseier, H., and Lindenmann, J. Aliotypic antibodies. *Transplant. Rev.* 10:57, 1972.

120. Schöne, G. Über Transplantationsimmunität. *Munch. Med. Wochenschr.* 59:459, 1916.

121. Schwartz, R. S., and Dameshek, W. Drug induced immunological tolerance. *Nature* (Lond.) 183:1682, 1959.

122. Seigler, H. F., Gunnells, J. C., Robinson, R. R., Ward, F. E., Amos, D. B., Rowlands, D. T., Burkholder, P. M., Klein, W. J., and Stickel, D. L. Renal transplantation between HL-A identical donor-recipient pairs: Functional and morphological evaluation. *J. Clin. Invest.* 51:3200, 1972.

123. Shellam, G. R. Mechanism of induction of immunological tolerance: VI. Tolerance induction following thoracic duct drainage or treatment with anti-

lymphocyte serum. *Immunology* 17:267, 1969.

124. Simmons, R. L., Moberg, A. W., Gewurz, H., Soll, R., and Najarian, J. W. Immunosuppression by anti-human lymphocyte globulin: Correlation of human and animal assay systems with clinical results. *Transplant. Proc.* 3:745, 1971.

125. Sjögren, H. O., Hellstrom, I., Bansal, S. C., and Hellstrom, K. E. Suggestive evidence that the "blocking antibodies" of tumor-bearing individuals may be antigen-antibody complexes. *Proc. Natl. Acad. Sci. U.S.A.* 68:1372, 1971.

126. Smith, R. T. Possibilities and problems of immunologic intervention in cancer. *N. Engl. J. Med.* 287:439, 1972.

127. Smith, T. Active immunity produced by so-called balanced or neutral mixtures of diphtheria toxin and antitoxin. *J. Exp. Med.* 11:241, 1909.

128. Snell, G. D., and Stimpfling, J. H. Genetics of Tissue Transplantation. In Green, E. L. (Ed.), *Biology of the Laboratory Mouse.* New York: McGraw-Hill, 1966. P. 457.

129. Starzl, T. E. *Experiences in Renal Transplantation.* Philadelphia: Saunders, 1964.

130. Starzl, T. E., Boehmig, H. J., Amemiga, H., Wilson, C. B., Dixon, F. J., Giles, G. R., Simpson, K. M., and Halgrimson, C. G. Clotting changes, including disseminated intravascular coagulation during rapid renal-homograft rejection. *N. Engl. J. Med.* 283:383, 1970.

131. Starzl, T. E., Groth, C. G., Putnam, C. W., Corman, J., Halgrimson, C. G., Penn, J., Husberg, B., Gustafsson, A., Cascardo, S., Gus, P., and Iwatsuki, S. Cyclophosphamide for clinical renal and hepatic transplantation. *Transplant. Proc.* 5:511, 1973.

132. Strayer, D. S., Lee, W. M. F., Kohler, H., and Rowley, D. A. Depletion of a clone in neonatal mice using anti-receptor antibody. *Fed. Proc.* 33:808, 1974. (Abstract.)

133. Strober, S., and Gowans, J. L. The role of lymphocytes in the sensitization of rats to renal homografts. *J. Exp. Med.* 122:347, 1965.

134. Thiersch, C. Über Hautverpflamzung. *Verh. Ges. Chir.* 15:17, 1886.

135. Turcotte, J. G., Feduska, N. J., Carpenter, E. W., McDonald, F. D., and Bacon, G. E. Rejection crises in human renal transplant recipients. Control with high dose methylprednisolone therapy. *Arch. Surg.* 105:230, 1972.

136. Uhr, J. W., and Moller, G. Regulatory effect of antibody on the immune response. *Adv. Immunol.* 8:31, 1968.

137. Walker, S. M., and Lucas, Z. J. Cytotoxic activity of lymphocytes: II. Studies of mechanism of lymphotoxin-mediated cytotoxicity. *J. Immunol.* 109:1233, 1972.

138. Walker, S. M., and Lucas, Z. J. Role of soluble cytotoxins in cell-mediated immunity. *Transplant. Proc.* 5:137, 1973.

139. Ward, P. A., Remold, H. G., and David, J. R. The production by antigen stimulated lymphocytes of a leucotactic factor distinct from migration inhibitory factor. *Cell. Immunol.* 1:162, 1970.

140. Weigle, W. O. The induction of autoimmunity in rabbits following injection of heterologous or altered homologous thyroglobulin. *J. Exp. Med.* 121:289, 1965.

141. Weigle, W. O. Immunologic unresponsiveness. *Adv. Immunol.* 16:61, 1973.

142. W.H.O. Terminology Report. In Dausset, J., and Colombani, J. (Eds.), *Histocompatibility Testing 1972.* Copenhagen: Munksgaard, 1973. P. 3.

143. Wigzell, H. Studies on the regulation of antibody synthesis. *Cold Spring Harbor Symp. Quant. Biol.* 32:507, 1967.

144. Williamson, A. R., and Askonas, B. A. Senescence of an antibody-forming cell clone. *Nature* (Lond.) 238:337, 1972.

145. Willoughby, D. A., Boughton, B., and Schild, H. O. A factor capable of increasing vascular permeability present in lymph node cells. A possible mediator of the delayed reaction. *Immunology* 6:484, 1963.

146. Wilson, D. B. Quantitative studies on the mixed lymphocyte interaction in rats: I. Conditions and parameters of response. *J. Exp. Med.* 126:625, 1967.

147. Witz, I. P., Yagi, Y., and Pressman, D. IgG associated with microsomes from autochthonous hepatomas and normal liver of rats. *Cancer Res.* 27:2295, 1967.

148. Woodruff, M. F. A., and Anderson, N. A. Effect of lymphatic depletion by thoracic duct fistula and administration of anti-lymphocytic serum on the survival of skin homografts in rats. *Nature* (Lond.) 200:702, 1963.

149. Yunis, E. J., and Amos, D. B. Three closely linked genetic systems relevant to transplantation. *Proc. Natl. Acad. Sci. U.S.A.* 68:3031, 1971.

VII

Healing of the Wound

INTRODUCTION

Whether tissue has been damaged by external or internal factors, and whether attempts are made to modify the response by surgery or not, the natural and marvelous response known as healing will begin, certainly as soon as causative agents are removed and sometimes while they are still present.

This section presents in detail the mechanism of healing of those tissues which as reconstructive surgeons we work with at all times. Intimate knowledge of the mechanism is essential in order to understand how the best surgical result may be obtained, and it also becomes a guide to possible reasons for modification of surgical techniques. Moreover, armed with such knowledge the reconstructive surgeon will also be best equipped to make the decision often thought to be the mark of any mature surgeon: when not to operate.

18

General Aspects and
Healing of Skin

Norman E. Hugo

Wound healing is one of those miracles of nature that works so well, so consistently, that we often pay it little attention. Only when it fails and we get delayed healing of wounds or dehiscence do we become concerned. The senior surgeon details wound closure to a junior member demonstrating the confidence with which wounds are expected to heal.

Wound healing is a complex, kinetic, metabolic coordination between various cells and tissues which finally results in sealing off the body from the external environment and reinstituting structural integrity. All the tissues and cells participate simultaneously, but for convenience we shall divide the process into three facets: epithelialization, mesenchymal healing, and wound contraction.

INITIAL EVENTS

Antecedent to repair of the wound by the above mechanisms, inflammation of varying degrees and duration occurs. Immediately after injury both polymorphonuclear cells and mononuclear cells migrate from the vessels by insinuating pseudopodia through the interendothelial junctions [57]. They leave in a ratio of 5:1 regardless of the intensity of the stimulus although the ratio may change with the type of stimulus, a bacterial challenge eliciting a greater polymorphonuclear response [46]. In human wounds polymorphonuclear neutrophils migrate through the wound, undergo lysis during the first 48 hours, and release their contained hydrolytic granules throughout the extracellular matrix. This action may prepare the extracellular matrix for subsequent phagocytosis and partially stimulate the succeeding fibroplasia. While the neutrophils exhibit slight phagocytic activity, the monocytes perform the major phagocytic role. They ingest granules, fibrin, and cellular debris. After a few days the diapedesis of neutrophils declines markedly while that of the monocytes remains relatively constant, perhaps in response to an additional stimulus [76].

EPITHELIALIZATION

In the rhesus monkey, if the epidermis is incised to the dermis, the area fills with threads of fibrin, erythrocytes, and exudate. Within a few hours leukocytes invade the area and by 12 to 18 hours are arranged in a thick compact layer demarcating the dermis from the wound. Presently the threads of fibrin arrange themselves in a centripetal fashion to serve as conduits for the subsequent epithelial migration [32]. Meanwhile, the individual epithelial cells are responding by active mitosis [11]. For the epidermis to respond it must be injured. If the dermis beneath the epidermis is injured, but the epidermis is untouched, no epidermal response follows [14]. Only those epidermal cells within 2 ml of the wound edge increase their mitotic rate [13], but the increase reaches a level as high as 40 times that of uninjured tissue [17]. The cells undergoing rapid mitosis do not migrate; the cells that are migrating do not resume mitosis until they have ceased migrating and come to rest.

What causes this sustained burst in mitotic activity? It was perhaps natural that earlier concepts would invoke a wound hormone. Critical evaluation has not confirmed this.

More recently another concept has gained favor [14]. Bullough and Laurence found that epidermal reaction to wounding was more in keeping with an absence of a restraining influence than with the presence of a stimulating substance. Finegold later came to a similar conclusion [29].

A water-soluble glycoprotein with a molecular weight near 30,000 and capable of inhibiting epidermal mitosis has been identified [10, 12, 16]. This substance is apparently synthesized by the cells of the epidermis with an increasing concentration as the cells progress toward keratinization. It is also tissue-specific; that is, it inhibits the mitotic activity of similar cells. It has been postulated that this chalone programs the genetic structure of cells to following the aging process. In its absence, the genetic programming is changed to that of mitosis.

That mitotic activity in the uninjured epidermis is diurnal, being greatest during the resting or sleeping phases and least during the times of wakefulness or stress, is well established [15]. It is only natural to consider what role, if any, the stress hormones, epi-

nephrine and the glucocorticoids, play in inhibiting mitosis. If the epinephrine is removed from small strips of epidermis by placing them in saline solution, the epidermal chalone is ineffective. Adding a dilute solution of epinephrine restores the activity of the epidermal chalone. Yet epinephrine is not by itself a mitotic inhibitor. Thus, epinephrine seems to be a cofactor enabling the epidermal chalone to exert its effect in some unknown way.

Hydrocortisone by itself likewise has no inhibitory effect; it has some inhibitory effect when coupled with epinephrine, multiplying the antimitotic effect of the epidermal chalone. The combination of hydrocortisone, epinephrine, and chalone results in a marked mitotic depression. Thus, the glucocorticoids also act to enhance the effect of the epidermal chalone.

With the cellular recruitment that ensues after injury sheets of epidermal cells are produced at the wound margin. The cells pierce (*invade*) the uninjured dermis and migrate toward the wound to reach the deeper fibrin "guidelines," which are arranged centripetally. They then advance beneath the leukocytic barrier, along the fibrin strands, so that the wound is epithelialized [32]. This lining up occurs on the third day after wounding. While a fibrin network is unnecessary for epithelial coverage of a wound, it is necessary for orderly coverage.

Production of collagenase by the epidermal cells parallels the increased migratory and proliferative activity. In humans, as compared to guinea pigs, increased levels of collagenase are also seen in the new mesenchymal elements of healing wounds [38]. This enzyme presumably allows not only for the penetration of the dermis by the epidermal cells but also for the freeing of the epithelial cells for migration. Why should the epithelial cells choose to travel such a difficult route instead of migrating via a more superficial and direct route? Winter has shown that it may be a question of preventing dehydration [82]. In wounds kept moist, as contrasted to wounds that were allowed to dry, cells migrated at a much more superficial level and faster.

Epithelial cells migrate as sheets, attached to one another by desmosomes, not as individual cells [73]. In addition, they appear to be actively phagocytic, having reverted to a less differentiated state [74].

MESENCHYMAL HEALING

Connective tissue repair is initiated as soon as injury is sustained and is designed to replace the damaged tissues with collagen, commonly referred to as *scar*. It is this phase of healing that imparts strength to the wound. A period of time passes, however, between appreciable gain in tensile strength and the wounding. Originally called the *lag phase*, this period has more recently been called the *substrate phase* in realization of the many metabolic happenings that prepare the wound for elaboration of collagen [23].

The substrate phase is characterized by changes in the ground substance. The ground substance is composed of mucopolysaccharides and protein polysaccharides. There are approximately eight mucopolysaccharides containing carbohydrate, usually hexosamine and uronic acid, associated with protein [7], although one of them, heparin, is not found in ground substance. Indeed, they may not exist as discrete entities but as hybrids [30]. Early interest in the mucopolysaccharides stemmed from the observation that they appeared to peak at around the fourth to sixth day after wounding and from then declined as collagen production increased, the interpretation being that they were somehow necessary for collagen production [24]. Later, Edwards et al. found the hexosamine content very high in subcutaneously implanted sponges as early as six hours after wounding [25]. The conclusion was that the immediate high hexosamine concentrations were due to serum glycoprotein and that previous theories concerning mucopolysaccharides were not valid. Since then, fractionation methods have given us a better idea of the

happenings with mucopolysaccharides. Many theories attempt to explain the role of the mucopolysaccharides but none does so completely. Bentley has summarized them: Different mucopolysaccharides are synthesized at different rates in different tissues; they may control the synthesis of other tissue components; they may determine the size and orientation of collagen fibers; or their production may reflect the differentiation of the fibroblasts in the wound [7].

Collagen is produced by the fibroblasts that appear three days after wounding. It was originally felt that the fibroblasts were circulating pluripotential monocytes transformed into fibroblasts after reaching the wound. However, two experiments have given strong support to the contention that the fibroblasts are derived from local tissue mesenchyme. After an area of skin was irradiated with 1000 rads to a depth of 5 ml, standard wounds were made in animals and these exhibited the normal inflammatory reaction. Yet microscopically there was a paucity of fibroblasts [76]. In a second experiment, two parabiotic rats were irradiated to destroy the hematopoietic organs except in the leg of one. After clamping of the anastomosing flap, tritiated thymidine was injected into the rat with the intact hematopoietic organ while wounds were made in both rats. After the clamp was removed on the anastomosing flap, labeled blood cells appeared in the circulation of both rats. Fibroblast production in both wounds was abundant although none of the fibroblasts were labeled [63]. Mitotic activity is usually sporadic in dermal fibrocytes [34], but after wounding there is heightened mitotic activity of the fibrocytes of the loose connective tissue in the area between the dermis-epidermis and dermis-subcutaneous tissues [33, 60].

The movement of these fibroblasts into the wound area is of considerable interest. The direction they follow is not unlike that of migrating epithelial cells (see above), being determined by centripetally oriented fibrin strands [81]. These cells move by means of a *ruffled membrane* which develops at their leading edge [3]. When the ruffled membrane abuts upon a similar cell, it ceases to move and the cells adhere. The cell may subsequently develop another ruffled membrane and migrate again, stopping only when its ruffled membrane juxtaposes another fibroblast. However, it is not always so neat and tidy. In some instances cells grown in tissue culture will overlap at junctional areas, or when the concentration or composition of the nutrient medium is changed [19, 21]. The character of the contact between fibroblasts has interested many, but its exact nature has not been fully defined.

The major tissue of repair is collagen produced by the fibroblasts. It is a complex molecule composed of three polypeptides arranged in a superhelical fashion with a molecular weight of 300,000 [40]. In most collagen molecules the chains differ slightly in amino acid composition, giving rise to alpha-1 and alpha-2 chains. There are approximately 1000 amino acid residues in each alpha chain, which upon hydrolysis yields roughly 330 glycine, 130 proline, 100 hydroxyproline, and 110 alanine residues. Collagen does not contain cysteine or tryptophan but does contain hydroxyproline and 5 to 10 residues of hydroxylysine, the latter hydroxy amino acids not being found in significant amounts in any other animal protein. Collagen, like other proteins, is synthesized on polyribosomes but interestingly it is 10 times longer than the polyribosome.

Stetlen [77] discovered that the hydroxyproline comes only from hydroxylation of proline and suggested that this occurred after incorporation of the proline. Confirmation has subsequently been made by others [50, 51, 65, 67].

An understanding of wound healing is inextricably linked to a knowledge of the biosynthesis of collagen and its structure. The biosynthesis is initiated within the fibroblasts on ribosomal complexes resulting in production of a polypeptide precursor, *protocollagen.* Protocollagen differs from collagen, being rich in proline and lysine but containing no hydroxyproline, hydroxylysine, or glycosylated hydroxylysine. The ribosomal complexes contain an RNA (messenger ribonucleic acid) which has a molecular weight of nearly a million, making it one of the largest [35]. The alpha chains of collagen are very large, and it was originally felt that protocollagen was composed of subunits joined after their release from the ribosomal complexes. Fernandez-Madrid postulated that small polyribosomes might be involved in the synthesis of these subunits [28]. Subsequently, Vuust and Piez, using β-aminopropionitrile and pulse-labeling with radioactive glycine, found that the time required for completion of one alpha chain of about 1040 amino acids was slightly less than five minutes and these were synthesized as single chains by sequential amino acid addition and not as subunits later joined [78].

It remains unclear whether the triple helical structure of protocollagen is formed on the ribosomes or after its release. Equally unresolved is the location of hydroxylation of protocollagen. It has been established that hydroxylation is not necessary for its release from the ribosomal complexes. On in vivo experiments with mouse fibroblasts, the major site of proline hydroxylation was found to be the nascent collagen peptide chains prior to their release [54]. Using ribosomes from guinea pigs, experimenters found the extent of hydroxylation of nascent polypeptide chains to be 50 percent of that for completed granuloma collagen, indicating that one-half of the hydroxylation was accomplished before release [58]. Finally, other experiments with mouse fibroblasts suggested that little or no hydroxylation occurs in the nascent collagen chains but rather with released completed collagen chains [5].

Conclusive evidence is lacking on whether the triple helix is formed while the polypeptide chains are being synthesized on ribosomes or later. There are theoretical difficulties with either concept. Recently it has been suggested that the initial polypeptide chains are longer than alpha chains and contain disulfide bonds and that while the growing chains are still attached to ribosomes the triple helix is formed [35].

One of the important events in the biosynthesis of collagen is the hydroxylation of protocollagen. Prockop et al. [66] using $O_2{}^{18}$, established that the oxygen for the reaction was atmospheric, not derived from water.

When unossified chicken tibias were used, very low concentrations of ferrous or ferric ion reversed the inhibition of proline hydroxylation produced by ethylenediaminetetraacetate (EDTA), but high concentrations of cupric, manganous, magnesium, cobaltous, zinc, and calcium ions would not do so [65]. Ascorbic acid also appears necessary for the hydroxylation of proline, and exogenous sources are required for the guinea pig and

requirement, as has been suggested [63], requires further investigation. It is currently accepted that ascorbate under normal circumstances is necessary in the hydroxylation of proline. The hydroxylation of proline requires α-ketoglutarate [48]. Dialyzed preparations of proline hydroxylase are unable to hydroxylate proline until α-ketoglutarate is added. Pyruvate and oxalacetate also exhibit some activity but only 6 and 8 percent that of α-ketoglutarate. Subsequent experiments have revealed the absolute necessity for α-ketoglutarate. The synthesis of one mole of hydroxyproline involves the stoichiometric conversion of α-ketoglutarate to succinate and carbon dioxide, and it was postulated that α-ketoglutarate serves as a specific electron donor in proline hydroxylation [69]. Thus the reaction has been postulated as follows:

$$\text{Peptidyl proline} + \alpha\text{-ketoglutarate} + O_2 \xrightarrow[\text{ascorbate}]{Fe^{++}} \text{peptidyl hydroxyproline} + \text{succinate} + CO_2.$$

primates. In experiments with ascorbic acid and collagen proline hydroxylase, it was found that ascorbic acid or any one of several other reducing agents was required for the enzymatic conversion of peptidyl proline to peptidyl hydroxyproline. Isoascorbic acid was equally effective in this role while the enediols, dihydroxymaleate and piperidinohexose reductase, were only 20 percent as active. The reduced pteridines, tetrahydrofolate and tetrahydropteridine, were able to function as cofactors in the place of ascorbic acid, but even in concentrations two to three times greater the reaction was significantly less rapid than with ascorbate [48]. Mussini et al. found that lung and skin from scorbutic fetal guinea pigs contain only a third as much proline hydroxylase as normal [59]. Whether this finding means that ascorbate is the essential cofactor in the hydroxylation process or is required only during rapid collagen synthesis while other reducing agents may substitute during times of low

The enzyme responsible for proline hydroxylation [70], known as *protocollagen proline hydroxylase*, has been recently identified in pure form from chick embryos and characterized by electron microscopy to be 85 × 85 A by 40 × 85 A on top and side views with subunits of 40 A in diameter and a molecular weight of 240,000 [8]. The enzyme most readily hydroxylates a sequence of -Gly-X-Pro- and it may do so by moving laterally along the substrate [35].

Lysine must also be hydroxylated in the conversion of protocollagen, and this reaction requires iron [47], atmospheric oxygen [68], ascorbate, and α-ketoglutarate [43]. However, the enzyme lysine hydroxylase differs from proline hydroxylase [80].

After release from the ribosomal complexes the collagen peptides probably pass into the cisternae of the endoplasmic reticulum. Two theories have been postulated to explain its extracellular extrusion. Ross and Benditt [72], studying guinea pig wound fibroblasts, suggested that the collagen peptides were extruded directly from the ergastoplasmic cisternae to the cell exterior, while Cooper and Prockop [20], using embryonic chicken cartilage, found no activity in the Golgi vacuoles or cisternae and felt that the completed collagen molecules pass directly from the ground cytoplasm to their extracellular destination. Data by Salpeter [75], working with regenerating limbs of adult newts, suggested that a fraction of the collagen is extruded by the endoplasmic reticulum and then the Golgi vacuoles, but most of it leaves the cell directly from the ground cytoplasm. The evidence now available also indicates that selective hydroxylysyl residues

blast is estimated to form 40 to 50 micromicrograms of collagen [52].

The microfibrils that are spontaneously formed by tropocollagen have little tensile strength and are soluble in saline and later acid solutions. This is immature collagen. As it matures it gains tensile strength and becomes insoluble because of the formation of cross-linkages, covalent bonds, between adjacent tropocollagen molecules in the microfibrils and possibly between adjacent microfibrils. The first step in the cross-linking of collagen is the removal of the terminal amino groups of several lysyl or hydroxylysyl residues in tropocollagen to produce aldehydes which form cross-links by two reactions:

$$(1) \quad R_1 - CHO + H_2N - CH_2 - R_2 \;\rightleftharpoons\; R_1 - CH = N - CH_2 - R_2 + H_2O$$

$$(2) \quad R_1 - CH_2 - CHO + \begin{array}{c} CHO \\ | \\ CH_2 \end{array} \Big/ R_2 \longrightarrow R_1 - CH_2 \Big/ \begin{array}{ccc} CH & CHO \\ | & \backslash & | \\ OH & & CH \end{array} - R_2$$

must be glycosylated before extrusion into the extracellular matrix [71].

After extrusion the soluble tropocollagen is aggregated into insoluble microfibrils, ma-

The bond produced by the first reaction is not entirely stable, but that produced by the second reaction is very stable [36]. Its stability is increased further by dehydration to give

$$R_1 - CH_2 - \begin{array}{ccc} CH & & CHO \\ | & - & | \\ OH & & CH \end{array} - R_2 \rightarrow R_1 - CH_2 - CH = C\,(CHO) - R_2$$

ture collagen. To protect against immediate conversion of the tropocollagen into insoluble microfibrils and incarceration of the fibroblasts, the first collagen peptides are actually larger than tropocollagen, with different properties of solubility [22]. They have been termed a *modified form of collagen*, with a greater number of alpha-2 chains, and may function in the transport of collagen from cell to fiber [53]. Collagen accumulation ceases when approximately 7 mg per cubic centimeter has been formed. A single fibro-

WOUND CONTRACTION

Carrel and Hartmann (1916) called attention to the importance of contraction in the repair of a wound [18]. A wound will contract until the elasticity of the surrounding skin prevents further reduction in size. They stated that this process is dependent on contraction of granulation tissue. Abercrombie et al. [1] did not know whether it was due to contraction of collagen fibers or fibroblasts. Abercrombie et al. later reported that wound contraction was essentially normal in scorbutic guinea pigs, thereby belying the idea that collagen contraction was responsible [2]. Their finding has been confirmed by others [37]. It was known that granulation tissue must be present before wound remodeling would occur [49]. Grillo et al. felt this was a specialized part of the granulation tissue in juxtaposition to the wound margin [39]. They postulated that the mass of granulation tissue did not act as a unit but the region of active contraction was in a rim of newly formed tissue next to the skin. Subsequently they observed a "picture frame" of connective tissue beneath the wound edge, strongly adherent, which moved with this edge during contraction [79]. Excising the central granulation mass but leaving this area intact produced wound contraction. Excision of the "picture frame" or detaching it from the wound margin produced inhibition of contraction. They speculated that this zone was rich in fibroblasts and that their mass migration pulled the wound margins together. In an equally impressive series of experiments, with rabbits, quite the opposite was found [4]. Ten days after wounding and splinting of the wounds to keep them open, removal of the splint resulted in a rapid, visible contraction of the wound. Excision of the central core of granulation tissue just prior to removal of the splint retarded the contraction process. If the central granulation core was isolated by incisions in the splinted wound, it would contract. If this process was repeated in an unsplinted contracted wound, the central granulation mass would contract further while the wound edges retracted. Lindquist, in an earlier observation, found that the central granulation contracted when freed from the periphery [55]. It should be pointed out that all experimenters worked with different animals—Grillo and Watts with guinea pigs, Abercrombie et al. with rabbits [4], and Lindquist with rats. The differences may be due to the type of animal employed. Peacock and van Winkle have suggested that a single hypothesis might explain these results [62].

They feel that the "picture frame" cells may migrate toward the center and then contract while mutually adhering to one another and to the wound edge and base.

More recently, there has been increasing evidence that the fibroblast itself, contained within and throughout the granulation tissue, may be the active contractile agent. Hirschel et al. employed the human antismooth muscle serum produced by patients with autoimmune hepatitis [41]. They found it was bound to smooth muscle cells of rats, to fibroblasts of granulation tissue of rats, but not to "normal" fibroblasts. Thus it suggested a similarity between fibroblasts in contractile granulation tissue and smooth muscle cells. It has been known for a long time that glycerol-extracted fibroblasts contract when stimulated with adenosine triphosphate (ATP) [42]. Granulation tissue produced by various methods and from various sites will contract as smooth muscle does when stimulated with various smooth muscle excitatory agents—e.g., 5-hydroxytryptamine, bradykinin, angiotensin, vasopressin, epinephrine, and norepinephrine—if the granulation is old enough (around 11 days) and conditions are aerobic. Papaverine will cause relaxation [56]. Electron microscopy of fibroblasts in granulation tissue from a variety of sites and caused by a variety of agents reveals characteristics typical of smooth muscle such as an extensive cytoplasmic fibrillar system, nuclear folds and indentations suggesting cellular contraction, and cell-to-stroma and cell-to-cell attachments. Similar quantities of actomyosin can be extracted from granulation tissue and from pregnant rat uterus. It has been recently suggested, therefore, that under certain conditions (development of granulation tissue) fibroblasts can differentiate into a cell-type-like smooth muscle. The resulting *myofibroblast* may play the central role in wound contraction [31].

Many factors influence the rate of wound healing. It is generally accepted that wound healing proceeds at an optimal rate and that addition or deletion of substances only impedes the healing rate rather than accelerating it. An exception may be the more rapid wound healing of second, separate wounds. Second, separate wounds created in rabbits 9 and 12 days after primary wounding and tested at 12 days exhibited a statistically significant increase in their tensile strength. Thus, secondary wounds made during the collagen phase of the primary wound and tested during their collagen phase show a secondary wound acceleration. Whether this effect is due to substance(s) produced by the primary wound or to a systemic reaction to the wound remains conjectural [44]. The secondary wound is different from a wound that is resutured after having been disrupted. This will heal faster, bypassing the lag phase. The acceleration can be abolished if instead of being separated the primary wound is excised as a 1 cm strip [61].

Anemia has no significant effect upon wound healing, whether it is caused by iron deficiency [6], hemolysis [45], or hemorrhage [83], providing plasma volume is maintained.

Peacock and van Winkle have reviewed the literature on the effects of steroids on wound healing [64]. They point out that ACTH, cortisone, hydrocortisone, and prednisolone decrease wound healing by inhibiting fibroplasia. However, they wisely stress that the doses used to achieve these effects were generally higher than the doses employed in humans. In addition, analysis of the literature is confusing because of the different species, drug dosages, duration of treatment, and varied parameters employed to test the effect.

β-Aminopropionitrile causes lathyrism. In this disease cross-linking of collagen is prevented by interference with the amine oxidase enzyme that allows the reaction in which terminal amino groups of several lysyl or hydroxylysyl residues are removed: $R - CH_2 - NH_3^+ \rightarrow R - CHO + NH_4^+$. This reaction is the first step in the formation of cross-linkages. The fact that amine oxidase contains copper may explain why copper deficiency also produces a lathyritic type of condition. If aldehydes were produced from this reaction, they would form cross-links in the manner described above. Penicillamine, by reacting with the aldehyde groups before they produce cross-linkages, can cause a lathyritic-type disease too [36].

Vitamin E has been shown to significantly retard collagen synthesis in the rat. Its action is thought to be due to a lysosomal stabilizing effect [26].

Vitamin A has been shown to reverse the inhibiting effects of glucocorticoids by reestablishing inflammation and fibroplasia [29].

REFERENCES

1. Abercrombie, M., Flint, M. H., and James, D. W. Collagen formation and contraction during repair of small excised wounds in the skin of rats. *J. Embryol. Exp. Morphol.* 2:264, 1954.
2. Abercrombie, M., Flint, M. H., and James, D. W. Wound contraction in relation to collagen formation in scorbutic guinea pigs. *J. Embryol. Exp. Morphol.* 4:167, 1956.
3. Abercrombie, M., and Heaysman, J. E. M. Observations on the social behavior of cells in tissue culture: II. Monolayering of fibroblasts. *Exp. Cell Res.* 13:276, 1954.
4. Abercrombie, M., James, D. W., and Newcome, J. F. Wound contraction in rabbit skin, studied by splinting the wound margins. *J. Anat.* 94:170, 1960.
5. Bachra, B. N., and van der Eb, A. J. Site of proline hydroxylation during collagen synthesis in mouse fibroblasts. *Biochemistry* 9:3001, 1970.
6. Bains, J. W., Crawford, D. T., and Ketcham, A. S. Effect of chronic anemia on wound tensile strength. *Ann. Surg.* 164:243, 1966.
7. Bentley, J. P. Mucopolysaccharide Synthesis in Healing Wounds. In Dunphy, J. E., and van Winkle, W. (Eds.), *Repair and Regeneration.* New York: McGraw-Hill, 1969. P. 151.
8. Berg, R. A., Olson, B. R., and Kivirikko, K. I. The quaternary structure of protocollagen proline hydroxylase. *Fed. Proc.* 31:479, 1972. (Abstract 1491.)

9. Billingham, R. E., and Medawar, P. B. Contracture and intussusceptive growth in the healing of extensive wounds in mammalian skin. *J. Anat.* 89:114, 1955.

10. Boldingh, W. H., and Laurence, E. B. Extraction, purification, and preliminary characterisation of the epidermal chalone: A tissue specific mitotic inhibitor from vertebrate skin. *Eur. J. Biochem.* 5:191, 1968.

11. Bullough, W. S. Mitotic and functional homeostasis. *Cancer Res.* 25:1683, 1965.

12. Bullough, W. S., Hewett, C. L., and Laurence, E. B. The epidermal chalone: A preliminary attempt at isolation. *Exp. Cell Res.* 36:192, 1964.

13. Bullough, W. S., and Laurence, E. B. A technique for the study of small epidermal wounds. *Br. J. Exp. Pathol.* 37:273, 1957.

14. Bullough, W. S., and Laurence, E. B. The control of epidermal mitotic activity in the mouse. *Proc. R. Soc. Lond. [Biol.]* 151:517, 1960.

15. Bullough, W. S., and Laurence, E. B. Stress and adrenaline in relation to the diurnal cycle of epidermal mitotic activity in adult male mice. *Proc. R. Soc. Lond. [Biol.]* 154:540, 1961.

16. Bullough, W. S., and Laurence, E. B. Mitotic control by internal secretion: The role of the chalone-adrenaline complex. *Exp. Cell Res.* 33:176, 1964.

17. Bullough, W. S., and Laurence, E. B. The cycle in epidermal mitotic observation and its relation to chalone and adrenaline. *Exp. Cell Res.* 43:343, 1966.

18. Carrel, A., and Hartmann, A. Cicatrization of wounds: I. The relation between the size of a wound and the rate of its cicatrization. *J. Exp. Med.* 24:429, 1916.

19. Carter, S. B. Principles of cell motility: The directional control of cell movement. *Nature* (Lond.) 168:787, 1965.

20. Cooper, G. W., and Prockop, D. J. Intracellular accumulation of protocollagen and extrusion of collagen by embryonic cartilage cells. *J. Cell Biol.* 38:523, 1968.

21. Curtis, A. S. G. Control of some cell contact reactions in tissue culture. *J. Natl. Cancer Inst.* 26:256, 1961.

22. Dehm, P., and Prockop, D. J. Synthesis and extrusion of collagen by freshly isolated cells from chick embryo tendon. *Biochim. Biophys. Acta* 240:358, 1971.

23. Dunphy, J. E., and Jackson, D. S. Practical application of experimental studies in the care of the primarily closed wound. *Am. J. Surg.* 104:273, 1962.

24. Dunphy, J. E., and Udupa, K. N. Chemical and histochemical sequences in the normal healing of wounds. *N. Engl. J. Med.* 253:847, 1955.

25. Edwards, L. C., Pernokas, L. N., and Dunphy, J. E. The use of a plastic sponge to sample regenerating tissue in healing wounds. *Surg. Gynecol. Obstet.* 105:303, 1957.

26. Ehrlich, H. P., Tarver, H., and Hunt, T. K. Inhibitory effects of vitamin E on collagen synthesis and wound repair. *Ann. Surg.* 175:235, 1972.

27. Ehrlich, H. P., Tarver, H., and Hunt, T. K. Effects of vitamin A and glucocorticoids upon inflammation and collagen synthesis. *Ann. Surg.* 172:222, 1973.

28. Fernandez-Madrid, F. Biosynthesis of collagen, biochemical and physicochemical characterization of collagen-synthesizing polyribosomes. *J. Cell Biol.* 33:27, 1967.

29. Finegold, M. J. Control of cell multiplication in epidermis. *Proc. Soc. Exp. Biol. Med.* 119:96, 1965.

30. Fransson, L. A., and Roden, L. Structure of dermatan sulfate: II. Characterization of products obtained by hyaluronidase digestion of dermatan sulfate. *J. Biol. Chem.* 242:4170, 1967.

31. Gabbiani, G., Hirschel, J., Ryan, G. B., Statkov, P. R., and Majno, G. Granulation tissue as a contractile organ. A study of structure and function. *J. Exp. Med.* 135:719, 1972.

32. Giacometti, L., and Montagna, W. Healing of Skin Wounds in Primates. In Dunphy, J. E., and van Winkle, W. (Eds.), *Repair and Regeneration.* New York: McGraw-Hill, 1969. Pp. 47–55.

33. Gillman, T., and Penn, J. Studies on

the repair of cutaneous wounds. *Med. Proc.* 2 (Suppl.):121, 1956.

34. Gluckmann, A. Mesenchymal Healing. In Montagna, W., and Billingham, R. E. (Eds.), *Advances in Biology of Skin.* New York: Pergamon, 1964.

35. Grant, M. E., and Prockop, D. J. The biosynthesis of collagen. (Second of three parts.) *N. Engl. J. Med.* 286:242, 1972.

36. Grant, M. E., and Prockop, D. J. The biosynthesis of collagen. (Third of three parts.) *N. Engl. J. Med.* 286:291, 1972.

37. Grillo, H. C., and Gross, J. Studies in wound healing: III. Contraction in vitamin C deficiency. *Proc. Soc. Exp. Biol. Med.* 101:268, 1959.

38. Grillo, H. C., McLennan, J. E., and Wolfort, F. G. Activity and Properties of Collagenase from Healing Wounds in Mammals. In Dunphy, J. E., and van Winkle, W. (Eds.), *Repair and Regeneration.* New York: McGraw-Hill, 1969. Pp. 185–197.

39. Grillo, H. C., Watts, G. T., and Gross, J. Studies in wound healing: I. Contraction and the wound contents. *Ann. Surg.* 148:145, 1958.

40. Harrington, W., and von Hippel, P. The Structure of Collagen and Gelatin. In Anfinsen, C. B. (Ed.), *Advances in Protein Chemistry.* New York: Academic, 1961.

41. Hirschel, B. J., Gabbiani, G., Ryan, G. B., and Majno, G. Fibroblasts of granulation tissue; immunofluorescent staining with antismooth muscle serum (35920). *Proc. Soc. Exp. Biol. Med.* 138:466, 1971.

42. Hoffman-Berling, J. Adenosintriphosphate als Betriebstoff von Zellbewegungen. *Biochim. Biophys. Acta* 14:182, 1954.

43. Housmann, E. Cofactor requirements for the enzymatic hydroxylation of lysine in a polypeptide precursor of collagen. *Biochim. Biophys. Acta* 133:591, 1967.

44. Hugo, N. E., Epstein, L., Cone, A., and Bennett, J. E. The effect of primary wounding on the tensile strength of secondary wounds. *Surg. Gynecol. Obstet.* 131:516, 1970.

45. Hugo, N. E., Thompson, L. W., Zook, E. G., and Bennett, J. E. Effect of chronic anemia on the tensile strength of healing wounds. *Surgery* 66:741, 1969.

46. Hurley, J. U., Ryan, G. B., and Friedman, A. The mononuclear response to intrapleural injection in the rat. *J. Pathol. Bacteriol.* 91:575, 1966.

47. Hurych, J., and Nordwig, A. Inhibition of collagen hydroxylysine formation by chelating agents. *Biochim. Biophys. Acta* 140:168, 1967.

48. Hutton, J. J., Tappel, A. L., and Udenfriend, S. Cofactor and substrate requirements of collagen proline hydroxylase. *Arch. Biochem. Biophys.* 118:231, 1967.

49. James, D. W. Wound Remodeling. In Dunphy, J. E., and van Winkle, W. (Eds.), *Repair and Regeneration.* New York: McGraw-Hill, 1969. P. 169.

50. Kivirikko, K. I., and Prockop, D. J. Hydroxylation of proline in synthetic polypeptides with purified protocollagen hydroxylase. *J. Biol. Chem.* 242:4006, 1967.

51. Kivirikko, K. I., and Prockop, D. J. Enzymatic hydroxylation of proline and lysine in protocollagen. *Proc. Natl. Acad. Sci. U.S.A.* 57:782, 1967.

52. Lampiaho, K., and Kulonen, E. Metabolic phases during the development of granulation tissue. *Biochem. J.* 105:333, 1967.

53. Layman, D. L., McGoodwin, E. B., and Martin, G. R. The nature of the collagen synthesized by cultured human fibroblasts. *Proc. Natl. Acad. Sci. U.S.A.* 68:454, 1971.

54. Lazarides, E. L., Lukens, L. N., and Infank, A. A. Collagen polysomes: Site of hydroxylation of proline residues. *J. Mol. Biol.* 58:831, 1971.

55. Lindquist, G. The healing of skin defects. An experimental study of the white rat. *Acta Chir. Scand.* 94 (Suppl. 1071):1, 1946.

56. Majno, G., Gabbiani, G., Hirschel, B. J., Ryan, G. B., and Statkov, P. R. Contraction of granulation tissue in vitro: Similarity to smooth muscle. *Science* 173:548, 1971.

57. Marchesi, V. T. The site of leukocyte

emigration during inflammation. *Q. J. Exp. Physiol.* 46:115, 1961.

58. Miller, R. L., and Udenfriend, S. Hydroxylation of proline residues in collagen nascent chains. *Arch. Biochem. Biophys.* 139:104, 1970.

59. Mussini, E., Hutton, J. J., and Udenfriend, S. Collagen proline hydroxylase in wound healing, granuloma formation, scurvy, and growth. *Science* 157:927, 1967.

60. Ordman, L. J., and Gillman, T. Studies in the healing of cutaneous wounds. *Arch. Surg.* 93:857, 1966.

61. Peacock, E. E. Some aspects of fibrogenesis during the healing of primary and secondary wounds. *Surg. Gynecol. Obstet.* 115:408, 1962.

62. Peacock, E. E., and van Winkle, W. Contraction. In Peacock, E. E., and van Winkle, W. (Eds.), *Surgery and Biology of Wound Repair.* Philadephia: Saunders, 1970. P. 49.

63. Peacock, E. E., and van Winkle, W. Structure, Synthesis, and Interaction of Fibrous Protein and Matrix. In Peacock, E. E., and van Winkle, W. (Eds.), *Surgery and Biology of Wound Repair.* Philadelphia: Saunders, 1970.

64. Peacock, E. E., and van Winkle, W. The Biochemistry and the Environment of Wounds and Their Relation to Wound Strength. In Peacock, E. E., and van Winkle, W. (Eds.), *Surgery and Biology of Wound Repair.* Philadelphia: Saunders, 1970. P. 129.

65. Prockop, D. J., and Juva, K. Synthesis of hydroxyproline in vitro by the hydroxylation of proline in a precursor of collagen. *Proc. Natl. Acad. Sci. U.S.A.* 53:661, 1965.

66. Prockop, D. J., Kaplan, A., and Udenfriend, S. Oxygen-18 studies in the conversion of proline to collagen hydroxyproline. *Arch. Biochem. Biophys.* 101:499, 1963.

67. Prockop, D. J., Peterkofsky, B., and Udenfriend, S. Studies on the intracellular localization of collagen synthesis in the intact chick embryo. *J. Biol. Chem.* 237:1581, 1962.

68. Prockop, D. J., Weinstein, E., and Mulveny, T. Hydroxylation of lysine in a polypeptide precursor of collagen. *Biochem. Biophys. Res. Commun.* 22:124, 1966.

69. Rhoads, R. E., and Udenfriend, S. Decarboxylation of α-ketoglutarate coupled to collagen proline hydroxylase. *Proc. Natl. Acad. Sci. U.S.A.* 60:1473, 1968.

70. Rhoads, R. E., and Udenfriend, S. Purification and properties of collagen proline hydroxylase from newborn rat skin. *Arch. Biochem. Biophys.* 139:329, 1970.

71. Rosenbloom, J., and Prockop, D. J. Biochemical Aspects of Collagen Biosynthesis. In Dunphy, J. E., and van Winkle, W. (Eds.), *Repair and Regeneration.* New York: McGraw-Hill, 1969. P. 133.

72. Ross, R., and Benditt, E. P. Wound healing and collagen formation: V. Quantitative electron microscope radioontographic observations of proline-H^3 utilization by fibroblasts. *J. Cell Biol.* 27:83, 1965.

73. Ross, R., and Odland, G. The fine structure of human skin wounds. *Q. J. Surg. Sci.* 3:2, 1967.

74. Ross, R., and Odland, G. Fine Structure Observations of Human Skin Wounds and Fibrogenesis. In Dunphy, J. E., and van Winkle, W. (Eds.), *Repair and Regeneration.* New York: McGraw-Hill, 1969. Pp. 100–115.

75. Salpeter, M. M. H^3-proline incorporation into cartilage: Electron microscope autoradiographic observations. *J. Morphol.* 124:387, 1968.

76. Spector, W. G. Inflammation. In Dunphy, J. E., and van Winkle, W. (Eds.), *Repair and Regeneration.* New York: McGraw-Hill, 1969. P. 3.

77. Stetlen, M. R. Some aspects of the metabolism of hydroxyproline studied with the aid of isotopic nitrogen. *J. Biol. Chem.* 181:31, 1949.

78. Vuust, J., and Piez, K. A. Biosynthesis of the α chains of collagen studied by pulse-labelling in culture. *J. Biol. Chem.* 245:6201, 1970.

79. Watts, G. T., Grillo, H. C., and Gross, J. Studies in wound healing: II. The

role of granulation tissue in contraction. *Ann. Surg.* 148:153, 1958.

80. Weinstein, E., Blumenkrantz, N., and Prockop, D. J.   Hydroxylation of proline and lysine in protocollagen involves two separate enzymatic sites. *Biochim. Biophys. Acta* 191:747, 1969.

81. Weiss, P., and Garber, B.   Shape and movement of mesenchymal cells as functions of the physical structure of the medium: Contributions to a quantitative morphology. *Proc. Natl. Acad. Sci. U.S.A.* 38:264, 1952.

82. Winter, G. D.   Wound Healing. In Anfinsen, C. B. (Ed.), *Advances in Biology of Skin,* Vol. 5. New York: Pergamon, 1964.

83. Zederfeldt, B.   Studies in wound healing and trauma, with special reference to intravascular aggregation of erythrocytes. *Acta Chir. Scand.* 224:1, 1957.

19

The Healing of Cartilage

Hunter J. H. Fry

Mature cartilage is a skeletal tissue with a number of important properties, including viscoelasticity, immunological privilege, and an inbuilt system of forces that is capable of causing distortion of shape. These properties are of practical importance to the reconstructive surgeon.

Cartilage is elastic. A piece of cartilage will return to its neutral position after it has been deformed by an external stress. It is also viscous, for the maintenance of such deformation requires a lesser force once the original deformation has been produced; that is, there is "creep" as though the tissue were behaving like a thick fluid [1].

Hyaline cartilage enjoys immunological privilege because the chondrocytes of a homograft are protected by the matrix from the antibody-containing cells of the recipient. A homograft of cartilage needs no protection by immunosuppressive drugs [14, 15, 22].

A complex and balanced system of forces within cartilage [5, 7, 13] is described later in this chapter. Its importance to the reconstructive surgeon lies in the fact that operative procedures involving cartilage may fail in some way if these potentially deforming forces locked within cartilage are not understood and respected.

CHEMICAL COMPOSITION

Hyaline cartilage is mainly water and two proteins [16]. The protein polysaccharide complexes are long-chain, large-molecular-weight structures with a protein core and negatively charged polysaccharide side chains. These negatively charged side chains repel each other, and, in fact, in a 3% saline solution the molecules are touching each other. In cartilage, therefore, there is considerable interlocking of the molecules creating an expansile force.

The collagen fibrillar network accounts for some 13 percent wet weight of hyaline cartilage. This appears to exert a "binding" effect and act as a skeleton for the tissue. It is intimately concerned with the maintenance of shape of the tissue [6].

It has been shown that the combination of these two proteins—protein polysaccharide and collagen—can bind more water than the sum of the two proteins by themselves [23]. This factor, when taken in conjunction with the interlocking of protein polysaccharide complexes, is important in understanding the origin of so-called swelling pressure, referred to below.

MICROSCOPICAL ANATOMY

Hyaline cartilage itself has no blood supply. The perichondrium does have a blood supply, and substances diffuse to and from the chondrocytes through the matrix. The oxygen demand of the tissue is quite low, and only molecules of a certain size will penetrate the matrix effectively.

The perichondrium is a fibrous capsule around the cartilage. Continuity of some of its fibers with the collagen fibrillar network of the cartilage itself can be demonstrated.

The arrangement of the chondrocytes within the matrix is of considerable importance. It has been known for some time that the chondrocytes nearest the surface of cartilage present a flattened appearance and on section seem to be aligned parallel to the surface. The significance of the cellular arrangement has been appreciated only recently, however, in that it reflects lines of tensile stress (see below). In the more central parts of the cartilage, as seen in both costal cartilage and nasal septal cartilage, the cells tend to be arranged in columns. Some of them may be aligned at right angles to the surface or at various angles to it. The pattern varies from one part of the cartilage to another [7] (Figs. 19-1, 19-2).

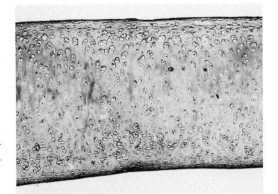

FIGURE 19-1.

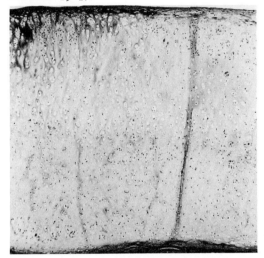

FIGURE 19-2.

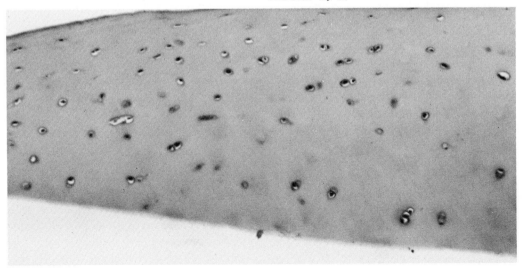

FIGURE 19-3.

FIGURE 19-1. *Histological section of nasal septal cartilage showing parallel arrangement of cells in the outer surface layers.*

FIGURE 19-2. *Section of nasal septal cartilage lacking the degree of differentiation in surface parallel layers shown in Figure 19-1.*

FIGURE 19-3. *Histological section of cartilage facing of the lower end of the radius, showing little tendency toward parallel arrangement in the surface layers.*

Articular cartilage shows a unique modification of this cellular arrangement: there is only one external surface. The cartilage attached to the bone end presents the appearance of "central" cartilage while the surface layers have flattened cells. It is almost as though the bone itself represented the other "half" of the cartilage (Figs. 19-3, 19-4).

The collagen fibrillar network is demonstrated in Figures 19-5 to 19-8. This is seen as a delicate lacework, though the appearance is that of the fibers being stretched taut by an expansile force. There is no real difference in the disposition of the fibers in the inner and outer zones of the cartilage. The stress alignment shown by the cellular arrangement is not mirrored in any way by the collagen network. Fiber continuity can be shown at the junction of cartilage and its perichondrium [9].

If cartilage is breached by injury or by surgery, healing occurs by undifferentiated fibrous tissue and not by cartilage [7] (Fig. 19-9). The only possible exception seen by the writer was that of a nasal septal cartilage in an infant shortly after death; there was a right-angle bend with complete cartilage continuity near the lower border of the nasal septal cartilage. Histology was compatible with an externally imposed change of shape of the cartilage or a breach in the cartilage which had closed by cartilage regeneration.

THE ORGANIZATION OF FORCES WITHIN HYALINE CARTILAGE

In 1958 Gibson and Davis first demonstrated the presence of "interlocked stresses" within costal cartilage [13]. These forces are dramatically demonstrated by the distortion occurring in a cartilage graft after it has been shaped by carving. In 1966 Fry showed the presence of such intrinsic deforming forces within nasal septal cartilage which could lead to deformation of the cartilage after injury or surgery [5, 7] (Fig. 19-10).

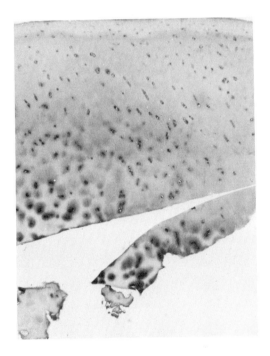

FIGURE 19-4. *Section of articular cartilage from metacarpal head showing more specific arrangement of surface layers than is shown in Figure 19-3.*

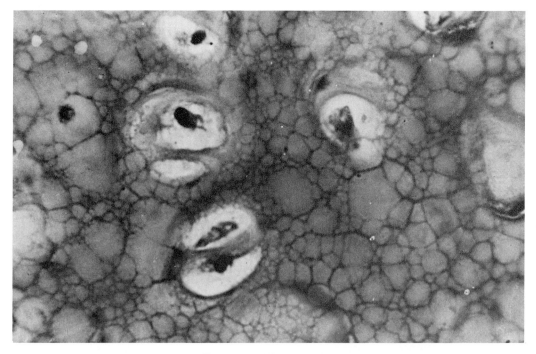

FIGURE 19-5.   *The collagen fibrillar network of nasal septal cartilage.*

FIGURE 19-6.   *Low-power view of collagen fibrillar network of nasal septal cartilage. Although this cartilage does show some parallel alignment of the chondrocytes in the more superficial layers, there is no change in the arrangement of the collagen fibrillar network to correspond with it.*

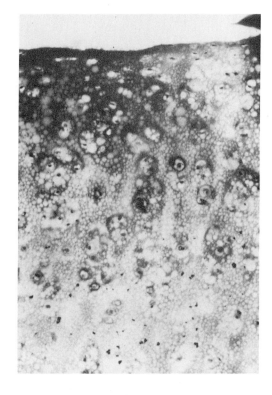

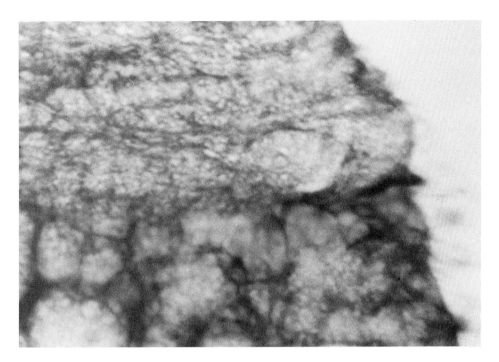

FIGURE 19-7.   *High-power view of junction of cartilage and perichondrium.*

FIGURE 19-8.   *Fibrillar network of nasal septal cartilage teased outside main section.*

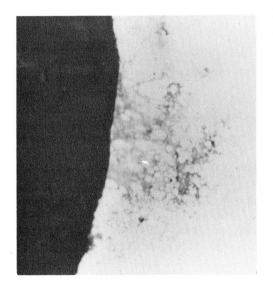

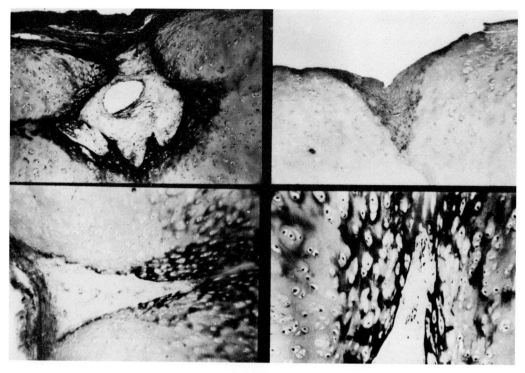

FIGURE 19-9.   *Once cartilage is fractured, it heals by fibrous tissue and not by cartilage. Figure shows four incomplete fractures in nasal septal cartilage that have been healed by undifferentiated fibrous tissue.*

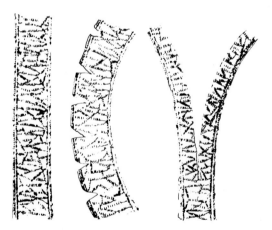

FIGURE 19-10.   *Diagram of forces within nasal septal cartilage as represented by tiny springs under tension. At* left *the forces are in balance. At* center *the inside layer has been interrupted allowing the other unopposed tensile layer to shorten and so deforming the cartilage. At* right *the cartilage is split so each tensile layer is intact but no longer opposed by the other.*

It was shown that the layers of cartilage just beneath the perichondrium were maintained in lines of tension parallel to the surface so that in the intact cartilage these tensile forces are in balance. The cellular arrangement in the area has already been described. In the case of costal cartilage distortion of a graft occurs if the tensile surfaces are randomly interrupted by surgical carving [13]. The more nearly intact surfaces are released from the influence of the opposing tensile layers and can shorten, causing distortion of the cartilage. In the case of nasal septal cartilage a buckling stress, such as would be applied by nasal injury, predictably causes more damage to one surface than to the other [7, 10] because cartilage is weaker in tension than in compression. Buckling of the cartilage increases tension on the convexity while the concavity is thrust into relative compression. Surface damage from incomplete fractures is

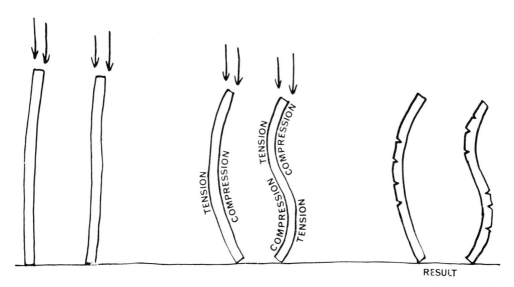

FIGURE 19-11. *Diagram showing mechanism of production of active intrinsic distortion of the nasal septal cartilage. At* left *is seen buckling stress applied to two pieces of cartilage. At* center *the deformities result in sides of tension and relative compression. At* right *is shown damage on convexities in tension. The passive deformity shown at center is now perpetuated by the damage to the surface of the cartilage (see Fig. 19-12).*

not uncommon after nasal injury, and these will perpetuate the deformity that originally caused the fracture (Figs. 19-11, 19-12).

The histology of articular cartilage implies that it is stressed like half of an intact section of costal or nasal septal cartilage and that it is anchored and stressed against the bone. If articular cartilage is detached from the underlying bone, its deformation clearly indicates that this is the case [12] (Figs. 19-13 to 19-16).

"Septal deflections" have been experimentally produced in the rabbit. Surgical interruption of the surface layers of one side in the immature animal leads to a predictable distorted growth pattern similar to the human septal deflections [8] (Fig. 19-17).

Such "interlocked stresses," or at least the manifestation of them, can be abolished effectively by an enzymatic attack on the protein core or the polysaccharide side chains of the protein polysaccharide complexes. Cartilage thus altered shows little reduction in its elasticity, and the collagen network remains intact. An enzymatic attack upon the collagen

network itself by highly purified collagenase, if sufficiently prolonged, will cause a complete dissolution of the cartilage. Well before that point, however, the cartilage loses its elasticity and may be deformed passively. Where the cartilage has been incubated with collagenase, analysis of the incubation medium shows collagen breakdown products and protein polysaccharide breakdown products, exactly in the proportion seen in intact cartilage even though collagenase does not attack the protein polysaccharide itself. This is an indication of the "binding" capacity of collagen as well as its apparent function of maintaining the shape of the tissue [6].

If a new shape is imposed on the cartilage by an external force such as occurs in an untreated nasal injury—whether intrinsic deforming forces are released or not—the collagen will remold over a period of 6 to 12 months. This new shape is then accepted as neutral or "normal."

A graft of costal cartilage is often used for an augmentation rhinoplasty. Gibson and Davis have showed that cartilage grafts will

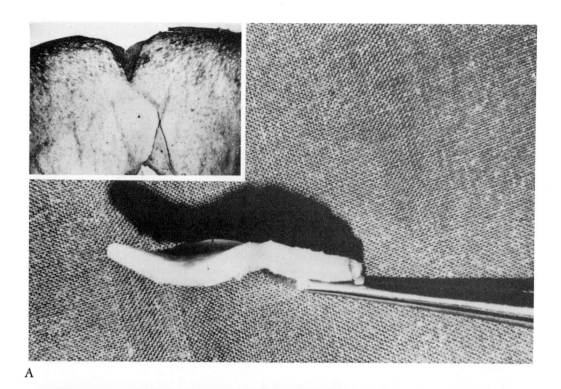

A

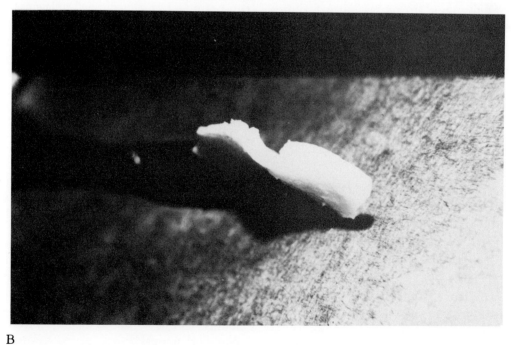

B

FIGURE 19-12.   *A. Distortion of piece of nasal septal cartilage from incomplete fracture. Insert shows its histology. B. Complete fracture of nasal septal cartilage ending in an incomplete fracture causing conical distortion.*

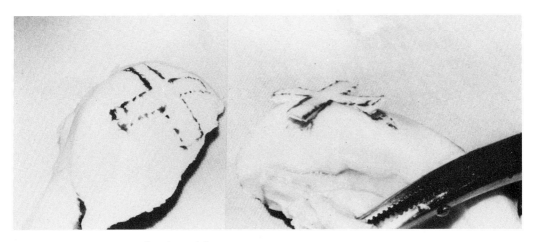

FIGURE 19-13. *Articular face of femoral condyle; ink markings for incision.*

FIGURE 19-14. *A deformation shown after cartilage has been separated from the bone up to the junction of the limbs.*

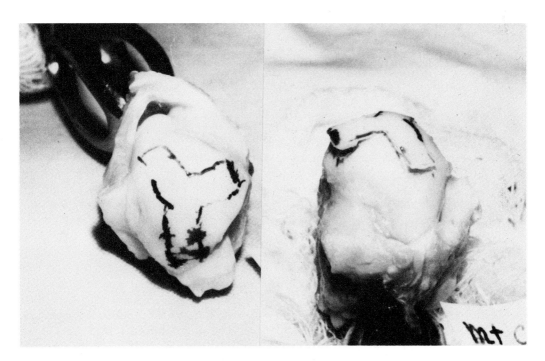

FIGURE 19-15. *Articular face of metacarpal head with incision lines marked out as in Figure 19-13.*

FIGURE 19-16. *Deformation occurring after separation of cartilage from underlying bone up to the junction of the limbs. Such deformation is stable within 5 to 10 minutes.*

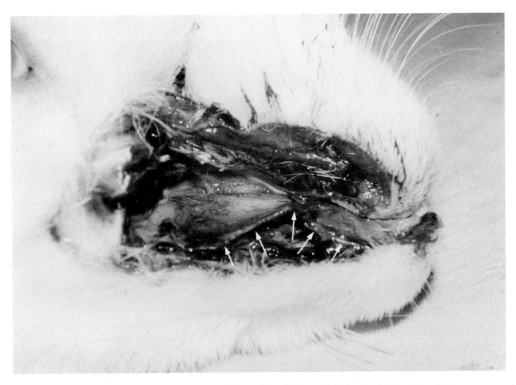

FIGURE 19-17. *Experimentally produced "septal deflection" in the rabbit.*

not "distort" if the balance of forces in the cartilage is preserved. It is important not to carve the external layers much, in order to avoid an imbalance in these outer tensile layers and deformation of the cartilage. Some pieces of cartilage may be used without any external carving at all except at the ends where all tensile surfaces are removed. Another reliable way of employing this useful tissue as a graft is by cutting a deep D-shaped section so as to leave a stable situation which will not lead to deformation [13].

When a reconstructive surgeon rectifies the deformed nasal septal cartilage to correct airway obstruction and external deformity, it is well to distinguish between recent and remote injury. In recent injury the buckling stress, as already explained, invariably damages the convex side of any curve thus produced much more than the concave side. So long as the cartilage was straight before the injury, the deformity can be made good by breaching the tensile layers on the other side

[7]. In old injury, however, the deformity is "fixed" since the remolding of collagen has already occurred. It is a disappointing exercise to breach the concave, more nearly intact, surface in an attempt to straighten it because the original injury caused damage to the outer layers of the convex side. This cannot, therefore, act as an effective tensile layer to straighten the cartilage since the cartilage has healed by fibrous tissue and not by cartilage. In such instances it is better to resect the septum leaving an L-shaped dorsal and columellar strut which is adequate for skeletal support. If the residual strut itself is deformed, it should be corrected separately without further resection of cartilage. A suitable technique for correction has been described elsewhere [10]. It is indeed important that an adequate strut be left behind to avoid "post-SMR collapse" (Fig. 19-18). Such saddling of the bridge line may occur some time after the submucous resection. The available evidence suggests that the tissue

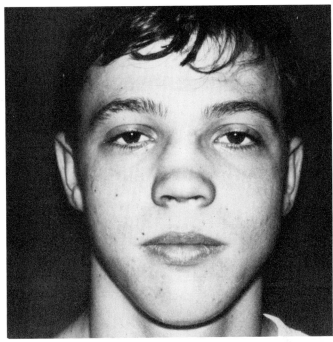
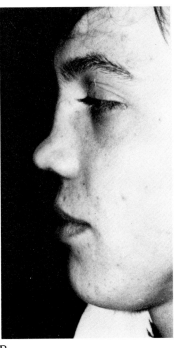

A   B

FIGURE 19-18.   *A, B. Collapse of the cartilaginous bridge line after radical submucous resection of the septum.*

tensions alone are sufficient to cause a gradual saddling of the remaining dorsal cartilage strut, and with time this change of shape becomes permanent as the collagen remolds and gives biological approval.

A difficult problem in the patient with facial paralysis is the paralyzed eyelid. One useful technique, or at least an adjunct to relieve the eye problem, is designed to stiffen the lower eyelid with a large crescentic piece of material with some support inferiorly to hold the lower eyelid against the globe (Fig. 19-19). Nasal septal cartilage is a practical material for this operation (Fig. 19-20), and if one surface is shaved off it will curve concave toward the intact surface so it can be made to fit the contour of the globe snugly.

The interlocked stresses are differentially oriented tensile stresses, their total effect being to thrust the whole tissue into compression. This must clearly be balanced by an equal and opposite expansile force, almost certainly provided by the so-called swelling pressure [20, 21]. Swelling pressure has been

referred to above and is produced at least to some degree by the way collagen and polysaccharide combine and the expansile force implicit in a 7% solution of protein polysaccharide. Under compression load cartilage will lose fluid and will develop a similar pressure in order to regain that fluid. Thus the expansile and compression forces are in balance and the tissue is stable. Only when the forces are interfered with in some way will the shape of the cartilage change. Since water is incompressible, a change in shape of the cartilage (by breaching the surface tensile layers of the cartilage) must involve rapid transfer of water through the matrix, for such deformation can occur in a matter of minutes [6].

BEHAVIOR OF CARTILAGE AS A GRAFT

A cartilage graft will "take" and remain viable whether it is transplanted with its perichondrium or without it. When a cartilage graft is used with perichondrium intact it

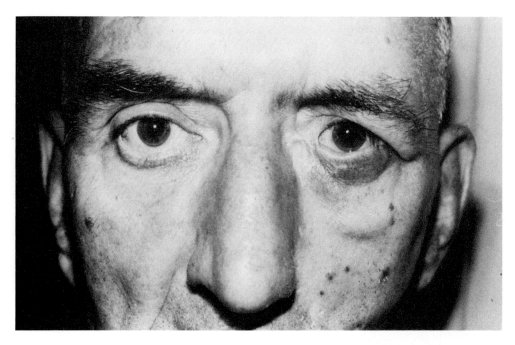

FIGURE 19-19.   *Patient with facial palsy left side. A graft of nasal septal cartilage supports the left lower eyelid against the globe.*

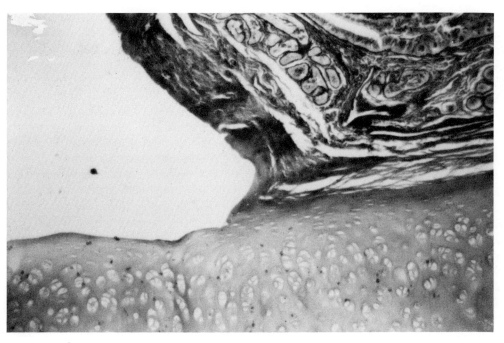

FIGURE 19-20.   *The clean plane of separation between mucoperichondrium and nasal septal cartilage as is used in the operation of submucous resection of the septum, or septoplasty.*

is undoubtedly the perichondrium that actually "takes." The mechanics of nutrition are therefore virtually unchanged from those the cartilage enjoyed in its original donor site. When a cartilage graft is transplanted without perichondrium, later histological section reveals a condensation of fibrous tissue around the cartilage closely resembling perichondrium. It is probably better to use the cartilage with its perichondrium intact if possible so as to cause the least possible disturbance to the graft in the transplantation. It is important, however, not to have any excessive soft tissue such as aponeurosis or muscle on the outside of the cartilage as this will place a greater demand on the revascularization process.

The revascularization of the perichondrium, or, in the case of a naked cartilage graft, reestablishment of its nutrition, depends on intimate apposition of the cartilage graft and the tissues in its recipient site. In this respect it is just like any other graft, and hematoma (which may not be clinically obvious) is the greatest risk. When a hematoma largely prevents the "taking" of the graft, some months may pass before the clinical result is seen to be compromised. Slow absorption of some or all of the tissue occurs. So long as this complication is avoided, a cartilage autograft will last indefinitely.

The problem of distortion in a carved cartilage graft has already been referred to. The point to be emphasized here is that it is sometimes difficult to find a rib tip which is absolutely straight. It is not recommended that bent rib tip be made straight by removal of some of the surface layers on the concave side; the result is not predictable. Instead, one of the higher straighter cartilages should be used, if necessary by resorting to the deep D-shaped section.

Growth of Immature Cartilage Grafts

Some immature cartilage grafts may clearly show growth while others fail to do so after transplantation. The literature on the subject tells us little more than this simple fact. It would seem reasonable to suppose that the immature tissue must be transplanted in the optimal and least disturbing manner possible if its growth capability is to be retained. Transplantation of cartilage into the anterior chamber of the eye allows for "instant" nutrition by diffusion from the aqueous fluid. Some cartilage grafts appear to lose their growth capability, possibly because of delayed establishment of nutrition or for mechanical reasons such as occult hematoma or failure of complete apposition of the surrounding tissues. The role of the perichondrium in the growth of transplanted cartilage is still not clear. The reader is referred to the many outstanding works of Lyndon Peer and more recently the work of Furnas [12].

Cartilage Homografts

A cartilage homograft has relative immunological privilege because the cartilage matrix acts very much like a millipore chamber, preventing immunological confrontation between graft and host cells. The size of molecules which can diffuse into the matrix is also limited. The matrix of a homograft is only weakly antigenic, but over a long period of time a little of the outer portion of such a homograft may become replaced with host fibrous tissues. This action appears not to compromise the clinical result [15, 22]. Some auricular cartilage has been reported as being alive (by sulfur 35 uptake studies) after 23 years [15]. One is often unprepared to use a young child's own cartilage as a graft for a saddle nose from childhood injury. Instead it is more sensible to put the child on an operating list to follow an adult who is having cartilage taken for that or another purpose. Under these circumstances one might wisely use the cartilage homograft without perichondrium. With progressive growth of the face and other parts of the nose the child's nasal cartilage graft may be replaced with his own cartilage at a later age.

Use of Preserved Cartilage Grafts

A preserved cartilage graft differs from a fresh autograft or homograft only in one respect. If the "storing" process results in death of chondrocytes, a "graft" will gradually be absorbed over a period of time because the integrity of the matrix can no longer be sustained by dead chondrocytes. The most obvious example of a graft altered in this way is one that has been boiled. Such grafts were used earlier in the century in the hope that their tendency to warp would thus be averted. The graft is a serviceable strut for a time, but its fate is inevitable.

Since cartilage is generally utilized in small quantities as a graft and for specific purposes, it is probably better to use fresh autografts in an adult and, if need be, homografts for a child.

Cartilage Heterografts

Cartilage heterografts have some biological interest but little clinical application today. The matrix is more antigenic than that of the same species, and slow absorption is inevitable. Their use as an immunological model is an interesting possibility. Earlier in this part of the century surgical experiments with them yielded generally unfavorable results because of the now predictable absorption and replacement. However, some pertinent observations were recorded. For example, one heterograft of Sir Harold Gillies which persisted was surrounded by a bursa. The graft could actually be turned through 180 degrees within the bursa. The immunological explanation is too obvious to need stating.

Elastic Cartilage

Elastic cartilage is somewhat different from hyaline cartilage. Its behavior as a free graft is very similar, but the arrangement of its inbuilt stresses and its histology show variation. Although there is a similar pattern of flattened cells in the surface layers, the matrix is permeated by heavy elastic fibers that continue into the perichondrium. It is difficult to separate perichondrium from elastic cartilage, in contrast to the situation in hyaline cartilage. The perichondrium is much more

bound to the superficial cartilage layers and could almost be regarded as a continuation of it.

When the intrinsic distortional forces are examined, it becomes evident that breaching one surface causes the cartilage to curl concave toward the intact side. Bergman and Stenstrom claim that this reaction is due to the perichondrium rather than the cartilage [3]. While it is difficult to exclude the presence of perichondrium from the experimental pieces used, the conclusion that the perichondrium is totally responsible for the deformation might be going beyond the limits of the data. Indeed, Bergman and Stenstrom's sections tend not to support this view, but rather the reverse, in that splitting of auricular cartilage causes "curling" in the pieces near the surface where there is no perichondrium [see 3, p. 432, Fig. 2A]. It seems rather extravagant to conclude further that such a hypothesis must apply to hyaline cartilage, in which the deformation occurs without any perichondrium [7, 13] (see Figs. 19-13 to 19-16). Moreover, elastic cartilage and hyaline cartilage probably do not differ so radically in terms of basic organization.

The forces in elastic cartilage may be partially liberated in the clinical situation for surgeons to make an antihelix in the outstanding ear [4, 17, 24]. Standard techniques for ear operations have evolved independently and empirically.

FIBROCARTILAGE

Fibrocartilage is seen in the intervertebral disk and the intra-articular disks of knee joint and temporomandibular joint. Clinical interest has been limited to excisional procedures. Histology and behavior of this tissue do not indicate any differentially oriented surface tensile layers; rather, the structure has been modified for "shock absorbing" and gliding functions. Again the fibers (collagen) are dense, and there is a "shading off" into the perichondrium rather than the sharp division seen in hyaline cartilage.

SUMMARY

The mechanical characteristics and biological properties of cartilage, together with its clinical applications for the reconstructive surgeon, require that these be understood if one is to gain optimum results from surgery. This chapter is an attempt to correlate these properties with clinical practice. For comprehensive information and references the reader is referred to the excellent review by Barrett [2].

REFERENCES

1. Abrahams, M., and Duggan, T. C. The Mechanical Characteristics of Costal Cartilage. In Kenedi, R. M. (Ed.), *Biomechanics and Related Bioengineering Topics.* Proceedings of Symposium Held in Glasgow, September 1964. New York: Pergamon, 1965.
2. Barrett, A. J. *Comprehensive Biochemistry.* Amsterdam: Florkin & Stotz, 1962. Vol. 26B, chap. 6, p. 425, and addendum p. 593.
3. Bergman, F. O., and Stenstrom, S. J. Curling Tendency of Various Types of Distortionable Cartilages. In Hueston, J. (Ed.), *Transactions of the 5th International Congress of Plastic and Reconstructive Surgery.* London: Butterworth, 1971.
4. Chonchet, V. A method of antihelix reconstruction. *Br. J. Plast. Surg.* 16:268, 1963.
5. Fry, H. J. H. Interlocked stresses in human nasal septal cartilage. *Br. J. Plast. Surg.* 19:276, 1966.
6. Fry, H. J. H. Cartilage and cartilage grafts: The basic properties of the tissue and the components responsible for them. *Plast. Reconstr. Surg.* 40:426, 1967.
7. Fry, H. J. H. Nasal trauma and the interlocked stresses of the nasal septal cartilage. *Br. J. Plast. Surg.* 20:146, 1967.
8. Fry, H. J. H. The aetiology of so-called "septal deviations" and their experimental production in the growing rabbit. *Br. J. Plast. Surg.* 21:419, 1968.
9. Fry, H. J. H. Applied histology of the nasal septal cartilage. *Aust. N.Z. J. Surg.* 36:311, 1968.
10. Fry, H. J. H. The residual distorted cartilage strut after submucous resection of the nasal septum. *Br. J. Plast. Surg.* 21:170, 1968.
11. Fry, H. J. H. Articular cartilage: The interlocked stresses and their manifestations. *Br. J. Plast. Surg.* 27:363, 1974.
12. Furnas, D. W. The growth of cartilage transplants in baby rabbits. *Plast. Reconstr. Surg.* 45:356, 1970.
13. Gibson, T., and Davis, W. B. The distortion of autogenous cartilage grafts: Its cause and prevention. *Br. J. Plast. Surg.* 10:257, 1958.
14. Gibson, T., and Davis, W. B. *Transactions of the International Society of Plastic Surgeons (Second Congress), London, 1959.* Edinburgh: Livingstone, 1960. P. 452.
15. Gibson, T., Davis, W. B., and Curran, R. C. The long term survival of cartilage homografts in man. *Br. J. Plast. Surg.* 11:177, 1958.
16. Goh, A. J. W., and Lowther, D. A. Effect of age on the composition of bovine nasal cartilage. *Nature* (Lond.) 210:1270, 1966.
17. Ju, D. M. C., Li, C., and Crickelair, G. F. The surgical correction of protruding ears. *Plast. Reconstr. Surg.* 32:283, 1963.
18. Lewis, P. R., and McCutchen, C. W. Experimental evidence for weeping lubrication in mammalian joints. *Nature* (Lond.) 184:1285, 1959.
19. Lowther, D. A. Personal communication, 1972.
20. McCutchen, C. W. Sponge-hydrostatic and weeping bearings. *Nature* (Lond.) 184:1284, 1959.
21. McCutchen, C. W. Animal joints and weeping lubrication. *New Scientist* 15:412, 1962.
22. Peer, L. Sex chromatin study to determine the survival of cartilage homografts. *Trans. Bull.* 5:404, 1958.
23. Schubert, M. *Structure and Function of Connective and Skeletal Tissue.* London: Butterworth, 1965.
24. Stenstrom, S. J. A "natural" technique for correction of congenitally prominent ears. *Plast. Reconstr. Surg.* 32:509, 1963.

20

The Healing of Bone
·
Donald A. Nagel

BONE HEALING

Disruptions of bone vary significantly in their severity, from the taking of a small bone graft by a surgeon to an open comminuted fracture with damage to adjacent muscle, arteries, and nerves. The systemic response will be minimal to the first procedure but maximal to the compound, comminuted fracture, producing shock and possibly even causing renal shutdown and death.

When considering bone healing, one should remember that this is a process of regeneration as well as repair. Bone is not healed by scar tissue unless nonunion occurs. In most instances a fracture is replaced by normal bone and such regeneration is different from that which occurs in many other tissues in the body.

The process is affected not only by the variable of the severity of the injury but also by the variables of age of the individual with the fracture, type of immobilization of the fracture, presence or absence of infection in the fracture, and diabetes or Cushing's disease in the patient. These factors must be kept in mind as we try to understand bone healing.

Historical Data

The earliest medical writings contain references to practical methods of treating fractures, but the basic science approach to understanding the healing of fractures had to await such men as Duhamel. In 1741 he noted that the dye "madder" stained the bone that was laid down as the animal was fed the dye and that the underside of the periosteum was stained in a healing fracture in such an animal. Several decades later Hunter, following the treachings of Haller, indicated that he believed that vascularization of a blood clot in a fracture was the first important step in the formation of repairing callus and that only arteries could form bone. Controversy has reigned since then as to whether fractures healed by periosteal new bone formation or by a vascular tissue growing into the fracture gap. In 1835 Syme entered the conflict. He resected 1¾ inch of bone from both radii of dogs and noted that bone healed on the left where the periosteum was intact and did not heal on the right where periosteum was removed.* In 1867 Ollier published his

*The stories of Duhamel, Hunter, Haller, and Syme, and

367

findings, based on many experiments [47]. He found that in a young animal the periosteum was the greatest source of cells in fracture healing, that the marrow presented only a small number of cells to the process, and that the bone itself gave the least number of cells.

Histological Data

According to Ham, the reason for his experiments on fracture repair was the confusion that existed in his mind after reading about the subject in the late 1920s. Some of the chaos in the literature is the result of the difference in the species studied, the age of the animal, the type of fracture, and the type of immobilization following the fracture. The definitions of such terms as *periosteum* and *fibrocyte* have also led to confusion. In his experiments on rabbits' fractured ribs Ham noted that associated with a fracture to a bone there is tearing of the blood vessels in the periosteum and in the haversian system [33]. A blood clot forms between the bone ends, but, in addition, circulation ceases in the haversian vessels for some distance each side of the fracture and there is osteocyte death. Contrary to others, he found no ingrowth of new young capillaries into the blood clot that formed in the fracture gap. Pritchard believes the blood clot is debrided by macrophages that enter the blood clot [50]. Ham describes the histological formation of the callus as occurring by the proliferation of cells from the underside of the periosteum and from cells of the marrow endosteum as well as from undifferentiated cells of the bone marrow [33]. In his view the cells differentiate into osteoblasts when they are close to capillaries and those farther from capillaries form chondrocytes. In the course of the healing of the fracture, he notes, bony trabeculae are firmly cemented into the bone fragments close to the fractured ends and to each other. Thus the fracture is immobilized and remodeling

of other early contributors to our knowledge of the musculoskeletal system, are well told in Keith's book *Menders of the Maimed* [36].

can occur. Recent studies by Craft et al. [24] would indicate that membranous bone has the same histological healing pattern as Ham has described for ribs.

Studying human fractures under clinical conditions, Urist and Johnson, in 1943, felt there was "complete similarity in general pattern of bone repair in man and animals" [63]. However, they noted two differences: (1) Human fractures differed somewhat from experimental fractures surgically produced and immobilized in that soft tissue was interposed to some extent between the fracture ends in all human cases. This became a problem only if the interposed tissue was viable and in large quantity. (2) The calcification of the osteoid of the callus was delayed in human compared with animal fractures. They studied 48 cases that were thought to represent normal human callus at varying stages and described the general pattern of fracture healing as consisting of a procallus, a fibrocartilaginous callus, and a bony callus. The procallus, an "organizing hematoma and highly vascular granulation tissue that develops in the first weeks of healing," contains pieces of injured tissue and fragments of dead bone. Aseptic inflammation is part of this process. Developing almost simultaneously, a fibrocartilaginous callus is produced by differentiation of "granulation tissue or primitive connective tissue cells" to a "translucent mass of dense, fibrous connective tissue, fibrocartilage, and cartilage which is seen from the second or third week of healing until the time of union." Bony callus originates in some fractures as early as the first week when osteoblasts from the inner layer of the periosteum and from the endosteum of fracture ends deposits new bone on the periosteal and medullary surfaces of the injured cortex. This is an example of intramembranous bone formation. Enchondral bone formation is also seen as the fibrocartilaginous callus is replaced, beginning in the third to fourth week after fracture.

Figure 20-1 shows a histological longitudinal section of a 31-day-old closed fracture of

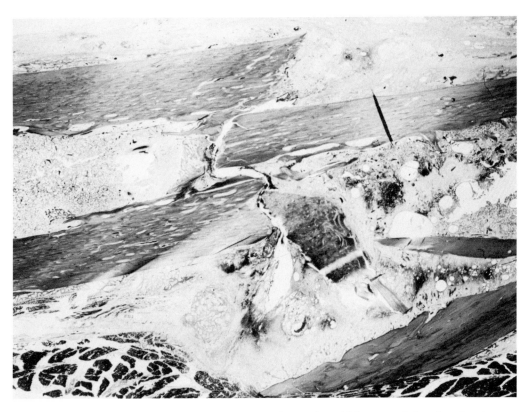

FIGURE 20-1. *Histological longitudinal section of a 31-day-old fracture of the tibia showing new bone formation in the fibrocartilaginous callus and resorption with enlargement of the haversian canals in the cortical bone.*

the tibia of a 19-year-old male. The injury was sustained as he crossed a freeway and was hit by a car. Death resulted from a head injury received at the same time, and he was in coma with flaccid paralysis until the time of his death.

There is proliferation of cells under the periosteum throughout the entire section but it is most marked over the fracture ends. New bone formation is noted in the fibrocartilaginous callus under the periosteum in this area. The lacunae in the cortical bone in both the fragments and the shaft are devoid of cells. Resorption, revascularization, and new bone formation take place in the haversian canals. In the endosteal fibrocartilaginous callus a great deal of new bone formation is seen.

A different type of histological picture of fracture healing occurs when there is little or no gap between the fractured ends of the bone. This type of healing has been called primary bone healing and was described by Groves [31] in 1914 and popularized by Shenk [55] in 1964. It consists in healing of the fracture without x-ray or histological evidence of the significant amount of callus. The repair is accomplished almost entirely by remodeling of the cortical bone. In the remodeling, formation of resorption canals through the cortex across the fracture is followed by formation of osteons in the canals as new blood vessels course through them and new bone is laid down.

What is the origin of the cells that heal bone? Tonna, using tritiated thymidine, tritiated glycine, and tritiated proline, attempted to answer this question [60]. He concluded that they come from progenitive cells found in the periosteum, the endosteum, and the mesenchymal pool. According to Pritchard [50], there is evidence from studying histological sections of repairing fracture to support three possibilities:

1. "Differentiation from a perivascular reserve of cells having their ultimate origin in the deep periosteum and bone marrow."
2. "Recruited from fibroblasts of the fibrous part of the callus by the process of induction."
3. "Predetermined" fibroblasts which form osteoblasts on some signal.

Other theories have not been disproved. In 1941 Bloom, Bloom, and McLean reported evidence that myeloid reticular cells were transformed to bone in pigeons during the egg-laying cycle [13]. Algöwer feels that one of the blood cells, either a lymphocyte or a monocyte, multiplies to give rise to the early callus [4]. Trueta and Little believe the cells come from the vascular endothelium [61].

Metabolism of Fracture Healing

Recently, Brighton and Krebs using an oxygen probe, have found that initially there is low oxygen tension in the fracture hematoma and in the newly formed callus around the fracture [19]. This returns to normal levels when healing is complete. It would appear, then, that in the area of the fracture early anaerobic metabolism later shifts to aerobic metabolism. Wray studied the metabolic activity of healing fractures of the rabbit tibia and found large amounts of mucopolysaccharides in the fracture callus at first [67]. They diminished as ossification increased. As might be expected, fracture callus utilized large quantities of glucose in the healing period. There is evidence that animals on diets deficient in protein and carbohydrates do not heal fractures as well as animals on normal diets [35]. In a previous publication Wray postulated that the changes in pH, lactic acid, phosphorus, and alkaline phosphatase, which he found in human fracture

aspirations, may be attributed to red cell metabolism in the hematoma [66].

Other Factors Influencing Bone Healing

Blood Flow

Of the many factors influencing bone healing, perhaps the most important is blood flow. Existence of a hyperemic response to fracture has been assumed since the pioneering work of Lexer, which was reported in 1922 [43]. Subsequent work by Wray and Lynch [68], using vascular injection techniques, and by Rhinelander and Baraguy [54], using microangiography, beautifully demonstrated that after a fracture, there is an opening of the existing arterial tree, with both medullary and periosteal circulation increasing by the development of new blood vessels. It is their contention that the medullary blood supply, when intact, plays a major role in nutrition of the uniting callus and revascularization of necrotic bone around the fracture. Laurnen and Kelly, using a dilution technique, also noted an increase in blood flow which reached its peak, two weeks after fracture in dogs, of six times normal flow and then gradually returned to normal at the time the fracture healed [42]. They found no difference in oxygen content, PO_2, PCO_2, or pH when blood from the fractured limb was compared with the control limb. Kruse and Kelly have observed that a venous tourniquet increases the amount of periosteal callus in a healing fracture [41].

Ham emphasized that with every fracture there is death of the osteocytes at the end of the fracture fragments. This is due to the disruption of a portion of the endosteal and periosteal blood supply and in turn a disruption of the blood vessels of the haversian canals which are derived from the periosteal and endosteal blood vessels. A more severe injury will destroy a greater portion of this blood supply. Every fracture surgeon has noted that nonunions occur more frequently in the markedly displaced fracture, with consequently greater tearing of the periosteum than in nondisplaced fractures. Since surgical treatment of fractures will also lessen the blood supply, it must be balanced by markedly improved apposition and fixation if it is to be justified. Finally, infection, particularly with coagulase-positive *Staphylococcus aureus*, will cause thrombosis of vessels which may lead to delayed union or nonunion.

Minerals

Most investigators would agree with Key and Odell that the availability of minerals does not greatly influence bone healing [37]. Goldsmith et al., however, feel that the presence of phosphates in large amounts may shorten the time required for bone healing [30].

Hormones

There is some disagreement as to which hormones influence bone healing. Growth hormone and thyrotropin are said by Koskinen to have an osseous anabolic effect [39]. This is denied by Wray [66]. These two writers do agree that orchiectomy and thyroidectomy seem to have little effect on bone healing [40]. It is not certain that calcitonin has any effect on bone healing. Cortisone inhibits all aspects of bone healing, at least in rabbits [58], and diabetes also delays bone healing [35].

Induction Substances

There has been tremendous interest in the last few years in "induction" substances that will speed the rate of bone repair. Chondroitin sulfate [20] and a "macromolecule" found in decalcified bone matrix probably bound to bone collagen [62] have been said to increase fracture healing. "Induction" substances need further study before they are clinically applicable.

Mechanical Factors

Throughout the years the response of bone to the mechanical stresses applied to it has been studied with interest. In 1892 Wolff noted that bone adapts its external form and internal architecture to the stresses to which it is subjected [64]. The remodeling that occurs or how the cells behave in the bony callus with fracture healing is believed today by most investigators to be due to the mechanical stress applied by muscles and gravity. Mechanical factors also play a role in the amount of periosteal response to fracture. People dealing with fractures daily have found that the periosteal response is greater when the fracture is poorly immobilized provided the periosteum is intact (shown experimentally by Groves [31]). Mechanical factors, then, have something to do with proliferation of cells. Finally, mechanical factors may also have something to do with the kind of cell that is derived from the pluripotential cells present in the early stages of fracture healing. Bassett and Herrman have shown that in tissue culture 20-day-old chick embryo tibial cortex explants will produce osteocytes if allowed to compact and fibrocytes if placed under tension [10]. Both experiments were conducted under high O_2 tension. If the O_2 tension was low, chondrocytes formed with compaction.

The experimental work of Groves provides the basis for the operative treatment of fractures and is recommended reading for all surgeons who treat fractures [31]. Groves showed the superiority of intramedullary pegs of steel over various types of bone pegs and the superiority of long plates with good fixation over short plates with poor fixation. He wrote, "Bones firmly and accurately fixed will heal by first intention." Bones weakly joined by a method that allows more and more movement between them will not join at all, or their junction will be long delayed. He believed that motion in surgical wounds led to sepsis by the formation of a great amount of fluid which escaped through the wound and subsequently became infected.

Effects of Electricity

Becker and Murray have demonstrated that a fracture in a bullfrog changes the polarity in the bone [11]. They have also shown that nucleated red cells in the amphibian are part of the repair process, changing from red blood cells to fibroblasts to osteoblasts. Furthermore, they have taken the same red blood cells and subjected them to 100 to 400 microamperes voltage outside the body and produced the same changes seen in cells in fracture healing in vivo. Is the flow of electrons the regulating mechanism of fracture healing?

In addition to the piezoelectric production of current in bone that is bent (by *piezoelectric* we mean a charge separation produced by a force that causes molecular deformation), there are other sources of electricity within the human body. Streaming potentials are formed by a hydraulic mechanism in blood vessels. Exercise produces both piezoelectrical potentials and streaming potentials by bending bone and by increasing the blood supply. Bassett has recently found that muscle injury is the most effective way yet found to raise potential in bone [9]. These three means and perhaps another involving nerves certainly do change the electrical environment around a fracture.

Bassett has been able to induce current in bone by creating an electrical field outside the bone. Animals subjected to such a field produced less callus but a stiffer callus which appears to be more mature than the control fracture. This technique is now being used in a few selected human cases for treatment of pseudarthrosis. The implantation of a cathode into the nonunion of a fracture has also been reported by Brighton to stimulate bone healing [18].

It would appear that both biological and physical processes are intermingled in the repair of fractures. One cannot help feeling a certain excitement in anticipation of a breakthrough which may change the approach to fracture treatment—an approach that, since the time of Hippocrates, has been primarily one of immobilization.

BONE GRAFTING

Bone grafts are being used at present to induce healing in delayed union and nonunion of fractures; to bridge gaps in bones caused by compounding wounds, disease, or tumor surgery; to help bring about arthrodesis of a joint; to restore entire missing units such as a finger, usually along with the transference of other tissue; and to improve facial contour. Ray and Sabet estimate that over 200,000 bone grafting procedures are done in the United States in a single year [53].

Terminology

At the outset, terminology should be clarified because the newer terms that have been accepted by international agreement are somewhat different from some of those used in older writings. An *autograft* is a transplant of tissue from one portion of an individual to another portion of the same individual. This is the same meaning as in the older terminology. An *isograft* is a transplant of tissue from one individual to another individual having the same genetic makeup, such as transplantation between identical twins or between inbred animals. This is a new term, not used in the past. An *allograft* is a transplant of tissue from one individual to another of the same species who does not have the same genetic background. This term replaces the term *homograft* used in the past. A *xenograft* is a transplant of tissue from an individual of one species to an individual of another species, such as the transplantation of bone from calf to human. This word replaces *heterograft*, which is the term used to describe such transplantation in the past.

Early Experiments

Bick has written, "The transference of animal bone to replace defects in the human skeleton has been attempted since the earliest eras of surgery" [12]. Such transferences were, in modern parlance, xenografts (heterografts in the older language). It was Hunter (1728–1793), however, who applied scientific methods of experimentation to surgical problems. He is credited with the first written account of the use of an autograft when he described the transfer of a chicken's spur to its head.

Ollier was also a scientific surgeon, who in 1835 attempted to reconstruct a nose by transplanting a piece of tibial periosteum under the skin of the forehead. The graft became infected and when it was removed it was found to be adherent at several points and beginning to grow. Ollier published in 1867 his observations on experimental studies done and clinical results concerning the regeneration of bone [47]. Experiments performed on very young dogs and rabbits conclusively showed that at least in young animals the transplanted periosteum grew. He also noted that a flap of periosteum, if scraped on its deep surface, did not produce bone. He further felt that transplanted fragments of bone even without the periosteum would live.

Barth published his first paper in 1893, describing experiments placing bone grafts in holes in dogs' skulls, and reported there was no difference in the behavior of dead and living bone grafts [7]. It was his feeling that all bone grafts with or without periosteum—autografts, allografts, and xenografts—acted alike; all died and simply provided a passive scaffolding through which bone from the host provided new bone substance.

Considerable controversy arose as to whether the periosteum was important in the transplantation of bone and also over the question of whether the transplanted bone lived or died. In 1912 Axhausen published the results of his experiments on rats, rabbits, and dogs wherein he transferred pieces of bone as autografts, allografts, and xenografts with and without periosteum to beds of bone and into soft tissues [6]. He reported new cells forming under the periosteum of a living bone graft and announced that the marrow tissue of the graft showed new bone formation when it was in contact with living vascular tissue of the host. He also noted that the cells in compact bone always seemed to be absent from the lacunae of the bone within several weeks after transplantation. Certain cells close to the periosteum and marrow did maintain their staining characteristics, how-

ever. The compact bone of the graft was rebuilt by absorption of its surface and its haversian system, revascularization, and then apposition of new bone. Axhausen believed that bone grafts taken without periosteum were inferior to those taken with periosteum and that allografts were less viable than autografts. Xenografts, he commented, became encapsulated or absorbed and had no viability.

Another scientific surgeon, Macewen wrote his book *The Growth of Bone* in 1912 [44]. After describing numerous experiments on dogs, he recorded an operation in 1880 wherein he had transplanted wedges of bone taken from the tibia of one child into the humerus of another child whose shaft was missing because of osteomyelitis. This had been treated surgically some two years previously. Three bone grafting procedures were carried out at two month intervals. "These all fused together and to the condyles of the humerus, filled the gap in the arm to the extent of four and a quarter inches; the humerus then measured six inches in length." This allograft (in older terminology, a homograft) appears to be the first written account of such a procedure in humans in the English language. Macewen did not agree with Axhausen's views of the importance of the periosteum. In his experimental work he used dogs in "the developmental period" and showed that periosteal flaps and transplants did not produce bone and that periosteum was not necessary for the production of bone to fill in defects. He demonstrated that allografts placed in the gap in the bone without periosteum filled the gap in seven weeks. Furthermore, shavings of allograft bone grew in the neck and in the omentum, as revealed by examination at six and seven weeks. Transplanted bone dust did not produce bone. Macewen thought of periosteum as being only a "limiting membrane" without osteogenic potential.

In 1917 Groves reviewed the writings of the previous investigators mentioned and reported his own experiments [32]. Ollier himself observed, he noted, that "periosteum formed no new bone in an adult after resection" and that periosteum without its deeper layer (cambium layer) produced no bone. Further, Macewen felt that when a superficial portion of the bone was raised with the periosteum this transplanted periosteum formed bone. The differences between the opinions of Ollier and Macewen lay in their definitions of the exact location of the cells taking part in osteogenesis following transplantation of autografts. Ollier thought that these cells went with the periosteum, as indeed they do in the young animal. Macewen thought that they were not part of the periosteum but simply the outer surface of the bone; hence their conflict over the ability of the periosteum to produce bone. Concerning the marrow, both Ollier and Macewen put tubes into the marrow canal and noted new bone filling these tubes, thereby proving that marrow contributed to osteogenesis. Both Ollier and Macewen believed that compact bone could live and produce new bone. Axhausen and Barth pointed out that with most cases of compact bone transplantation bone cells die. The important factor is how soon do the cells in transplanted compact bone obtain satisfactory nourishment? If compact bone is put into a vascular bed as small chips, the osteocytes receive blood and live. If the transplant is put in as a large piece of compact bone, the blood supply does not penetrate the material surrounding the osteocytes in time for them to survive. Having discerned what the main facts established by previous investigators really were, Groves conducted experiments on his own to find the "best methods of transplanting bone tissue so as to make good, defects left by trauma or disease."

Using adult cats, Groves found that both full-thickness struts of an entire autogenous bone and split-section struts of autogenous bone provided a good means of filling in gaps in the cat's tibia. Intramedullary grafts, however, if fitted as tightly as possible, seemed to block the ingrowth of bone from the endosteum so that the gap was not filled and the graft subsequently broke. Where the peg graft lay loose in the marrow cavity, it did not provide stability. The intramedullary pegging with live or dead bone seemed to be of little value. In previous experiments on fracture healing Groves found that, if a portion of the tibia was removed, broken up in small pieces, and placed back in the gap that remained, very little new bone formed. This was an entirely different matter from the massive bone formation that occurred in comminuted fractures when periosteum remained attached to the fragments. Repeating his previous experiments and finding, again, that "after six weeks the pieces of bone are still quite distinct and not very firmly united to one another or to either main fragment," he concluded that full-thickness bones or split whole bones were better for filling gaps than filling them with bone fragments. He also removed a piece of tibia and "reduced it [to powder] by a small grinding machine." "The dust was placed in the periosteal tube and after six weeks the bone dust had been completely absorbed and replaced by blood stained connective tissue. There is no evidence of new bone formation." His experiments showed, he believed, that insecure fixation resulted in failures with bone grafts. Furthermore, "properly applied metal sutures or pins" do not prevent bone formation by their presence. In fact, because of the firm fixation of the graft to the graft bed, they help with its incorporation. Comparing the placement of living grafts and dead grafts into a defect in a cat's tibia, he demonstrated the superiority of the living graft over the dead bone graft. However, the dead graft might actually become inseparably united to its bony bed and was practical if no living material was available for grafting. It was important, moreover, for the grafted limb to be immobilized for the shortest period of time and then subjected to motion. "In this way, nutrition of the muscles and the flexibility of the tendons and joints are preserved while the formation of new bone is encouraged."

Histological Data

In 1955 Chase and Herndon, after reviewing 1500 papers relating to the fate of bone grafts, concluded, "Our present day knowledge of histological fate of bone following transplantation is but little changed from the views originally presented by Axhausen" [23]. They emphasized that the process of reorganization of bone is by resorption and apposition. Phemister introduced the term "creeping substitution" into the English language in 1914, translating it from Barth's work to describe this process [48]. Phemister's views on the fate of autogenous bone graft to defects in the ulna of dogs are based on extensive histological study (recorded in English) and summarized as follows: At three days microscopic examination revealed no changes in the bone cells or periosteum of the transplanted bone, but beginning proliferation of the inner layer of the periosteum was noted. At 10 days there was periosteal fibrous callus and endosteal callus, which was beginning to ossify, at the point of proximation of the graft to the host bed. About half the cells of the cortical bone transplant either had disappeared or were shrunken and stained poorly. At 26 days the bone cells of the cortex of the transplant were all dead, leaving the lacunae vacant. "The periosteum along the transplant away from its end is alive and one side has formed a thin callus which was largely ossified." At 51 days, "From the periosteum of the surfaces of the transplant and from the callus of the medullary canal, blood vessels have grown into many of the old haversian canals. The medullary canal of the graft at either end is filled with a bony callus." At 132 days, "Revascularization of the transplant has occurred with absorption of portions of the dead cortex and deposition of new bone in its place so that about one half the old compact is substituted by new bone." At 350 days there was no gross evidence where the graft had been placed through the ulna. Microscopic examination revealed that new bone had almost completely replaced the old cortical bone. However, haversian canals were not yet oriented in a longitudinal direction as they were in the host bone.

Enneking and Morris have obtained quantitative data concerning the rate at which bone transplants are replaced and how it is related to the physical strength of the transplants [26]. On the basis of five human cortical onlay tibial transplants studied, they postulated that there was 80 percent viable new bone in the graft at one year. Animal studies have been presented by Enneking and his associates [27]. Studying a dog's fibula, they noted that resorption of bone is already present at two weeks and reaches its maximum at six weeks. Porosity of bone reached its maximum between 6 and 12 weeks, and the strength of the bone tested at this time was only 40 percent of the strength of the original fibula. Apposition of new bone began at 8 weeks and reached its maximum at 12 weeks, continuing throughout the 48 weeks of the experiment. From the twenty-fourth week on, strength of the transplant of the fibula gradually increased, until at 48 weeks it was almost normal.

Cancellous bone, as distinct from cortical or corticocancellous bone graft, is replaced much more rapidly than cortical bone. The osteoblasts on its surface quickly line the edges of the dead trabeculae, and new bone takes over.

Studies of allografts reveal that periosteal new bone may occur within the first two weeks, but by three weeks this bone frequently undergoes necrosis and absorption in association with the peak of the host inflammatory reaction to the allograft. The inflammatory reaction involves numerous lymphocytes and macrophages and scattered eosinophils. Simultaneously the host vascular connective tissue surrounds the allografts and produces absorption of the cortex, rather than uniting the graft to the host. It has been noted that frozen allografts produce less intense inflammatory reaction, but such is still present. Bonfiglio and Jetter believe that the character and timing of the exudate may indicate a delayed type of hypersensitivity reaction [15]. Their studies suggest that immunization procedures "with soluble extracts of bone in adjuvant may cause the appearance of a blocking factor (possibly antibody) which prevents the inflammatory reaction and enhances somewhat the opportunity for the homograft acceptance to occur." Axhausen, in his early studies, noted that healing of allografts takes place in the same way as it does with autogenous grafts but that the healing process is slower. With regard to the use of dead bone, most experimenters feel that complete reorganization of dead bone may be delayed for years. Xenografts have also been studied histologically, and, in spite of the various procedures attempting to take away their antigenicity, an inflammatory reaction develops around these grafts and destroys them.

Figure 20-2 is a photomicrograph of a cross section taken from the midportion of a tibial cortical strut autograft placed from the trochanter to the ilium to induce arthrodesis of the hip. The graft was removed 14 months after the original transplant as arthrodesis failed to occur. The histological section of the graft used for this figure was then prepared. Note the remains of the original graft with the empty lacunae indicating dead bone (labeled *a*). New bone formation is also seen in cross section (labeled *b*) at the periphery of haversian canals (labeled *c*).

Figure 20-3 is a photomicrograph of the cancellous portion of a corticocancellous autograft that had been taken from the tibia and transplanted over the lamina of the thoracic vertebrae. The bone for this section was taken from the end of the graft at the time of extension of the fusion nine days after the initial transplant. The trabecula of the graft (labeled *a*) shows a few pyknotic cells still

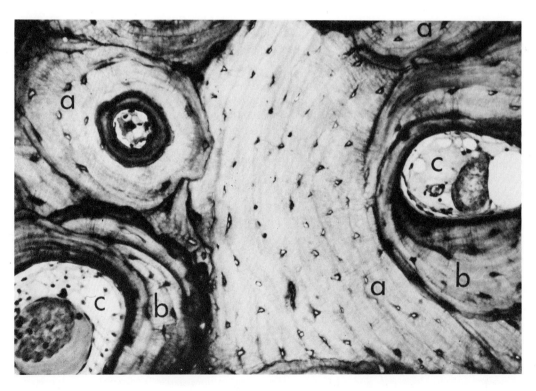

FIGURE 20-2.   *Transverse histological section of a cortical strut autograft that has been in place for 14 months.* (a) *Original bone with empty lacunae;* (b) *new bone formation at the outside of* (c) *haversian systems.*

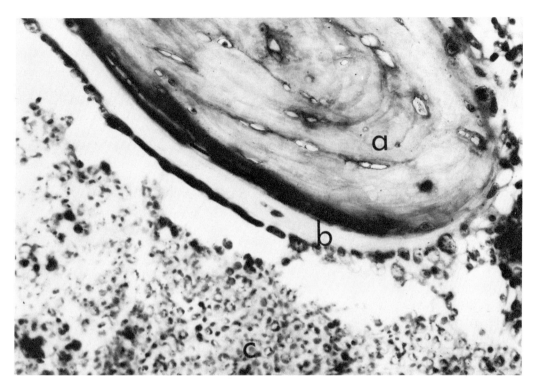

FIGURE 20-3. *High-power photomicrograph of cancellous bone nine days after transplant.* (a) *Trabecula of graft with some lacunae still containing pyknotic cells;* (b) *new bone formation;* (c) *marrow.*

present in some lacunae while others are empty. New bone (*b*) is already formed on the surface of the trabecula. Viable marrow is labeled *c*.

More Recent Studies

The questions raised by previous investigators concerning the importance of the periosteum and whether the cells of the bone graft really live have been answered by modern investigation techniques. In 1974 Knize showed that autogenous bone grafts with intact periosteum placed in a young rabbit's nasal bone underwent less resorption than bare bone grafts [38]. Resorption was even further diminished if the rabbits were given calcitonin. In 1964 Arora and Laskin reported their experiments using sex chromatin as a cellular label for osteogenesis following bone grafts [5]. They used isografts from male to female and from female to male rab-

bits and, studying the transplant histologically at intervals from 1 to 16 weeks, found that in 75 percent of the animals cells from the transplant had formed bone to fill the gap. In 25 percent of the animals the cells forming the new bone were from the host. This was confirmation of the work by Ray and Sabet, who in 1963 reported their results using tritiated thymidine as a cellular label [53]. They had shown that when the femora of inbred newborn mice were transplanted as isografts the cells of both the graft and the host contributed to the new bone formation.

How does a transplanted bone induce new bone formation in the host? In 1961 Goldhaber reported osteogenic induction across a millipore filter causing new bone formation on the host side of the chamber [29]. This was done in mice immunized against allograft tissues. Goldhaber postulated that if by chance any cells had crossed the millipore filter they would have been destroyed by the immune reaction, and that the new bone formed on the host side of the filter was therefore caused by a diffusible osteogenic factor from within the chamber rather than from undetected escaping cells. The question of just how this induction occurs has been of interest for many years. A review of the subject of induction is contained in a paper by Burwell in 1966 [21]. At that time, he concluded, "the evidence of osteogenic inductions obtained from the use of devitalized implants of adult bone tissue, though suggestive, is still controversial."

Factors Influencing Bone Grafting Procedures

Types of Grafts

Ghormley and Stuck, after reviewing the literature on bone grafting, set out to determine the healing rates of grafts taken from bone of different regions [28]. The experimental animals were adult dogs, and the spine was the area of transplantation of autogenous periosteal, cortical and endosteal, or cancellous grafts. The animals were fed alizarin red for supravital staining. From their studies, reported in 1934, they concluded that "periosteal transplants in all animals do not produce new bone." "Cortical transplants do not completely die but unite slowly with the bone of their hosts." "Cancellous bone unites more quickly and more firmly than cortical bone whether taken from the cancellous bone of the ilium or from the endosteum of the tibia."

In 1947 Abbott et al. reported the results of their studies on young rabbits and dogs [1]. In all of their experiments the superiority of cancellous bone over cortical bone was shown. Cancellous bone "presents a very extensive endosteal surface and numerous accommodation spaces which allow for osteogenesis." In 1955 Siffert, using rabbits, found that autogenous iliac bone produced the best results when placed in ulnar defects [56]. "Shaved grafts of tibial bone incited ex-

tensive osteoplastic and fibroplastic reaction and then were almost completely destroyed before healing of the defect occurred." Allografts were usually well incorporated in the defects, but healing was not as rapid as with autogenous iliac bone. Further, all iliac bone and callus transplanted to muscle became necrotic.

Boyne reported the results of his experiments using autogenous cancellous bone and marrow transplants in gaps in the mandibles of adult dogs in 1970 [17]. He found that particulate grafts containing marrow within a Vitallium implant produced more bone and fewer nonunions than did the solid autogenous iliac crest graft.

One should be careful in applying these experimental results directly to humans. Although cancellous grafts have been shown to heal faster than cortical grafts, the use of cancellous grafts to fill a defect in a nonunion of the tibia without some device for stabilization would probably end in disaster. There still is a time and place for stability added by a cortical graft.

With the development of the bone bank in 1942, interest in the use of allografts and xenografts revived. In 1963 Heiple, Chase, and Herndon reported their experiments on 116 adult dogs [34]. Grafts of various types were taken and placed in varying defects in the ulna, and an autogenous control graft was placed in the opposite ulna. A freeze-dried allograft was slower in healing than an autogenous graft; otherwise it healed as well. The freeze-dried allograft was better than the frozen allograft, which was better than the decalcified allograft, which was better than the frozen irradiated allograft, which was better than the freeze-dried irradiated allograft. All of these were better than the fresh allograft, and all allografts were better than the deproteinized xenografts except for the deproteinized allograft. Attempts were being made to remove the antigens from the allografts and xenografts by freeze-drying, by washing out the red cells, and by other means, but most investigators agree that the autogenous bone graft is far superior to any kind of allograft or xenograft.

Care of the Graft

As it has been shown that cells can live in transplanted bone and contribute significantly to the new bone formed after transplantation, one must pay attention to keeping the cells viable during the process of transplantation. There is a marked decrease in cell viability if a graft is exposed to air for one hour [14]. According to Bassett, exposure to physiological saline solution for prolonged periods will kill bone cells, as will an elevation of temperature above 42°C which might result from exposure to operating room lights [8]. Various antibiotics have the potential for killing cells as well as for killing bacteria, and bone wax will also kill cells. Bassett recommends that bone taken for grafts be wrapped in a blood-soaked sponge and placed in a container the top of which is covered by saline-moistened sponges.

Vascular Supply for Bone Grafts

Siffert and Barash have shown that there is greater survival of cells from fresh autologous cancellous grafts if they are placed in a bed where there are actively proliferating blood vessels [57]. The bed is prepared three to four weeks ahead of time. Albee emphasized that it is advantageous if cancellous bone tissue is put in contact with cancellous bone of the bed [3]. Although it is not necessary for the survival of cancellous grafts, if they are so placed they have available to them better sources of blood supply. Phemister [48] and others have emphasized that one must eliminate as much as possible interposing hematoma between the bone graft and the bone graft bed. Stringa recommends limiting the thickness of the cancellous graft to a maximum of 5 mm if a central zone of necrosis is to be prevented [59]. Bassett advises that the cumulative mass of grafts should not be "so thick and dense that perfusion from the underlying bony bed and overlying soft tissue is rendered ineffective [8]".

In 1957 Stringa reported his studies on the vascularization of autografts, allografts, and xenografts in rabbits and guinea pigs [59]. He found the average vascular perforation of autografts to be 2 to 3 mm per week. Vascularization was slower for the isograft, and there was almost none for xenografts. In 1972 Ray described a "surge" type of vascularization between the fourth and fifth days of an embryonic femur transplanted subcutaneously [52].

Mechanical Factors

Phemister reemphasized that bone grafts placed in an area where they are subjected to some mechanical stress will grow [48]. If they are placed in soft tissues where no force is applied, they will atrophy and disappear after a prolonged period of disuse. On the other hand, it has been noted that if grafts are placed in a position where there is too much motion between the grafts and the host bed they too will not survive because vasculature will not be able to bridge from the host to the graft material.

An understanding of the basic science of bone grafting is essential for the reconstructive surgeon, but he should also know the clinical experience of such men as Albee [2, 3] (inlay graft), Campbell [22] (onlay graft), Delagenière [25] (osteoperiosteal graft), Phemister [49] (corticocancellous onlay graft), Boyd [16] (dual onlay graft), Mowlem [45] (cancellous chip graft), and Nicoll [46] (cancellous inlay grafts with metal plates). All experienced clinicians would agree with Nicoll, who wrote, "It is a first principle of grafting, whether of bones or roses, that there must be intimate and undisturbed contact between graft and host until union is achieved."

REFERENCES

1. Abbott, L. C., Schottstaedt, E. R., Saunders, J. B., and Bost, F. C. The evaluation of cortical and cancellous bone as grafting material. *J. Bone Joint Surg.* 29:381, 1947.

2. Albee, F. H. *Bone Graft Surgery.* Philadelphia: Saunders, 1915.

3. Albee, F. H. Principles of the treatment of non union of fracture. *Surg. Gynecol. Obstet.* 51:289, 1930.

4. Algöwer, M. *The Cellular Basis of Wound Repair.* Springfield, Ill.: Thomas, 1956.

5. Arora, B. K., and Laskin, D. M. Sex chromatin as a cellular label of osteogenesis by bone grafts. *J. Bone Joint Surg.* [Am.] 46:1269, 1964.

6. Axhausen, G. Ueber den histologischen Vorgang bei der Transplantation von Gelenkenden. *Arch. Klin. Chir.* 99:1, 1912.

7. Barth, F. Histologischen Befunde nach Knochen Implantation. *Arch. Klin. Chir.* 46:418, 1893.

8. Bassett, C. A. L. Clinical implications of cell function in bone grafting. *Clin. Orthop.* 87:49, 1972.

9. Bassett, C. A. L. Personal communication, 1973.

10. Bassett, C. A. L., and Herrman, I. Influence of oxygen concentration and mechanical factors on differentiation of connective tissues in vitro. *Nature* (Lond.) 190:460, 1961.

11. Becker, R. O., and Murray, D. G. The electrical control system regulating fracture healing in amphibians. *Clin. Orthop.* 73:169, 1970.

12. Bick, E. *Source Book of Orthopaedics.* Darien, Conn.: Hafner, 1968.

13. Bloom, W., Bloom, M. A., and McLean, F. C. Calcification and ossification. Medullary bone changes in reproductive cycle of female pigeons. *Anat. Rec.* 81:443, 1941.

14. Bohr, H., Raun, H. O., and Werner, H. The osteogenic effect of bone transplants in rabbits. *J. Bone Joint Surg.* [Br.] 50:866, 1968.

15. Bonfiglio, M., and Jetter, W. Immunological responses to bone. *Clin. Orthop.* 87:19, 1972.

16. Boyd, H. B. Treatment of difficult and unusual non-union. *J. Bone Joint Surg.* [Am.] 25:535, 1943.

17. Boyne, P. J. Autogenous cancellous bone and marrow transplants. *Clin. Orthop.* 73:199, 1970.

18. Brighton, C. T. Healing of non union of medial malleolus. *Trauma* 11:883, 1971.

19. Brighton, C. T., and Krebs, A. C. Oxygen tension of healing fractures in the rabbit. *J. Bone Joint Surg.* [Am.] 54:323, 1972.

20. Burger, M., Sherman, B., and Sobel, A. E. Observations of the influence of chondroitin sulfate on the rate of bone repair. *J. Bone Joint Surg.* [Br.] 44:675, 1962.

21. Burwell, R. G. Studies in the transplantation of bone: VIII. Treated composite homograft-autografts of cancellous bone: An analysis of inductive mechanisms in bone transplantation. *J. Bone Joint Surg.* [Br.] 48:532, 1966.

22. Campbell, W. Onlay graft for ununited fractures. *Arch. Surg.* 38:313, 1939.

23. Chase, S. W., and Herndon, C. H. The fate of autogenous and homogenous bone grafts. *J. Bone Joint Surg.* [Am.] 37:809, 1955.

24. Craft, P. D., Mani, M. M., Pazel, J., and Masters, F. W. Experimental study of healing in fractures of membranous bone. *Plast. Reconstr. Surg.* 53:321, 1974.

25. Delagenière, H. Repair of loss of bony substance and reconstruction of bones by osteo-periosteal grafts taken from the tibia. *Am. J. Surg.* 35:281, 1921.

26. Enneking, W. F., and Morris, J. C. Human autogenous cortical bone transplants. *Clin. Orthop.* 87:28, 1972.

27. Enneking, W. F., Puhl, J., and Burchardt, H. The Strength of the Remodeling Cortical Bone Grafts—An Exhibit at American Academy of Orthopedic Surgeons Annual Meeting, Dallas, 1974.

28. Ghormley, R. K., and Stuck, W. G. Experimental bone transplantation. *Arch. Surg.* 38:742, 1934.

29. Goldhaber, P. Osteogenic induction across millipore filters in vivo. *Science* 133:2065, 1961.

30. Goldsmith, R. S., Woodhouse, C. F., Ingbar, S. H., and Segal, D. Phosphate supplements in patients with fractures. *Lancet* 1:687, 1967.

31. Groves, E. W. H. An experimental study of the operative treatment of fractures. *Br. J. Surg.* 1:438, 1914.

32. Groves, E. W. H. Methods and results of transplantation of bone in the repair of defects. *Br. J. Surg.* 5:185, 1917.

33. Ham, A. W. *Histology* (6th ed.). Philadelphia: Lippincott, 1969.

34. Heiple, K. G., Chase, S. W., and Herndon, C. H. A comparative study of the healing process following different types of bone transplantation. *J. Bone Joint Surg.* [Am.] 45:1593, 1963.

35. Herbsman, H., Kwon, K., Shaftan, G., Gordon, B., Fox, L., and Enquist, I. The influence of systemic factors on fracture healing. *Trauma* 6:75, 1966.

36. Keith, A. *Menders of the Maimed.* Philadelphia: Lippincott, 1919.

37. Key, J. A., and Odell, R. T. Failure of excess minerals in diet to accelerate healing of experimental fracture. *J. Bone Joint Surg.* [Am.] 37:37, 1955.

38. Knize, D. M. The influence of periosteum and calcitonin on onlay bone graft survival. *Plast. Reconstr. Surg.* 53:190, 1974.

39. Koskinen, E. V. S. The effect of growth hormone and thyrotropin on human fracture healing. *Acta Orthop. Scand.* [Suppl.] 62:1, 1963.

40. Koskinen, E. V. S. The influence of hormonal treatment and orchiectomy, oophorectomy and thyroidectomy on experimental fractures. *Acta Orthop. Scand.* [Suppl.] 80:1, 1965.

41. Kruse, R. L., and Kelly, P. J. Acceleration of fracture healing distal to a venous tourniquet. *J. Bone Joint Surg.* [Am.] 56:730, 1974.

42. Laurnen, E. L., and Kelly, P. J. Blood flow, O_2 consumption, carbon dioxide production, blood calcium and pH changes in tibial fractures in dogs. *J. Bone Joint Surg.* [Am.] 51:298, 1969.

43. Lexer, E. Ueber die Entstehung von Pseudarthrosen nach Fracturen und nach Knochen Transplantation. *Arch. Klin. Chir.* 119:520, 1922.

44. Macewen, W. *The Growth of Bone.* Glasgow: Maclehose, 1912.

45. Mowlem, R. Cancellous chip bone-grafts. *Lancet* 2:746, 1944.

46. Nicoll, E. A. The treatment of gaps in long bones by cancellous insert grafts. *J. Bone Joint Surg.* [Br.] 38:70, 1956.

47. Ollier, L. *Traité experimentale et Clinique. Regeneration et la production artificielle du tissu osseux.* Paris: Masson, 1867.

48. Phemister, D. B. The fate of transplanted bone. . . . *Surg. Gynecol. Obstet.* 19:303, 1914.

49. Phemister, D. B. Splint grafts in the treatment of delayed and non-union of fractures. *Surg. Gynecol. Obstet.* 52:376, 1931.

50. Pritchard, J. J. Bone. In McMinn, R. (Ed.), *Tissue Repair.* New York: Academic, 1969. P. 148.

51. Puranen, J. Reorganization of fresh and preserved transplants. *Acta Orthop. Scand.* [Suppl.] 92:1, 1966.

52. Ray, R. D. Vascularization of bone grafts and implants. *Clin. Orthop.* 84:43, 1972.

53. Ray, R. D., and Sabet, T. Y. Bone grafts: Cellular survival versus induction. *J. Bone Joint Surg.* [Am.] 45:337, 1963.

54. Rhinelander, F. W., and Baraguy, R. A. Microangiography in bone healing. *J. Bone Joint Surg.* [Am.] 44:1273, 1962.

55. Shenk, R. Zur Histologie der primaren Knochen-heilung. *Arch. Klin. Chir.* 308:440, 1964.

56. Siffert, R. S. Experimental bone transplants. *J. Bone Joint Surg.* [Am.] 37:742, 1955.

57. Siffert, R. S., and Barash, E. S. Delayed bone transplantation: An experimental study of early host-transplant relationships. *J. Bone Joint Surg.* [Am.] 43:407, 1961.

58. Sissons, H. A., and Hadfield, C. J. The influence of cortisone on the repair of experimental fractures in the rabbit. *Br. J. Surg.* 39:172, 1951.

59. Stringa, G. Studies of the vascularization of bone grafts. *J. Bone Joint Surg.* [Br.] 39:395, 1957.

60. Tonna, E. A. The Source of Osteoblasts in Healing Fractures in Animals of Different Ages. In Robinson, R. (Ed.), *The Healing of Osseous Tissue.* Washington: National Academy of Sciences, National Research Council, 1967.

61. Trueta, J., and Little, L. The vascular contribution to osteogenesis: II: Studies

with electron microscope. *J. Bone Joint Surg.* [Br.] 42:367, 1960.

62. Urist, M. R., Dowell, T. A., Hay, P. H., and Strates, B. S.   Inductive substrates for bone formation. *Clin. Orthop.* 59:59, 1968.

63. Urist, M. R., and Johnson, R. W., Jr.   The healing of fractures in man under clinical conditions. *J. Bone Joint Surg.* [Am.] 25:375, 1943.

64. Wolff, J.   *Das Gesetz der Transformation der Knochen.* Berlin: Hirschwald, 1892.

65. Wray, J. B.   The influence of various hormones on the fracture healing process. *Clin. Orthop.* 50:324, 1967. (Abstracts.)

66. Wray, J. B.   A study of the biochemistry of human fracture hematoma. (In Proceedings of the American Orthopedic Association.) *J. Bone Joint Surg.* [Am.] 51:1674, 1967.

67. Wray, J. B.   Studies of metabolic activity in the healing fracture. (In Proceedings of the American Orthopedic Association.) *J. Bone Joint Surg.* [Am.] 51:1674, 1969.

68. Wray, J. B., and Lynch, C. J.   The vascular response to fracture of the tibia in the rat. *J. Bone Joint Surg.* [Am.] 41:1143, 1959.

21

The Healing of Tendon

Lawrence N. Hurst

One of man's greatest attributes is his ability to move. Purposeful active movement is dependent on many factors, but primarily on the ability of a myocyte to contract and thereby reduce its length. This motion is transmitted to the skeleton through a collection of longitudinally oriented collagen fibers: a tendon.

ANATOMY AND FUNCTION OF TENDON

Anatomy

A tendon is composed largely of collagen with a few interposed fibroblasts or tenocytes. The basic tropocollagen units are oriented parallel to each other and are laid down in such a manner that each molecule overlaps the adjacent ones by 10 to 25 percent of its length. Accumulations of the tropocollagen subunits form collagen filaments which have a characteristic banding recognized on light microscopy at 640 A [16]. These filaments accumulate into fibrils of approximately 2000 A diameter. Condensations of fibrils make up the basic collagen fiber found in skin and connective tissue. Fibers are condensed into fasciculi and surrounded by the endotenon, a loose, relatively acellular tissue carrying blood vessels. Fasciculi then accumulate to form the tendon.

The fascicles are surrounded by epitenon, a one- to three-cell fibroblastic layer on the surface of most tendons. The paratenon then surrounds the whole tendon and is closely applied to the epitenon (Figs. 21-1, 21-2).

Normal Blood Supply

The vascular supply reaches the tendon through the mesotenon. This is similar to the mesentery, through which blood vessels reach the intestine. In general, tendon has a longitudinally oriented blood supply fed segmentally through the mesotenon. The more central vessels are straight and parallel to each other, while toward the periphery superficial vessels show an arcuate and intercommunicating formation (Fig. 21-3) [18].

The blood supply is considerably modified in the fibro-osseous tunnel of the hand since it is no longer possible to maintain the segmental supply. The flexor profundus tendon, for example, has four major sources of vascular supply in its course through the tunnel. At

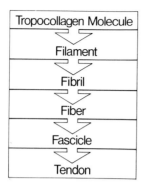

FIGURE 21-1.   *The structure of tendon.*

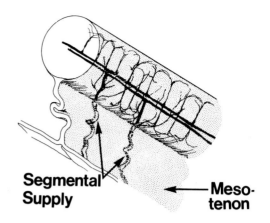

FIGURE 21-3.   *Segmental blood supply of tendon.*

the beginning, the longitudinally oriented segmental supply continues. The long mesotenon (vinculum longum) supplies blood over the proximal and middle phalanx. The short mesotenon (vinculum breve) supplies it near its termination. At its insertion, again there is a short longitudinal supply. Between these major sources of blood supply are zones of apparent avascularity (Fig. 21-4) [5].

Architecture

A tendon may assume various anatomical configurations depending on the dictates of its function and position. In the extensor mechanism of a digit, it forms a strong hood mechanism with multiple origins and inser-

tions. In the fibro-osseous sheath both tendons are flattened in the coronal plane to facilitate gliding one on top of the other. The more superficial tendon inserts first at the proximal end of the middle phalanx and splits to allow the deeper profundus tendon to continue. As well as inserting at each side of the profundus tendon, fibers decussate beneath the profundus and insert on the opposite side (Fig. 21-5).

Functional Adaptation

The tendon is generally well adapted to transmit the amplitude of movement generated by the muscle to the skeleton. Both the extensor and flexor tendons have a considerable breadth of movement and must glide freely to allow the phalanges a full range of motion. In contrast, musculotendinous units used primarily for stability, such as the brachioradialis, have a very limited amplitude of movement. Another consideration that governs the architecture of a tendon is the precision of the movement required. The major factor here is the number of neuromuscular end-plates fired by a single axon. In gross movements such as those of the leg, a single axon fires many neuromuscular end-plates. In the extremely precise movements of the eye or hand, a single axon fires very few neuromuscular end-plates. In

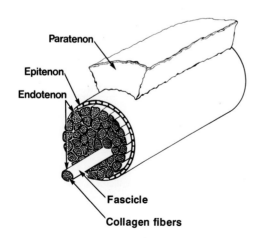

FIGURE 21-2.   *Tendon anatomy.*

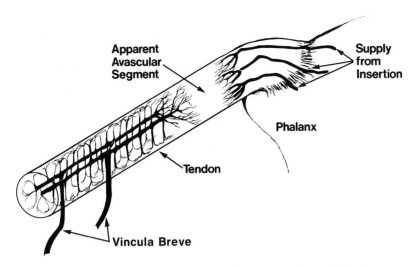

FIGURE 21-4.   *Blood supply of tendon in the digital sheath.*

general, the tendons responsible for precise delicate movements are more refined complex structures than those that subserve more powerful gross movement.

BIOLOGY OF REPAIR

Reaction to Injury

Disruption of a tendon prevents the force generated by a muscle from being transmitted, and active movement is lost. Regardless of the cause of the disruption—whether by trauma, spontaneous rupture, or ischemia with attendant necrosis—the objective of the healing process is to restore continuity. The magnitude of the response to injury varies directly with the amount of trauma. A traumatized tendon rarely regains full function. Experimental studies using the chicken, the closest practical experimental model to the human hand [4], show that with simple crushing of a tendon minimal function is lost. If the tendon is partially transected, a much brisker healing response ensues, and more function is lost. This is again increased if the tendon is completely transected and repaired [10]. Also, any further trauma inflicted during the operative repair again lessens the overall functional return (Fig. 21-6).

Tendon Softening

Tendon is relatively inert tissue but has a specific metabolic turnover and exceptionally

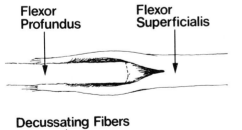

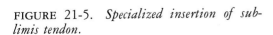

FIGURE 21-5.   *Specialized insertion of sublimis tendon.*

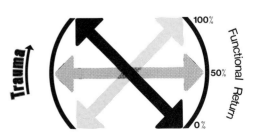

FIGURE 21-6.   *Increased trauma results in decreased functional return.*

high tensile strength. When a tendon is traumatized, a softening process occurs which reaches a peak at approximately five days [11]. During this time the tendon becomes friable and has greatly diminished tensile strength, not only over the traumatized segment but also over a segment both proximal and distal to it. Increasing the size of suture material beyond a given strength, therefore, simply serves to traumatize the tendon further and does not add strength to the repair. The suture material will cut through the softened tendon if the repair is stressed.

Cellular Response

Histological studies show that the healing response and fibroblastic proliferation seem to follow a set pattern [10]. Immediately after trauma an inflammatory cell exudate accumulates in the perisheath tissue and gap zone accompanied by a specific fibroblastic proliferation. In 48 hours the epitenon cells proliferate vigorously, contributing to the healing process. In another two days the endotenon cells, then the tenocytes themselves, take part in this proliferative reaction.

Cellular Migration

Controversy has arisen as to whether the proliferating cells are increasing in situ or the observed increase is due to the migration of extraneous cells. Radioactive thymidine, a DNA precursor, has been used to label the actively dividing cells and trace any migration [8]. The proliferating fibroblasts have been traced from their origin in the peritendinous tissue into the gap zone and traumatized tendon (Fig. 21-7).

This finding supports the theory that tendon healing is facilitated through fibroblasts originating in the peritendinous tissue. It is also apparent that any impervious interposition substance would block the migration and interfere with primary tendon healing.

Adhesions

A tendon does not heal in isolation; the "one wound" concept [15] has significantly

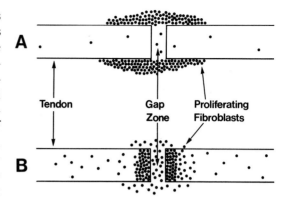

FIGURE 21-7. *Isotope-tagged fibroblasts migrate from peritendinous tissue into the gap zone and healing tendon. A. Cells tagged and specimen prepared on day of tendon laceration. B. Cells tagged on day of tendon laceration, specimen prepared on day 12.*

advanced our understanding of the healing process. The surrounding tissue heals in conjunction with and as an integral part of tendon healing. Revascularization occurs from the surrounding tissue, and new blood vessels together with migrating fibroblasts form adhesions. These are therefore not a complication of tendon surgery but an obligatory part of the healing response. The normal vascular pattern is replaced by an abundant but haphazard arrangement of small vessels with frequent cross-communications. During the process of resolution the vascular pattern changes to a more normal configuration, and by eight weeks the longitudinal supply has been reestablished [1].

Biochemical Considerations

Tendon is composed of a few cells (the fibroblasts) and the extracellular material (collagen, elastin, and reticulin) embedded in an amorphous material (ground substance) which contains mucopolysaccharides. The strength of collagen is dependent not only on its own cross-linkages but also on the surrounding environment, the most important part of which is mucopolysaccharides [14].

Studies using both isotope incorporation and quantitative biochemical analysis show that in a healing tendon collagen deposition commences about the fourth day while mucopolysaccharide concentration peaks at about four to eight days, then declines [2]. Thereafter, both substances generally accumulate in the healing area and reach a peak at about 21 days. Subsequently, they both gradually decline. The amount of new collagen deposition is directly related to the amount of trauma, being greatest in the most traumatized area. However, in a completely healed tendon the total amount of collagen present is not equal to the total amount in a normal tendon at the same area. Also, the collagen and mucopolysaccharide deposition in adhesive tissue closely parallels that of healing tendon. Unfortunately, no selective difference could be determined to differentiate the adhesions from the tendon.

Collagen Orientation

Normal tendon is composed largely of longitudinally oriented collagen fibers. In a healing tendon with no stress across the repair the new collagen is laid down in a random fashion, with no specific orientation. At this time it is almost impossible to differentiate tendon from adhesive tissue. When stress is placed across the healing area, the randomly oriented fibers assume a longitudinal orientation within 48 hours. The same type of polarization of collagen fibers has been observed in an electrical field; in fact, tendon is a piezoelectric substance [3], a material capable of converting mechanical stress into a measurable electrical potential. The origin of the effect is apparently the polarization or displacement of hydrogen bonds being formed in the polypeptide chains of collagen [6]. Work in this field is as yet in its infancy but shows great potential from both a research and a clinical point of view [7].

Resolution and Glide

The process of resolution and restoration of glide involves multiple factors. The total amount of collagen in the healing area gradually diminishes. The persisting collagen is longitudinally oriented and becomes more mature (less saline soluble) with ever increasing cross-linkages. The new vascular supply assumes a longitudinal orientation, and the vascularity of adhesions markedly decreases. In some patients the adhesions themselves attenuate and become filmy [17]; this type of adhesion no longer restricts movement, and glide is restored. In others, the adhesions retain their restrictive hold and incompletely resolve. This individual patient variable is largely responsible for the success or failure of any given tendon repair.

Tendon Grafts

The primary healing response is considerably modified by the addition of a tendon graft. Opinion has varied as to whether an isograft acts as a living transplant, supplementing the healing response, or merely as a strut through which living tissue can migrate. Histological studies separate the overall response into three merging processes [9]: (1) In areas of severe trauma, such as occur at the zone of suture or the zone of approximation of the cut ends, there is complete replacement of old lysed tendon elements by new fibers. This has been termed *regeneration*. (2) In areas of moderate trauma, somewhat removed from the zone of suture or the cut ends of tendon, repair is mediated through new fibroblasts producing new collagen, but the whole process is not nearly so voluminous. This is termed *reconstitution*. (3) In areas removed from the zone of injury fibroblasts already in the area contribute abundantly to the healing response. This process is termed *maintenance*.

Radioactive isotope studies have substantiated this histological picture [2]. Radioactive proline, an amino acid found almost exclusively in collagen, has been used to measure the rate and extent of incorporation into traumatized tendon. The uptake was directly proportional to the amount of trauma, being maximal in the zones of severe trauma and the junction-gap zone with minimal uptake in the central area of the graft (Fig. 21-8).

When the collagen was labeled prior to autogenous graft replacement and the disap-

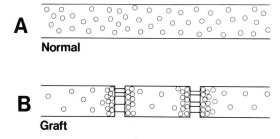

A
Normal

B
Graft

FIGURE 21-8. *Uptake of radioactive proline. A. Uptake of isotope by normal tendon. B. Uptake of isotope after tendon graft.*

pearance of isotope in the graft segment recorded, 70 percent of the labeled collagen was lost at the graft ends and 50 percent in the central portion. Therefore, 30 to 50 percent of the original collagen remained or was reutilized in the healed tendon [12]. An isograft thus acts as much more than an inert strut; rather, it is a viable transplant that adds significantly to the healing response.

This type of contribution to the healing response is not found in allografts, in which all cellular elements are lost and the tissue does function as an inert scaffold. A xenograft, on the other hand, evokes a marked inflammatory response in the host, and all donor tissue is replaced by host tissue.

FACTORS AFFECTING TENDON REPAIR

Aim of Repair

Disruption of a tendon prevents the force generated by a muscle from being transmitted to the skeleton. This deprivation leads not only to loss of active movements but also to deformity since the normal muscular balance is destroyed and the antagonist muscles have no equal force to oppose their pull. The prime aim of tendon repair is to restore the normal function of the tendon and with it regain balanced active motion.

Surgical Principles

The realization of this goal necessitates the scrupulous application of all established surgical principles: immediate attention to the wound, definitive repair as soon as possible, aseptic technique, adequate debridement, gentle handling of soft tissues, meticulous hemostasis—the list is well known to all involved in surgery. Of the many extraneous factors that affect the ultimate result, perhaps the age of the patient is the most important [13]. Excellent results can be achieved in children, when a similar situation would be disastrous in an adult.

Biological Principles

The foregoing material emphasizes that a tendon is a highly specialized structure, and its repair to produce functional healing requires a firm knowledge of the biological processes involved. Even minimal trauma during surgery augments the intensity of the evoked response and is detrimental. The size of suture material beyond a clear-cut limit does nothing to strengthen the repair. The injudicious use of interposition substances merely blocks cellular migration and impairs primary tendon healing.

It is well known that early guarded motion leads to a better overall functional outcome. It is exciting to speculate that the resultant stress on the tendon could set up an electrical field across the gap zone responsible for the early orientation of collagen molecules. Could this principle then be adapted to produce beneficial clinical results? Obviously, we have only just begun!

REFERENCES

1. Bergljung, L. Vascular reactions after tendon suture and tendon transplantation. *Scand. J. Plast. Reconstr. Surg.* Suppl. 4, 1968.
2. Birdsell, D. C., Tustanoff, E. R., and Lindsay, W. K. Collagen production in regenerating tendon. *Plast. Reconstr. Surg.* 37:504, 1966.
3. Cochran, G. V. B., Pawluk, R. J., and Bassett, C. A. L. Electromechanical characteristics of bone under physiologic moisture conditions. *Clin. Orthop.* 58:249, 1968.

4. Farkas, L. G., Thomson, H. G., and Martin, R. Some practical notes on the anatomy of the chicken toe for surgeon investigators. *Plast. Reconstr. Surg.* 54:452, 1974.

5. Freiberg, A., and Lindsay, W. K. The blood supply of the digital flexor tendon mechanism. Paper presented to the Canadian Society of Plastic Surgeons, 1971.

6. Fukada, E., and Yasuda, I. Piezoelectric effects in collagen. *Jap. J. Appl. Physiol.* 3:117, 1964.

7. Kappel, D., Ketchum, L. D., and Zilber, S. Observations on the Electrical Properties of Tendons and Healing Tendon. Plastic Surgery Research Council, St. Louis, May 3–4, 1973.

8. Lindsay, W. K., and Birch, J. R. The fibroblast in flexor tendon healing. *Plast. Reconstr. Surg.* 34:223, 1964.

9. Lindsay, W. K., and McDougall, E. P. Digital flexor tendons: An experimental study. Part III. *Br. J. Plast. Surg.* 13:293, 1961.

10. Lindsay, W. K., and Thomson, H. G. Digital flexor tendons: An experimental study. Part I. *Br. J. Plast. Surg.* 12:289, 1960.

11. Lindsay, W. K., Thomson, H. G., and Walker, F. G. Digital flexor tendons: An experimental study. Part II. *Br. J. Plast. Surg.* 13:1, 1964.

12. Lloyd, G. R., and Lindsay, W. K. The Fate of Collagen in an Autologous Free Tendon Graft. Plastic Surgery Research Council, Chicago, April 24–25, 1969.

13. McFarlane, R. M., Lamon, R., and Jarvis, G. Flexor tendon injuries within the finger. *J. Trauma* 8:987, 1968.

14. Munro, I. R., Lindsay, W. K., and Jackson, S. H. A synchronous study of collagen and mucopolysaccharide in healing flexor tendons of chickens. *Plast. Reconstr. Surg.* 45:493, 1970.

15. Peacock, E. E., Jr. Biology of tendon repair. *N. Engl. J. Med.* 276:680, 1967.

16. Peacock, E. E., Jr., and van Winkle, W., Jr. *Surgery and Biology of Wound Repair.* Philadelphia: Saunders, 1970.

17. Potenza, A. D. Tendon healing within the flexor digital sheath in the dog. *J. Bone Joint Surg.* [Am.] 44:49, 1962.

18. Smith, J. W. Blood supply of tendons. *Am. J. Surg.* 109:272, 1965.

22

The Healing of Nerve

William C. Grabb

The successful repair of peripheral nerves continues to be a challenge. The reanastomosis of these long electrical conduits has been the subject of laboratory and clinical investigation by physiologists, biochemists, anatomists, neurosurgeons, neurologists, orthopedic surgeons, general surgeons, and plastic surgeons. In vivo studies on peripheral nerves have been carried out for the past 80 years on mice, rats, rabbits, cats, dogs, goats, monkeys, baboons, chimpanzees, and humans. As normal function is seldom attained following repair of a severed nerve, there is no reason to believe that this evaluation will not continue unabated.

Reference must be made at this point to the comprehensive test by Sunderland on the subject of nerves and nerve repairs [27].

ANATOMY OF A PERIPHERAL NERVE

A peripheral nerve is primarily a composite of nerve tissue and its connective tissue covering. Sunderland found that the relative amount of each depends upon the level at which each nerve is examined [27]. The variations range from about 22 percent to 88 percent of the total. Most commonly, however, the connective tissue component constitutes from 30 to 75 percent of the cross-sectional area. Sunderland noted that there was more connective tissue at points where the neural components were small and numerous and less where the nerve bundles were large or relatively few in number. There was also a greater connective tissue concentration at any point where a peripheral nerve passed around a joint. The connective tissues surrounding the various parts of the nerve are the endoneurium, perineurium, and epineurium. Together they aid in isolating and insulating one part from another. Each component also has specific architectural and structural characteristics.

The endoneurium, which surrounds each axon–Schwann's cell complex, is composed mostly of collagenous tissue. It functions as a supporting connective tissue but also forms fine, intrafunicular septa that separate and subdivide nerve fibers inside a funiculus into even smaller component parts. These septa contain the interfunicular blood supply.

The perineurium invests each bundle or funiculus with a relatively thin but dense and distinctive sheath of fibrous tissue. It contains elastic and collagen fibers that intermesh by passing circularly, obliquely, and longitudinally. They form from 7 to 15 concentric lamellae or tubes, depending upon the size of the funiculus. Carefully examining the end of a freshly cut peripheral nerve, one sees that each funiculus can move back and forth within the perineurium independently of the others.

The third and outermost layer, the epineurium, serves as a sheath which surrounds all the component bundles in each peripheral nerve. Its loose areolar connective tissue framework contains collagen and elastic fibers, most of them running longitudinally. The epineurium can move back and forth along the surface of the nerve in a way completely independent of the other two structures.

The microcirculation to each funiculus runs in its adjacent perineurium. This internal circulation is piped in from without the nerve entirely through the mesoneurium by an anatomical relationship similar to that found in the intestine. As in the mesentery, all the nutrient vessels enter the nerve along a line where the mesoneurium attaches to the nerve. Its blood is supplied in a segmental fashion, being both dispersed and collected through a series of arcades with the mesoneurium. The grouping of arcades seems to change from one area to another to meet needs and requirements imposed by local anatomical variations. In the shoulder, elbow, and wrist, for example, where great mobility is required of the nerve, the mesoneurium is longer and more complex and contains a larger number of vessels. When there is little or no tension on these vessels, they contract in an accordion-like arrangement [26].

Two basic types of axons are found in peripheral nerves: sensory and motor. The motor fibers are efferent ones, while sensory axons can be either afferent or efferent. In some peripheral nerves there also appear to be axons from the autonomic system. Though they travel within peripheral nerves, most eventually terminate in blood vessel walls, etc., to provide the unconscious or autonomic control of these structures.

Because of the different types of axons it is important, from a clinical point of view, to know just what their interrelations might be in mixed peripheral nerves. The problem has been studied by Sunderland [27] and by Grabb, BeMent, Koepke, and Green [11]. Their findings show that in such peripheral areas as the hands and feet most small nerves and funiculi are predominately sensory or motor. However, mixed nerves, located more proximally in the extremity, characteristically contain more and more components rather

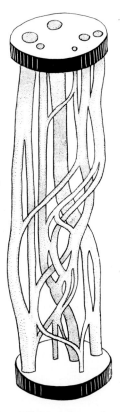

FIGURE 22-1. *The maximum length that the funicular pattern remains constant in a major nerve is about 15 mm (drawing after Sunderland [27]).*

than being purely of one type or the other, as they are in the periphery.

Sunderland [28, 29] has described the changes in funicular pattern, demonstrating the rapid changes in size, number, and arrangement of funiculi in cross-sectional studies. The maximum length that the funicular pattern remains constant in a major nerve is about 15 mm, the average length being much less than this (Fig. 22-1).

METABOLIC CHANGES FOLLOWING NERVE INJURY

Metabolic Changes in the Anterior Horn Cell

One of the many unique features of a nerve cell (or neuron) is that its cell body is located within the spinal cord (motor nerve cells) or the posterior root ganglion (sensory nerve cells) while its axons (or fibers) extend out into the arm for distances of over 3 feet. The nerve cell body and axon are parts of a single extremely long cell (Fig. 22-2).

When an axon is severed in a peripheral nerve injury, the nerve cell body progressively enlarges for 4 to 20 days, remains enlarged while active regeneration is taking place, and then slowly returns to normal size [8]. This nerve cell body enlargement is caused by an increased metabolism resulting in an increase in the total amount of protein in the cell body. The proteins in turn migrate through the cell's axon to the site of injury where they are utilized in axonal regeneration.

We can think in terms of a phase of *neuronal survival* followed by a phase of *neuronal regeneration* in discussing injuries of peripheral nerves. In injuries to the median and ulnar nerves around the wrist and hand, the phase of neuronal survival is 4 to 14 days long and the phase of neuronal regeneration begins at that time and lasts for 60 to 90 days. In more proximal injuries of the peripheral nerves in the arm, the phase of neuronal survival is 10 to 20 days and the phase of neuronal regeneration continues for a period

in the range of 300 days (Fig. 22-3). The severity of the trauma (e.g., knife cut versus gunshot wound) has a direct relationship to the number of days required for the phase of neuronal survival. These time intervals bear directly on the subject of primary versus secondary repair of peripheral nerves, as will be discussed subsequently.

The closer the peripheral nerve injury is to the cell body, the more pronounced are the metabolic changes within the cell body. There are two reasons. First, a greater amount of the cell mass is lost when the axon portion of the nerve cell is divided near the cell body. If the cut is very close to the cell body, the cellular insult may exceed the tolerance of the nerve cell to survive. Second, even if the nerve cell survives following trauma close to the spinal cord, the amount of axon that must be regenerated may exceed the metabolic capacity of the cell.

Metabolic Changes in the Nerve Distal and Proximal to the Point of Severance

After a nerve is cut, both nerve ends swell so that the cross-sectional area of each end increases three to four times. The swelling extends about 1 cm from the point of severance, both proximally and distally, and persists for a week or more before subsiding [7].

Wallerian Degeneration

Strictly speaking, wallerian degeneration occurs only in the portion of the nerve distal to the site of injury. The axon portion of the nerve cell, which has been separated from its cell body, undergoes physical disintegration. The myelin about the axon also disintegrates. Other structures in the nerve (e.g., sheath of Schwann, endoneurium, blood vessels) do not disintegrate but persist in the expectation of receiving and providing nutrition for regenerated axons. In about a week macrophages begin to phagocytize and remove the disintegrated axon and myelin. Disintegration and phagocytosis occur uniformly throughout the distal cut segment, so that

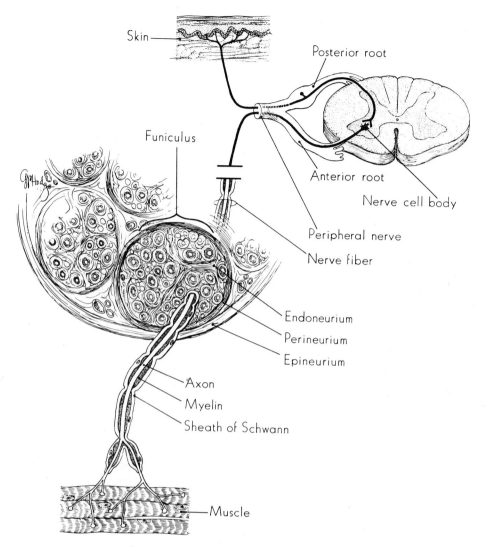

FIGURE 22-2. *Anatomy of a peripheral nerve.*

after two or three weeks most of the debris has been removed. By five to eight weeks the process is complete, leaving the empty and somewhat shrunken sheath of Schwann waiting in expectation [4, 27].

Traumatic Degeneration

The portion of the nerve proximal to the point of injury, assuming that the axon portion of the nerve cell is still in continuity with its cell body, undergoes what Cajal has termed *traumatic degeneration* [4]. This is essentially the same as wallerian degeneration in that it involves physical disintegration followed by phagocytosis of the axon and myelin, but it differs in that it extends only a few millimeters proximal to the point where the destruction of the axon ceases. For example, in a sharply cut nerve in the hand, the retrograde axonal destruction is so minimal that the traumatic degeneration extends but a few millimeters and axonal budding may begin at four days. In marked contrast, the nerves in the arm severed by a high-speed

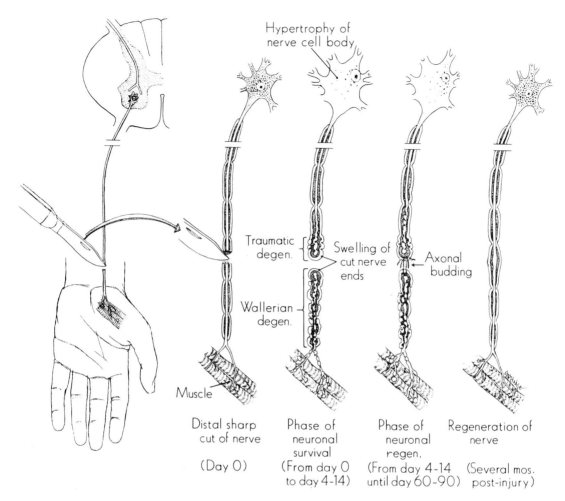

Hypertrophy of
nerve cell body

Traumatic
degen.

Swelling of
cut nerve
ends

Axonal
budding

Wallerian
degen.

Muscle

Distal sharp
cut of nerve

(Day 0)

Phase of
neuronal
survival

(From day 0
to day 4-14)

Phase of
neuronal
regen.

(From day 4-14
until day 60-90)

Regeneration of
nerve

(Several mos.
post-injury)

FIGURE 22-3. *Physiological changes that lead to regeneration of a severed peripheral nerve motor axon.*

missile may suffer traumatic destruction of the axon and myelin as well as disruption of their connective tissue sheaths for several centimeters both proximally and distally, and proximal axonal budding may not begin for 10 to 20 days. In the latter instance it is extremely important to know the proximal extent of axonal destruction before carrying out the nerve repair. Not until several days after injury can the extent of destruction be determined by operative inspection of the nerve and serial sectioning to identify a normal funicular pattern.

While the axon is regenerating, there is a vigorous outgrowth of cords of Schwann cells from both the proximal and distal cut ends of the nerve. These cells then become surrounded by endoneural and perineural cells, thus forming numerous small fascicles [30, 31].

Axonal budding begins at the end of the intact portion of the axon. The regenerating axons, growing at the rate of about 1 mm per day, eventually extend a distance of 3 mm to several centimeters to the point where the nerve was severed [16]. Ideally the regenerating axon and the rapidly proliferating supporting tissues will cross the site of nerve repair with such a timing that the axon bud can push into the intercellular spaces and into the cords of Schwann cells before the tissue laid down by mesenchymal proliferation becomes impermeable.

The axon then continues to regenerate down the tubular pathway of the empty shrunken sheath of Schwann until it reaches a muscle, where a motor end-plate forms, or an area, such as the skin, where the bare sensory nerve endings will perceive sensation even without the more elaborate sensory corpuscles. Because there is no way a motor axon can detect which Schwann sheaths lead to muscle instead of skin, it follows that in a mixed motor and sensory nerve perhaps 50 percent of the motor axons will grow down sensory pathways and the remaining, down motor pathways. When this factor is added to the known failure of all axons to successfully span the site of nerve repair and enter the tubular sheaths, the failure to regain normal sensory and motor function can be better understood.

The rate at which an axon will regenerate has stimulated the interest of many investigators. It is evident that following the severing of a peripheral nerve in the human there will first be a 4- to 14-day period of neuronal survival. The axon will then begin regenerating toward the site of injury at an unknown rate, probably 1 to 3 mm per day. Next, the axon must traverse the scar at the site of suture, taking 3 to 50 days but ordinarily 20 to 40 days. The axon then grows down the distal endoneural tubes at a rate of approximately 1 to 3 mm per day, a rate of growth that gradually slows as the length of the axon increases [27]. By testing for the Tinel sign at weekly or monthly intervals, (i.e., percussing distally to proximally over the course of the nerve in such a way that the neuroma itself is not disturbed and producing paresthesias referred to the area of sensory supply of the nerve), one can keep track of the rate of axonal growth.

Following nerve repair at the wrist in an adult, the first recovery of functional value occurs at about one year, but the final result requires five years [22].

CLASSIFICATION OF NERVE INJURIES

Sunderland has described a logical classification of five different degrees of injury to the internal structure of a peripheral nerve [27]. These are as follows:

1. *First-degree injury—interruption of conduction in the axons with preservation of the anatomical continuity of all components of the nerve.* This is Seddon's neuropraxia [25]. The etiology is usually ischemia of the nerve caused by pressure. Sensory and motor function may be lost from a few days to several months. Recovery will be complete.

2. *Second-degree injury—loss of continuity of the axons without loss of continuity of the endoneurium.* This is Seddon's axonotmesis [25]. Wallerian degeneration of the axon distal to the point of injury occurs. This is caused by minimal crushing of the nerve. Since the endoneural tubes are preserved, when the axon begins regeneration in a few days it is directed back to the end-organ originally innervated. Complete function returns over a period of months.

3. *Third-degree injury—loss of continuity of nerve fibers* (i.e., axon, myelin sheath, and sheath of Schwann). This more severe injury is limited, in that the perineurium and general funicular arrangement remain intact. The traumatic degeneration proximally is more marked, so that axon regeneration is delayed. Budding axons remain in the same funiculus, but as their endoneural tubes have been disrupted they will often grow into another tube. Intrafunicular fibrosis is more pronounced, and a fusiform swelling develops at the site of injury. Recovery is usually marked by a partial sensory and motor loss.

4. *Fourth-degree injury—preservation of continuity of the nerve trunk though the involved segment becomes a tangled strand of connective tissue, Schwann cells, and regenerating axons.* This is the type of injury that requires exci-

sion of the involved nerve segment and nerve repair.

5. *Fifth-degree injury—loss of continuity of the nerve trunk.* This is the completely severed peripheral nerve.

FACTORS INFLUENCING THE TIMING AND RESULTS OF NERVE REPAIR

Several well-identified factors have a definite bearing on the timing of nerve repair and the results of motor and sensory return following repair.

Age

A number of authors have reported on the increased rate and quality of recovery following nerve repair in children and even young adults [19, 24, 27]. Onne [24] reports that after median or ulnar nerve repair in children less than 6 years of age there was excellent recovery of sensibility in all cases. After the age of 6 years there was a steady decrease in functional return, the two-point discrimination value expressed in millimeters being about the same as the age of the patient up to 20 years (normal, 3 to 5 mm). Then from 20 to 31 years the sensory recovery varied but tended to be poor; and in those more than 31 years old all the results were poor, with a two-point discrimination near or above 30 mm.

Type of Trauma

Gunshot wounds, high-speed missile wounds, and trauma that stretches a nerve cause severe nerve injuries both at the site of wounding and extending several centimeters proximally and distally from this point. This type of trauma also causes gross destruction of nerve and other tissues, which leads to scarring and a poor bed for the repaired nerve. These injuries, most common in warfare, tend to occur in the upper arm and forearm as compared to injuries by knives and glass, most common in civilian life, which tend to occur in the wrist and hand. Nicholson and Seddon reported that 90 percent of

median nerve injuries treated in their civil practice were at a distal level [23].

Level of Nerve Injury

The rapidity and quality of sensory and motor function following high nerve injury are not as good as following lower level injury [12, 27]. The reasons are (1) the greater loss of nerve cell mass (as discussed in the section on metabolic changes of the nerve cell); (2) the more equal proportion of motor and sensory fibers at higher levels and thus the greater chance of cross-innervation, particularly in the median nerve; (3) the greater distance that motor axons must travel to reach muscle in high lesions, and hence the longer time for the denervation changes in muscle and the limited restoration of function; and (4) the more destructive types of trauma that are likely at higher levels.

Primary Versus Secondary Repair

Peripheral nerves severed by gunshot wounds, high-speed missiles, or stretching are best treated by secondary repair approximately two or three weeks after injury, particularly when the injury is high along the 3-foot-long pathway of a nerve in the upper extremity. It can also now be stated that peripheral nerves severed by sharp glass or knives or other well-localized trauma at a lower level are best treated on the day of injury or within the first 10 days [8, 10, 19, 27].

Grabb has shown in the monkey that median and ulnar nerves cut with a knife or crushed by a ball peen hammer at the wrist and repaired primarily have a statistically significant higher grade of motor reinnervation of the intrinsic muscles of the hand than those following secondary repairs [10]. There are a number of poorly controlled clinical studies of primary and secondary nerve suture in civilian life that will not be discussed here.

Epineural Versus Funicular Nerve Repair

Goto [9], Bora [1], Ito et al. [15], Hakstian [13], and Grabb et al. [11] have all reported a favoritism toward funicular suture in animal and human studies. It is my opinion that there is a suggestion but no statistically significant evidence that funicular nerve repair in humans produces better results than epineural repair.

The ability of the surgeon performing the nerve repair undoubtedly has a direct relationship to the results, although this has not been studied in a scientifically controlled manner.

Species

With the large volume of research being carried out in animals it should be noted that the higher the animal on the phylogenetic scale, the more difficult it is to obtain satisfactory return of function. Kline, Hackett, and May have shown that the chimpanzee, in comparison to the dog, rhesus monkey, and baboon, has more connective tissue proliferation and axonal disorganization at the repair site with less remyelination of the distal segment and thus more closely resembles humans [17].

Sensory Reeducation

Dillon, Curtis, and Edgerton have reported an exciting concept: teaching a patient whose nerve has regenerated to develop normal or near normal sensation [6]. In 9 adults with 12 injured nerves, sensory exercises involving the handling of various sizes of nuts and bolts, the pencil point and eraser, both with and without visual coordination, were carried out several times a day. After three or four weeks all patients with digital nerve lesions had recovered normal or near normal sensation, and three patients with a sutured median or ulnar nerve recovered normal or near normal functional sensation within a year after nerve suture.

NERVE GRAFTS

Long nerve gaps can be overcome by autogenous cable nerve grafts; autogenous, homogenous, or irradiated homogenous whole nerve grafts; nerve pedicle flaps from the same or the opposite arm; nerve crossing; or resection of bone.

The autogenous cable nerve graft is probably the best of these methods [20, 21, 26, 27]. Strands of a cutaneous nerve are of a small enough caliber so that they can be revascularized before central necrosis takes place. Sunderland is of the opinion that the sural nerve (14 to 35 cm in length before branching) and the superficial radial nerve (10 to 20 cm) are best for use as cable grafts [27]. The maximal length for successful cable grafts is 10 to 14 cm.

Millesi reported on 151 nerve grafts in 126 patients using mainly sural nerve interfascicular cable grafts [20, 21]. He obtained a 93 percent incidence of some return and an 85 percent functional recovery. Millesi pointed out that typically four grafts of the sural nerve are required when bridging ulnar nerve gaps, while five or six grafts are needed to accommodate the diameter of the median nerve. His technique involves making a sketch of the fascicular arrangement of each nerve stump. Then noting the size of the funiculi he endeavors to match the two stump ends so that the nerve graft will unite the same funicular bundles as were joined prior to injury. It is well known that the motor (thenar) branch of the median nerve is the largest discrete bundle and can usually be identified both proximally and distally. Using magnification, Millesi sutures the nerve graft in place without any tension, using one 10-0 nylon suture at each anastomosis.

Sunderland has described the technique of obtaining the sural nerve grafts, which can be up to 35 cm in length [27]. Rather than taking the nerve graft with the patient in the prone position before exploring the arm, it is better to have the patient on his back with the hip elevated on one side, so that the graft is removed only after inspection of the nerve in the arm.

There are instances in which full-thickness nerve trunks have survived and have given good results [27]. The use of irradiated nerve homografts has not been very successful in man.

RESULTS OF NERVE REPAIR

The functional aspects of motor and sensory return must be the basis for any study of the results of nerve repair. In my opinion the best available method of evaluating motor return is the determination of muscle power as described by Zachary and Holmes [32]. The best available method of evaluating sensory return is the two-point discrimination test as performed by Onne [24].

Reported Return of Function After Repair of the Median and Ulnar Nerves

This is a difficult subject to summarize, because the results of nerve suture are so clearly dependent upon the age of the patient, the type of trauma, the level of nerve injury, the timing and technique of repair, and the skill of the operator. In addition, since motor and sensory function can continue to improve for up to five years after nerve repair, the time of the evaluation is of importance.

Some of the best results were reported by McEwan following primary repair of civilian nerve injuries in children [19]. For example, 65 percent attained normal motor power and 86 percent attained normal sensation following median nerve repair. In a group of adults who had suffered similar trauma with repair, only 13 percent gained normal motor power; no one achieved normal sensation. Results following repair of peripheral nerves in wartime are less satisfactory than the results of civilian injuries.

SPECIAL PROBLEMS IN NERVE REPAIR

When to Explore a Repaired Nerve

One of the indications for exploration of a repaired nerve is failure of return of some voluntary muscle contractions or sensibility to pinprick within five months after median or ulnar nerve injury in the wrist or hand. For higher nerve repairs (i.e., upper arm or forearm) the time interval is seven months [27]. Serial electromyography provides even earlier evidence that motor fibers have reached the muscle. A decrease in the number of fibrillations and denervation potentials and the appearance of nascent motor units herald the onset of clinical function.

Another indication for exploration is knowing that the nerve repair was performed by a physician inexperienced in nerve suture. There are many known cases in which nerves have been sutured to tendons. When the nerve has been repaired by an inexperienced operator, some authorities recommend exploration without waiting the five months for evidence of motor or sensory return. In such a case the technique developed by Kline, Hackett, and May is very helpful [17]. It involves exposing the nerve at operation, placing bipolar electrodes on the nerve proximally and distally to the neurorrhaphy site, and then stimulating with an electrical current proximally and recording the presence or absence of nerve action potentials distally. The evoked nerve action potentials can be recorded as early as eight weeks following peripheral nerve repair in monkeys and provide objective evidence that axons are crossing the site of repair so that resection and resuture of the nerve are not indicated. This work has subsequently been applied successfully to humans.

Neurolysis

Internal Neurolysis

Curtis [5], Brown [2, 3], and Lewis [18] have all advocated the use of internal neurolysis for nerve lesions resulting in intraneural scarring. Traumatic crushing of the nerve, the injection of penicillin into a nerve, the carpal tunnel syndrome, and, of course, gunshot injuries can cause scarring within the nerve. Three to six longitudinal incisions, depending on the size of the nerve, are made in the thickened epineurium. The points of a pair of scissors are placed between the fascicles and then opened to tease the fascicles apart. By means of magnification a tiny fiber crossing from one fascicle to another can be preserved. Use of this technique has improved sensory and motor function and has even decreased causalgic pain.

External Neurolysis

External neurolysis is carried out by first identifying the nerve above and below the site of involvement and then carefully dissecting the scar from the nerve. It may be advisable also to transpose the nerve to a less scarred bed. The effectiveness of external neurolysis remains in doubt [27]. One instance in which it is effective is in a nerve showing evidence of recovery that has been proceeding satisfactorily and then abruptly stops.

REFERENCES

1. Bora, F. W.   Peripheral nerve repair in cats: The fascicular stitch. *J. Bone Joint Surg.* [Am.] 49:659, 1967.
2. Brown, H. A.   Internal neurolysis in treatment of traumatic peripheral nerve lesions. *Calif. Med.* 110:460, 1969.
3. Brown, H. A.   Internal Neurolysis in Treatment of Traumatic Peripheral Nerve Injuries. In Ojemann, R. G. (Ed.), *Clinical Neurosurgery.* Baltimore: Williams & Wilkins, 1970.
4. Cajal, S. R.   *Degeneration and Regeneration of the Nervous System.* London: Oxford University Press, 1928.
5. Curtis, R. M.   Internal neurolysis in nerve compression syndromes. Personal communications, 1970.
6. Dillon, A. L., Curtis, R. M., and Edgerton, M. T.   Re-education of sensation in the hand following nerve injury. *J. Bone Joint Surg.* [Am.] 53:813, 1971.
7. Ducker, T. B., and Hayes, G. J.   Experimental improvements in the use of Silastic cuff for peripheral nerve repair. *J. Neurosurg.* 28:582, 1968.
8. Ducker, T. B., Kempe, L. G., and Hayes, G. J.   The metabolic background for peripheral nerve surgery. *J. Neurosurg.* 30:270, 1969.
9. Goto, Y.   Experimental study of nerve autografting by funicular suture. *Arch. Jpn. Chir.* 36:478, 1967.
10. Grabb, W. C.   Median and ulnar nerve suture. An experimental study comparing primary and secondary repair in monkeys. *J. Bone Joint Surg.* [Am.] 50:964, 1968.
11. Grabb, W. C., BeMent, S. L., Koepke, G. H., and Green, R. A.   Comparison of methods of peripheral nerve suture in monkeys. *Plast. Reconstr. Surg.* 46:31, 1970.
12. Guttmann, E., and Guttmann, L.   Factors affecting recovery of sensory function after nerve lesions. *J. Neurol. Neurosurg. Psychiatry* 5:117, 1942.
13. Hakstian, R. W.   Funicular orientation by direct stimulation. *J. Bone Joint Surg.* [Am.] 50:1178, 1968.
14. Hyden, H.   The Neuron. In Brachet, J., and Mirsky, A. E. (Eds.), *The Cell.* New York: Academic, 1960. Vol. IV.
15. Ito, T., Hirotani, H., Goto, Y., and Tamura, T.   A study of funicular suture. Personal communication, 1967.
16. Jacobson, S., and Guth, L.   An electrophysiological study of the early stages of peripheral nerve regeneration. *Exp. Neurol.* 11:48, 1965.
17. Kline, D. G., Hackett, E. R., and May, P. R.   Evaluation of nerve injuries by evoked potentials and electromyography. *J. Neurosurg.* 31:128, 1969.
18. Lewis, D.   *Lewis's Practice of Surgery.* Hagerstown, Md.: Prior, 1948.
19. McEwan, L. E.   Median and ulnar nerve injuries. *Aust. N.Z. J. Surg.* 32:89, 1962.
20. Millesi, H.   The interfascicular nerve graft. *J. Bone Joint Surg.* [Am.] 53:813, 1971.
21. Millesi, H.   Microsurgery of peripheral nerves. *Hand* 5:157, 1973.
22. Moberg, E.   Nerve repair in hand surgery—an analysis. *Surg. Clin. North Am.* 48:985, 1968.
23. Nicholson, O. R., and Seddon, H. J.

Nerve repair in civil practice. *Br. Med. J.* 2:1065, 1957.

24. Onne, L. Recovery of sensibility and sudomotor function in the hand after nerve suture. *Acta Chir. Scand.* Suppl. 300, 1962.

25. Seddon, H. J. Three types of nerve injury. *Brain* 66:237, 1943.

26. Smith, J. W. Factors influencing nerve repair: 1. Blood supply of peripheral nerves. *Arch. Surg.* 93:335, 1966.

27. Sunderland, S. *Nerves and Nerve Injuries.* Edinburgh: Livingstone, 1968.

28. Sunderland, S. Anatomical Features of Nerve Trunks in Relation to Nerve Injury and Nerve Repair. In Ojemann, R. G. (Ed.), *Clinical Neurosurgery.* Baltimore: Williams & Wilkins, 1970.

29. Sunderland, S., and Bradley, K. C. Denervation atrophy of the distal stump of a severed nerve. *J. Comp. Neurol.* 93:401, 1950.

30. Thomas, P. K., and Jones, D. G. The cellular response to nerve injury. *J. Anat.* 100:287, 1966.

31. Thomas, P. K., and Jones, D. G. The cellular response to nerve injury: II. Regeneration of perineurium after nerve injury. *J. Anat.* 101:45, 1967.

32. Zachary, R. B., and Holmes, W. Primary suture of nerves. *Surg. Gynecol. Obstet.* 82:632, 1946.

Index

Index

Infections—*Continued*
  tetanus, 108–109
  transmitted by blood, 91–92
Inflammation
  acute, 131
  humoral mediators of, 170–172
Inhalation of fumes, 145
Inheritance. *See under* Genetic disorders
Injuries, 129–147
  burns, 149–160
  cold, 133–134
  electrical, 135–138
  radiation, 139–144
Insulin, 76, 80
  trauma and production of, 130
Interstitial fluid, 61
Intracellular fluid, 61
  maintenance of volume and composition, 66–67
Intravenous therapy
  burn wound infection, 158
  infusions, 84–85
  nutrition, 80–81
Isoimmunization and blood transfusions, 92
Isotonicity of solutions, 62
Isotope clearance methods, for viability of flaps, 256

Jowls, 226
Juvenile xanthogranuloma, 205
Juxtaglomerular apparatus, 70

Kallikreins, 170
Kanamycin, 123–124
Kaposi's sarcoma, 207–208
Kasabach-Merritt syndrome, 219–220
Keratinous cysts, 201
Keratoacanthomas, 201, 208
Keratosis
  actinic, 200
  seborrheic, 199–200
Ketones, 76
Kidneys
  congenital malformation, 41–42
  discoid, 41–42
  embryological basis, 30–33
  mechanisms for control of sodium balance, 69–70
  prolonged hypovolemic shock, 168
Kininogenases, 170
Kinins, 73, 170
Klebsiella species, 115, 122
Klippel-Trenaunay syndrome, 219

Leiomyomas, 207
Leiomyosarcomas, 207
Lentigo maligna (Hutchinson's freckle), 203–204
Leptomeningeal melanocytosis, 218

Lesch-Nyhan syndrome, 52
Leukemia, 141, 193
Limbs
  buds, 23, 28
  congenital defects, 25–30
    brachydactyly, 25, 30
    cleft hand and foot, 25
    clubfoot (talipes equinovarus), 30
    effect of thalidomide, 25
    embryological basis, 25–30
    hypoplasia of thumb, 30
    meromelia, 29
    polydactyly or supernumerary digits, 25, 30
    syndactyly or webbed digits, 25, 30
  development of, 23–25
    bones, 23, 28
    limb buds, 25, 28
    muscles, 23–25
    positional changes, 28
Lincomycins, 122–123
Lipogenesis and lipolysis, 76
Lips
  cleft, 21
  electrical burns, 138
Lungs
  postperfusion lung syndrome, 95
  pulmonary failure following trauma, 177–178
  in shock, 177–178
Lymph, 61, 220
  enlarged nodes, 144
Lymphadenitis, 108
  granulomatous, 144
Lymphangiomas, 220
Lymphangitis, 108
Lymphatic buds, 220
Lymphocytes
  activation in vitro, 297–300
  activation in vivo, 300–301
  antigen-sensitive, 295–296
  B- and T-lymphocytes, 294–295
  mixed lymphocyte culture (MLC), 288–289
Lymphocytopenia, 160
Lymphokines, 170–171
Lymphomas
  dermatological manifestations, 193
  malignant, 206
Lymphomatoid papulosis, 206
Lymphoplasia, cutaneous, 206
Lymporeticular lesions, 206

Macrolide antibiotics, 122
Maffucci's syndrome, 215, 220
Malaria, 92
Malignant melanoma. *See* Melanoma, malignant
Mandible
  hypoplasia, 21
  prominences, 16

Mandibulofacial dysostosis, 21
Marfan's syndrome, 49
Meissner's corpuscles, 188
Melanin, 187
Melanocytic tumors of skin, 202–205
  malignant melanoma, 203–205
  nevi, 202
  premalignant lesions, 203
Melanoma, malignant, 203–206
  depth of invasion, 204–205
  lentigo maligna melanoma, 203–204
  nodular, 204–205
  paradoxical ineffectiveness of tumor immunity, 326
  pathology report, 205
  prognosis and therapy, 205
  skin excision specimens, 208–209
  superficial spreading, 204–205
Melanosomes, 202
Meleney's synergistic gangrene, 112
Meleney's ulcer, 114
Meningomyelocele, 55
6-Mercaptopurine, 313
Metabolism, 75–87
  effects of trauma and stress, 75–78
  nutrition in surgical patient, 84–87
    hyperalimentation, 84–86
    normal diet, 87
    tubal nutrition, 86–87
  nutritional requirements, 78–84
    calories, 78–79
    proteins, 79–81
    vitamins, 81–84
  potassium balance, 78
  protein catabolic effect, 77–78
  rate of metabolic expenditure, 77
  storage of carbohydrate in normals, 76
Metacarpals, absence of, 29
Metastatic infections, 108
Methicillin, 121
Microbacterium tuberculosis, 125
Microorganisms and sepsis, 107–117
  antimicrobial therapy, 119–127
  clostridial myonecrosis, 109–112
  definitions, 107
  gas gangrene, 109–112
  hand infections, 115–117
  histotoxic clostridia, 109–112
  Meleney's ulcer, 114
  necrotizing fasciitis, 112–113
  osteomyelitis, 117
  progressive bacterial synergistic gangrene, 112
  rabies, 114–115
  synergistic necrotizing cellulitis, 113–114
  tetanus, 108–109